Case Studies in Palliative and End-of-Life Care

Case Studies in Palliative and End-of-Life Care

Edited by

Margaret L. Campbell, PhD, RN, FPCN

Associate Professor — Research
Office of Health Research
College of Nursing
Wayne State University
Detroit, MI

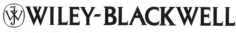
A John Wiley & Sons, Inc., Publication

This edition first published 2012 © 2012 by John Wiley & Sons, Inc.

Wiley-Blackwell is an imprint of John Wiley & Sons, formed by the merger of Wiley's global Scientific, Technical and Medical business with Blackwell Publishing.

Editorial Offices
2121 State Avenue, Ames, Iowa 50014-8300, USA
The Atrium, Southern Gate, Chichester, West Sussex, PO19 8SQ, UK
9600 Garsington Road, Oxford, OX4 2DQ, UK

For details of our global editorial offices, for customer services and for information about how to apply for permission to reuse the copyright material in this book please see our website at www.wiley.com/wiley-blackwell.

Library of Congress Cataloging-in-Publication Data

Case studies in palliative and end-of-life care / edited by Margaret L. Campbell.
    p. ; cm.
  Includes bibliographical references and index.
  ISBN 978-0-470-95825-4 (pbk. : alk. paper)
I. Campbell, Margaret L., 1954–
[DNLM: 1. Nursing Care–methods–Case Reports. 2. Palliative Care–methods–Case Reports.
3. Terminal Care–methods–Case Reports. WY 152.3]
  616.02'9–dc23

                2012011915
A catalogue record for this book is available from the British Library.

Wiley also publishes its books in a variety of electronic formats. Some content that appears in print may not be available in electronic books.

Set in 10/12pt Palatino by SPi Publisher Services, Pondicherry, India
Printed and bound in Malaysia by Vivar Printing Sdn Bhd

Disclaimer

1 2012

Table of Contents

Contributor List   **viii**

Introduction   **xii**
Margaret L. Campbell

| Section 1 | *Communication Case Studies* | 1 |

Case 1.1   **Communicating about a Progressive Diagnosis
and Prognosis**   **5**
Julia A. Walch

Case 1.2   **Diagnosis/Prognosis Uncomplicated Death at Home**   **12**
Constance Dahlin

Case 1.3   **Accommodating Religiosity and Spirituality in Medical
Decision-Making**   **18**
Jennifer Gentry

Case 1.4   **Discussing Cardiopulmonary Resuscitation When
it May Be Useful**   **26**
Kelli Gershon

Case 1.5   **Discussing CPR When it is a Non-Beneficial Intervention**   **33**
Judy Passaglia

Case 1.6   **Discussing Brain Death, Organ Donation, and Donation
after Cardiac Death**   **41**
Christine Westphal and Rebecca Williams

Case 1.7   **Discussing Physiological Futility**   **52**
Judy C. Wheeler

Case 1.8   **Wounded Families: Decision-Making in the Setting of
Stressed Coping and Maladaptive Behaviors in Health Crises**   60
Kerstin McSteen

Case 1.9   **Notification of an Expected Death**   68
Peg Nelson

Case 1.10   **Death Notification after Unexpected Death**   73
Garrett K. Chan

Section 2   *Symptom Management Case Studies*   83

Case 2.1   **Pain: Cancer in the Home**   87
Constance Dahlin

Case 2.2   **Treating an Acute, Severe, Cancer Pain Exacerbation**   98
Patrick J. Coyne

Case 2.3   **Pain and Advanced Heart Failure**   104
Margaret L. Campbell

Case 2.4   **Dyspnea and Advanced COPD**   110
Margaret L. Campbell

Case 2.5   **Dyspnea and Heart Failure**   117
Garrett K. Chan

Case 2.6   **Treating Dyspnea during Ventilator Withdrawal**   128
Margaret L. Campbell

Case 2.7   **Cough Associated with COPD and Lung Cancer**   138
Peg Nelson

Case 2.8   **Hiccups and Advanced Illness**   145
Marian Grant

Case 2.9   **Treating Nausea Associated with Advanced Cancer**   152
Judy C. Wheeler

Case 2.10   **Nausea Associated with Bowel Obstruction**   161
Terri L. Maxwell

Case 2.11   **Nausea Related to Uremia, Dialysis Cessation**   168
Linda M. Gorman

Case 2.12   **Opioid-Induced Pruritus**   176
Richelle Nugent Hooper

Case 2.13   **Pruritus in End-Stage Renal Disease**   183
Linda M. Gorman

Case 2.14   **Opioid-Induced Constipation**   **190**
Grace Cullen Oligario

Case 2.15   **Depression in Advanced Disease**   **198**
Todd Hultman

Case 2.16   **Treating Anxiety**   **205**
Darrell Owens

Case 2.17   **Terminal Secretions**   **213**
Terri L. Maxwell

Case 2.18   **Fungating Wounds and the Palliative Care Patient**   **220**
Laura C. Harmon

Case 2.19   **Pressure Ulcer Care in Palliative Care**   **229**
Laura C. Harmon

Case 2.20   **Treating Ascites**   **239**
Darrell Owens

Case 2.21   **Delirium Management in Palliative Care**   **247**
Kerstin McSteen

Section 3   *Family Care Case Studies*   257

Case 3.1   **Caring for the Family Expecting a Loss**   **259**
Patricia A. Murphy and David M. Price

Case 3.2   **Anticipatory Grief and the Dysfunctional Family**   **266**
Rita J. DiBiase

Case 3.3   **Acute and Uncomplicated Grief after an Expected Death**   **277**
Rita J. DiBiase

Case 3.4   **Bereavement after Unexpected Death**   **289**
Garrett K. Chan

Case 3.5   **Complicated Grief**   **300**
Rita J. DiBiase

Index   **309**

Contributor List

EDITOR

Margaret L. Campbell, PhD, RN, FPCN
Associate Professor—Research
Office of Health Research
College of Nursing
Wayne State University
Detroit, Michigan

CONTRIBUTORS

Garrett K. Chan, PhD, APRN, FPCN, FAEN, FAAN
Lead Advanced Practice Professional and Associate Clinical Director
Emergency Department Clinical Decision Unit
Stanford Hospital and Clinics
Stanford, California
Associate Adjunct Professor
School of Nursing
University of California, San Francisco
San Francisco, California

Patrick J. Coyne, MSN, ACHPN, ACNS-BC, FAAN, FPCN
Clinical Director of Thomas Palliative Program
Virginia Commonwealth University/Massey Center
Richmond, Virginia

Constance Dahlin, APRN, BC, ACHPN, FAAN
Palliative Care Service, North Shore Medical Center and
Massachusetts General Hospital
Associate Clinical Professor, Massachusetts General Hospital Institute
of Health Professions
Faculty, Harvard Medical School Center for Palliative Care
Boston, Massachusetts

**Rita J. DiBiase, MSN, RN(EC), ACNP-BC, ACNS-BC,
AOCNS, CHPCN(C)**
Palliative Care Nurse Practitioner
Windsor Regional Cancer Program, Windsor Regional Hospital
Windsor, Ontario
Canada

Jennifer Gentry, RN, ANP-BC, ACHPN, FPCN
Nurse Practitioner
Duke University Hospital Palliative Care Service
Durham, North Carolina

Kelli Gershon, FNP-BC, ACHPN
Nurse Practitioner
Symptom Management Consultant
The Woodlands, Texas

Linda M. Gorman, RN, MN, PMHCNS-BC, CHPN, FPCN
Palliative Care Clinical Nurse Specialist/Palliative
Care Consultant
Los Angeles, California

Marian Grant, DNP, RN, CRNP, ACHPN
Assistant Professor, Family and Community Health
University of Maryland School of Nursing
Baltimore, Maryland

Laura C. Harmon, ACNP, BC, CWOCN, CCRN
Nurse Practitioner
Internal Medicine and Wound Care
Detroit Receiving Hospital
Detroit, Michigan

Richelle Nugent Hooper, MSN, FNP, ACHPN
Director Palliative Care Clinical Operations
Four Seasons
Flat Rock, North Carolina

Todd Hultman, PhD, ACNP, ACHPN
Nurse Practitioner and Co-director, Inpatient Palliative Care
Consultation Service
Massachusetts General Hospital
Faculty, Harvard Medical School Center for Palliative Care
Boston, Massachusetts

Terri L. Maxwell, PhD, APRN
Vice President, Strategic Initiatives
Weatherbee Resources Inc. and the Hospice Education Network Inc.
Hyannis, Massachusetts

Kerstin McSteen, MS, ACNS-BC, ACHPN
Palliative Care Consultant
Abbott Northwestern Hospital
Minneapolis, Minnesota

Patrica A. Murphy, PhD, FAAN, FPCN
APN Ethics/Bereavement
University Medical and Dental of New Jersey-University Hospital
Newark, New Jersey

Peg Nelson, MSN, NP, ACHPN
Director, Mercy Supportive Care Palliative and Pain Services
St. Joseph Mercy Oakland
Pontiac, Michigan
Adjunct Faculty
Palliative Nurse Practitioner Track
Madonna University
Livonia, Michigan

Grace Cullen Oligario, MSN, FNP-C, ACHPN
Nurse Practitioner, Oncology and Palliative Care
John D. Dingell VA Medical Center
Detroit, Michigan

Darrell Owens, DNP, ARNP
Attending Provider and Director
Outpatient Palliative Care Services
Harborview Medical Center
Clinical Assistant Professor of Medicine and Nursing
University of Washington
Seattle, Washington

Judy Passaglia, APRN, ACHPN
Stanford Hospital and Clinics
Palliative Care and Supportive Oncology Program Manager
and APN
Palo Alto, California

David M. Price, M.Div, PhD
New Jersey Medical School
Ethics Faculty, retired
Newark, NJ

Julia A. Walch, RN, MSN, FNP-BC
Palliative Care
Detroit Receiving Hospital
Detroit, Michigan

Christine Westphal, MSN, NP, ACNS-BC, ACHPN
Director/Nurse Practitioner
Palliative and Restorative Integrated Services Model (PRISM)
Oakwood Healthcare System
Dearborn, Michigan

Judy C. Wheeler, MSN, MA, GNP-BC
Palliative Care Nurse Practitioner
Detroit Receiving Hospital
Detroit, Michigan

Rebecca Williams, BS, MA, HHCC
Hospital Services Associate
Gift of Life Michigan
Ann Arbor, Michigan

Introduction

Margaret L. Campbell

Case Studies In Palliative and End-of-Life Care is written for clinicians caring for patients and their families across diagnoses, illness trajectories, settings for care, and models of care delivery. All of the contributing authors are advanced practice nurses who bring their hands-on experience and join it with the evidence base for their respective chapters; hence, each chapter reflects the art and science of palliative care.

The conceptual framework for *Case Studies In Palliative and End of Life Care* is the Clinical Practice Guidelines for Quality Palliative Care produced by the National Consensus Project (NCP). For this book we embrace the definition of palliative care from the NCP as follows: "The goal of palliative care is to prevent and relieve suffering and to support the best possible quality of life for patients and their families, regardless of the stage of the disease or the need for other therapies. Palliative care is both a philosophy of care and an organized, highly structured system for delivering care. Palliative care expands traditional disease-model medical treatments to include the goals of enhancing quality of life for patient and family, optimizing function, helping with decision-making, and providing opportunities for personal growth. As such, it can be delivered concurrently with life-prolonging care or as the main focus of care."[1]

Each chapter begins with a case history followed by identification of a single clinical question raised by the case. A comprehensive, evidence-based discussion of the clinical problem follows and the chapter concludes by returning to the case for the outcomes of the treatment plan. Each case ends with "Take Away Points"—succinct summaries of the chapter.

Case studies rely on "story" to engage the learner and are an effective method for clinical teaching because they mimic the clinical encounter.

Stories are increasingly recognized as central to learning, facilitating a shared framework for understanding and enabling individuals to learn from one another. Stories also serve a purpose because people tell stories to make diverse information coherent, to give meaning and convey understanding, and to situate concepts in practice.[2]

Case Studies In Palliative and End-of-Life Care is comprised of three sections: Communication, Symptom Management, and Family Care, with a number of case studies in each section. The cases represent a cross-section of diagnoses including cancer, heart failure, chronic obstructive pulmonary disease (COPD), chronic kidney disease, and dementia. Illness trajectories discussed in the cases range from newly diagnosed to the moment of death. Settings of care are home or hospital. The cases may represent actual patients cared for by the author or may be a composite of similar cases. In no case can the identity of an actual patient or family be identified.

It is my hope that this collection of case studies will be employed for self-learning and for classroom teaching.

REFERENCES

[1] National Consensus Project for Quality Palliative Care. *Clinical Practice Guidelines for Quality Palliative Care*. 2nd edition. Pittsburgh, PA: National Consensus Project for Quality Palliative Care; 2009.

[2] Snowden L. Story-telling: an old skill in a new context. *Business Information Review*. 1999; 16(1):30–37.

Section 1

Communication Case Studies

Case 1.1   **Communicating about a Progressive Diagnosis and Prognosis**   **5**
Julia A. Walch

Case 1.2   **Diagnosis/Prognosis Uncomplicated Death at Home**   **12**
Constance Dahlin

Case 1.3   **Accommodating Religiosity and Spirituality in Medical Decision-Making**   **18**
Jennifer Gentry

Case 1.4   **Discussing Cardiopulmonary Resuscitation When it May Be Useful**   **26**
Kelli Gershon

Case 1.5   **Discussing CPR When it is a Non-Beneficial Intervention**   **33**
Judy Passaglia

Case 1.6   **Discussing Brain Death, Organ Donation, and Donation after Cardiac Death**   **41**
Christine Westphal and Rebecca Williams

Case 1.7   **Discussing Physiological Futility**   **52**
Judy C. Wheeler

Case 1.8   **Wounded Families: Decision-Making in the Setting of Stressed Coping and Maladaptive Behaviors in Health Crises**   **60**
Kerstin McSteen

Case 1.9   **Notification of an Expected Death**   **68**
Peg Nelson

Case 1.10   **Death Notification after Unexpected Death**   **73**
Garrett K. Chan

Overview

The effective communication of information to patients and their families is both evidence-based and artful. In the dominant U.S. culture, patients want to be told their diagnosis and prognosis. Because our society is multi-cultural, and not all members share the wish to know bad news, asking the patient about their preferences regarding information is the easiest way to avoid error and respect the patient's wishes. Breaking bad news to patients or their surrogates is one of the most difficult tasks clinicians face.

An early study identified two categories of spouse needs when the patient is dying in the hospital: relationship with the patient, and family needs for communication and support.[1] Successful communication is characterized by collaboration with the other members of the health care team, listening as much as speaking, and acknowledging patient or family emotions. In an early study of the needs of critically ill patients' families, five of the ten most important needs were for communication:[2]

- To be called at home about changes in the condition of the patient
- To know the prognosis
- To have questions answered honestly
- To receive information about the patient once a day
- To have explanations given in terms that are understandable

It is likely that the aforementioned needs of families of critically ill patients represent the needs of families in other settings, including the home or extended care facilities. In a study of the needs of spouses of patients dying in the hospital, these additional communication needs were identified:[1]

- Assurance of the comfort of the patient
- Information about the patient's condition
- Informed about the impending death

Ineffective communication about dying is frequently cited as a barrier to optimal care at the end of life.[3] In this first section about communication the cases are organized hierarchically from the types of communication that occur early in a diagnosis to those that occur at the time of death. The section opens in Case 1.1 with a case description about presenting a diagnosis and prognosis in a life-limiting illness (dementia). The skills presented can be applied across any condition. Each subsequent case has features that increase the communication complexity. In Case 1.2 the diagnosis and prognosis are presented in the context of the patient's imminent death. In Case 1.3 the clinician responds to family religiosity while attempting to provide information about a prognosis of imminent death.

The next cases (1.4 and 1.5) focus on routine discussions about resuscitation status and patient preferences. The euphemistic language that persists in clinician's discussions about cardiopulmonary resuscitation (CPR) and "do not resuscitate" (DNR) with each other, patients, and surrogates confuses medical decision-making; thus, the terms "code status" "coding," and "coded" have not been used. In the case in Case 1.4 CPR may be a useful intervention, whereas in the case in Case 1.5 CPR is not useful. The authors illustrate important concepts about discussing potentially beneficial and non-beneficial CPR.

Cases 1.6 through 1.8 present special communication circumstances. In Case 1.6 the complexities of discussing brain death and making organ donation decisions are illustrated. Communicating about physiological futility is addressed in Case 1.7 along with ethical considerations. The challenges of communicating with a maladaptive family are explained in Case 1.8.

This book section ends with two cases that describe how to inform the family that patient death has occurred. In Case 1.9 the family is expecting the death but in Case 1.10 the death is unexpected.

❗ TAKE AWAY POINTS

- Communicating about the end of life requires unique skills.
- Effective clinician communication is timely, honest, comprehensive, and comprehensible.
- Effective clinician communication entails listening as much as talking and acknowledging patient and family emotions.

📖 REFERENCES

[1] Hampe SO. Needs of the grieving spouse in a hospital setting. *Nursing Research*. 1975; 24:113–120.
[2] Molter NC. Needs of relatives of critically ill patients: a descriptive study. *Heart & Lung*. 1979; 8:332–339.
[3] Field MJ, Cassel CK, eds. *Approaching death: Improving care at the end of life*. Washington, DC: National Academy Press; 1997.

Case 1.1 Communicating about a Progressive Diagnosis and Prognosis

Julia A. Walch

HISTORY

Thomas was an 88-year-old African-American man who was admitted to the hospital for the third time in a month via the Emergency Department with fever and difficulty breathing; the admission diagnosis was urinary tract infection. He was discharged from the hospital just two days prior to the most recent admission after a prolonged hospitalization for health-care-acquired pneumonia which required intensive care and a short course of mechanical ventilation. He made slow but steady clinical improvements with the exception of his appetite, which remained poor. A percutaneous endoscopic gastrostomy (PEG) tube was being considered by the attending physician. Prior to recent admissions the patient had not been hospitalized in several years.

His past medical history included coronary artery disease status post coronary artery bypass graft surgery, atrial fibrillation, hypertension, Alzheimer's dementia (AD), and chronic kidney disease. He resided in a nursing home because his wife could no longer care for him at home. A palliative care consult was placed to discuss diagnosis, prognosis, and treatment goals with the patient's wife.

Thomas's wife reported that Thomas had been steadily declining over the past six to eight months, he was incontinent of bowel and bladder, and he was able to ambulate short distances and interact with her and other family members.

Case Studies in Palliative and End-of-Life Care, First Edition. Edited by Margaret L. Campbell.
© 2012 John Wiley & Sons, Inc. Published 2012 by John Wiley & Sons, Inc.

A geriatric assessment disclosed: needs assistance with activities of daily living (ADLs); dependent for instrumental activities of daily living (IADLs); able to remember three objects after five minutes; clock test abnormal; could not finish the Montreal Cognitive Assessment; able to draw a cube, name animals, recall four out of five words; and oriented to person and place but not time. Thus, he was categorized as being moderately impaired secondary to AD.

Further medical issues identified included malnutrition with hypo-albuminemia, depression with a geriatric depression scale score of 9/15, and debility. A speech language pathology evaluation revealed dysphagia related to pneumonia that may improve once pneumonia improves.

PHYSICAL EXAMINATION

Temperature: 36.9°C, heart rate: 70s, blood pressure: 110 to 150/60 to 70s
General: Elderly, cachectic male, sitting up in bed, appeared comfortable
Central nervous system: Alert, oriented to person and place, able to
    follow simple commands, recognized wife
Head, eyes, ears, nose, throat: Arcus senilis
Respiratory: Minimal bilateral basilar crackles, no accessory muscle
    use, on 2 liters nasal cannula
Cardiovascular: Irregularly irregular, no murmurs
Gastrointestinal: Soft, nontender, nondistended
Genitourinary: Voiding well 120 to 250cc/hour via urinary catheter
Extremities/skin: No pressure ulcers or deformities

DIAGNOSTICS

No diagnostic studies were conducted during this visit.

CLINICAL QUESTION

How should diagnosis and prognosis be discussed with the surrogate decision maker?

DISCUSSION

Most of what is known about communication of breaking bad news has focused on physician-patient communication in the oncology population at the end of life. Bad news is defined as any information which adversely and seriously affects an individual's view of his or her future and is always in the eye of the beholder.[1] Effective communication is the key to developing a relationship with the patient or family. This level of communication requires mutual respect and strong listening skills that allow for gathering and eliciting information and the implementation of a treatment plan. Doing this well can have a profound effect on how the patient or family approach their disease and its treatment. Effective communication can be achieved in the first meeting. In a first-person account a woman who had been a hospital patient explained how she changed hospitals and doctors three times during the course of her illness not because she was unhappy with the care, but because she was unhappy with the communication.[2]

Although physicians typically discuss diagnosis and prognosis, nurses are the constant, consistent health care providers, especially in the hospital or nursing home setting. Nurses are often the clinician who the patient or family asks to clarify questions or concerns after the multidisciplinary meeting is completed. Experienced nurses are more comfortable discussing prognosis compared to nurse with less experience.[3]

The communication strategy SPIKES (Setting, Perception, Invitation, Knowledge, Emotions and Empathic responses, and Strategies and Summary) is a mnemonic device developed to educate physicians on how to deliver bad news.[4] Communicating bad news or counseling a patient/family about a chronic, progressive, eventually terminal disease is an essential skill for nurses as well. The nurse can apply the SPIKES mnemonic device to discuss diagnosis and prognosis with patients or families.

Setting up the Interview

Before starting a family meeting, confirm the medical facts of the case and plan what will be discussed. Ascertain if the patient will be able to participate. The patient's preferences about which family members to include should be elicited. If uncomfortable with communicating the information, rehearse either mentally or to a colleague what you will say. Create the setting for the meeting, which should allow for privacy. A conference room is the ideal setting but if it is at the patient's bedside draw the curtains around the bed. Some families still prefer to meet at the patient's bedside even when the patient is unable to participate. Ensure there are enough chairs for everyone and that everyone is sitting down. This aids in relaxing the patient, gives the message that the focus is on the patient, gives an impression that time is not rushed, and prevents the psychological barrier of distance such as when one is seated and another is standing. Plan adequate time for discussion and alert nursing staff about the meeting to prevent interruptions.

Perception

Perception is assessing what the patient or family already understands about the patient's health. The meeting should start with asking the patient or family to describe the medical condition. The statement "Tell me what you understand about your condition" is an effective opening. A common misunderstanding among health care providers when caring for a patient with a chronic progressive medical condition is that the patient or family may be in denial. However, the real issue is that they do not understand the disease process. This is also the time for the nurse to assess the patient's or family's ability to understand and their readiness to accept information.

Invitation

Invitation involves finding out how much the patient or family wants to know. Ask, "Are you ready to talk about our impressions?" or "Is this a good time to talk?" This is also when the nurse establishes how much information the patient wants or whether the patient prefers his or her condition be discussed with someone else. Most people want to know the truth; more than 90% of people want to know the truth about their diagnosis even if it is grave.[4] Assessing the level of understanding the patient or family has about the disease helps the clinician to determine how much information/detail they need.

Knowledge

Sharing the information needs to be done in a straightforward, honest, yet sensitive manner. The information conveyed needs to be based on facts and evidence, not on personal opinion. Some families will ask, "What would you do?" A helpful response may be "It is important to base decisions on what your loved one would want." Information that is conveyed correctly to the patient or family allows them to cope with the situation and plan for the future. Avoid the use of medical terminology or technical jargon. There are times when a "warning shot" is needed to prepare the family that bad news is coming; for instance, the clinician might say "We have your results and I have bad news."

Emotions with Empathetic Responses

The clinician can display empathy while delivering bad news by saying "I am sorry to have to tell you this." It is best not to just say "I'm sorry" because this can be misinterpreted for pity or being responsible for the situation.

Patients and families respond to the news in a variety of ways such as through tears, sadness, love, anxiety, or other emotions. Some experience denial, blame, guilt, or disbelief. Some people walk out of a meeting or respond nonverbally. Patients who might not be able to walk away but do not want to participate any longer may turn away, close their eyes, or just stop speaking. In this case clarify with the patient that they want to stop meeting and ask permission to return at another time or day. It is important to acknowledge emotions by asking for a description about what is being displayed. "You appear to be....Can you tell me how you are feeling?" or "Tell me more about what you are feeling." Once the patient or family has worked through their emotions they are often able to make decisions in the best interests of themselves or their loved one. Patients or families who have good information and sufficient time are able to cope with the news and participate in decision making.

Strategy and Summary

The final step is planning and follow-up. This may include gathering further information from tests or procedures, setting up another family meeting, or making referrals to an outside agency such as hospice. This is also when the clinician explains treatment plans, addresses any concerns, and plans for follow-up. At the end of the meeting the patient and family should feel their concerns were addressed and not feel abandoned. A follow-up meeting should be made and contact information provided. Throughout the meeting, frequently allow the patient or family to ask questions, and assess whether they want to continue. Some people need to have the information repeated several times, whereas others need only to hear it once.

BACK TO OUR CASE

The primary goal for the meeting was to educate Thomas's wife about AD and its natural history and to counsel her that it is a progressive terminal illness. Other goals of the meeting included discussing resuscitation status, goals of care including hospice, and late stage care including recommendation for oral/hand feeding only in the end stage (no PEG). In this case the patient was not yet eligible for hospice; however, part of the education about a progressive illness is future planning.

Preparation for this meeting included a review of the medical record, examination of Thomas, and discussion with other health care providers. Thomas's wife was already in the his room and a meeting had not been formally set up, so the clinician introduced herself and the reason for the consultation by saying "I would like to speak with you about your husband's Alzheimer's. Is this a good time to meet?" The meeting was at the patient's bedside. Thomas' wife was asked her understanding of the patient's dementia. She had a basic understanding of the disease and gave a history of decline over the last six to eight months and recent nursing home placement. There was discussion about the natural course of AD, including late stage progression and feeding issues.

The following strategy was used to explain this to Thomas' wife: Alzheimer's is a disease of the brain that follows a pattern of decline, in which the brain stops sending out voluntary and involuntary signals. A patient with Alzheimer's does not stop walking because there is something wrong with their legs, the brain stops telling the person to get up and walk. They become incontinent not because there is an issue with the bladder or bowel but because the brain is no longer sending a signal that the bladder or bowel is full. Thomas's wife was able to comprehend the information and apply it to the changes she had seen in her husband.

Even though AD often lasts years, many families have limited knowledge of the disease and few understand that it is eventually fatal. Discussion with Thomas's wife about resuscitation status resulted in a decision to not resuscitate. Thomas's wife struggled with the discussion about hospice and the certainty of the disease progressing further. Thomas had a moderate stage dementia and by hospice guidelines was not eligible; however, he was declining and had a few recent hospitalizations including an intensive care unit stay for pneumonia. Thomas's wife declined to meet with hospice, but she had the knowledge that her husband's condition was expected to decline and that hospice was an available resource in the future.

! TAKE AWAY POINTS

- Take the time needed to gather information and prepare for the meeting.
- Patients and families want honest, evidence-based information, even when the prognosis is poor.
- Effective communication allows patients and their families to plan for the future.
- Effective communication is the key to developing a relationship with the patient or family. This level of communication requires mutual respect and strong listening skills that allow for gathering and eliciting information and the implementation of a treatment plan.

REFERENCES

[1] Buckman R. *Breaking Bad News: A Guide for Health Care Professionals*, 15th edition. Baltimore: Johns Hopkins University Press; 1992.
[2] Dias L, Chabner BA, Lynch TJ, Penson RT. Breaking bad news: A patient's perspective. *The Oncologist*. 2003; 8:587–596.

[3] Malloy P, Virani R, Kelly K. Beyond bad news: Communication skills of nurses in palliative care. *Journal of Hospice & Palliative Nursing.* 2010; 12(3):166–174.

[4] Baile WF, Buckman R, Lenzi R, Glober G, Beale EA, Kudelka AP. SPIKES—A Six-step protocol for delivering bad news: Application to the patient with cancer. *The Oncologist.* 2000; 5:302–311.

Case 1.2 Diagnosis/Prognosis Uncomplicated Death at Home

Constance Dahlin

HISTORY

Sundra was a 70-year-old Indian woman with a five-year history of dementia, diabetes, and debility. She had been admitted to the hospital three times in her last several months for infection. At her last hospital discharge, she indicated a preference for no future life-prolonging measures such as resuscitation, intubation/ventilation, or transfer to the intensive care unit. In fact, she wanted to avoid the hospital completely. She had talked with her family and they understood and respected her feelings.

Sundra was referred to hospice. Although she had lived in assisted living she moved to her daughter's house. Sundra had pain with movement and cried when she was touched. She disliked being cleaned or bathed because it hurt too much. In fact, she didn't like the finger sticks that were done to measure her glucose blood levels. After some discussion, these were discontinued because her blood sugar had been consistently low since she was not eating.

Her fatigue was profound. She had little energy to read, talk, or eat, the things she loved to do. She was, however, able to watch television. Her appetite had diminished, resulting in weakness and weight loss. She often coughed when she swallowed. She had no pruritis, shortness of breath, constipation, or discomfort from anything else.

Case Studies in Palliative and End-of-Life Care, First Edition. Edited by Margaret L. Campbell.
© 2012 John Wiley & Sons, Inc. Published 2012 by John Wiley & Sons, Inc.

PHYSICAL EXAMINATION

Temperature: 38.2°C, Blood pressure: 125/70, Heart rate: 80, respiratory rate: 14

Head, eyes, ears, nose, throat: Normocephalic; pupils equal, round, reactive to light and accommodation; extraocular movements intact; dry oral mucosa; no lesions; no defects; no abnormalities

Chest: Bilateral clear sounds, no extraneous sounds, unlabored breathing

Heart: S1 S2 no S3 or S4, no murmurs or rubs

Abdomen: Positive bowel sounds, soft, non-tender, soft,

Extremities: Thin, little muscle mass

Neurologic: Alert and oriented to person and place; flat affect

DIAGNOSTICS

No diagnostic studies were conducted during this visit.

CLINICAL QUESTION

How do you recognize imminent death and communicate it to the family?

DISCUSSION

In 1997, the Institute of Medicine described a good death as "one that is free from avoidable distress and suffering for patients, families, caregivers."[1] According the American Nurses Association Social Policy Statement, "Nursing helps patients experience a dignified death."[2] The essence of palliative care nursing is promoting death at home when possible and when desired by the patient. Death, like birth, can be predictable in its process although unpredictable as to the exact time. Death at home can be a healing process for patients and families. Many patients have an instinct about their time of death. Although a patient's instinct may not match their clinical condition, they may have more of a sense of when they will die.

The usual process in the last stage is very peaceful as the patient becomes more sleepy, then lethargic, obtunded, and comatose.[3] There are physical signs and symptoms of dying which can help offer some idea of time of death. Additionally, there are two conditions that may influence the time of death. First, there may be an emotional component that includes some closure that patients need to attend to. This may be an important milestone such as a birthday, anniversary, holiday, birth, graduation, or the like. Second, there are physiological aspects to time of death; for example, once patients stop receiving fluids in any form, it is unlikely that they will live more than two weeks.[4]

Signs and symptoms of dying have long been recognized, although in the literature signs and symptoms of dying now have been delineated as "syndrome of imminently dying." However, some signs and symptoms depend on the stage of disease from which the individual is dying as well as co-morbid illnesses. Some end-stage disease processes have fewer painful sequelae than others, although dying is similar no matter what the diagnosis. Dying from end-stage renal disease or dementia may be relatively painless because the patient may simply drift into unconsciousness. Dying from heart failure or amyotrophic lateral sclerosis or pulmonary failure may cause more discomfort due to the presence of more symptoms.[3]

There are a constellation of symptoms that signify that death is near. In terms of psychological and emotional aspects, patients may become more withdrawn. They may lack the energy to engage with people; they may not leave their room or their bed.

As a result, their social interactions diminish. They may also have visions of people close to them, some of whom may be deceased. They may also become restless or agitated.[3-5]

The signs of this weakness may be seen in changes in vital signs such as lowered blood pressure and higher heart rates and changing respiration rates. In the last stages of the dying process, patients are asleep more than they are awake. They may become obtunded and unable to be aroused. Their breathing may change and there may be secretions or congestion. This is more disturbing to family members than the patient.

Treatment

The key element is to listen to the patient. Often, the patient may say he is either done fighting or doesn't have the energy to do much more. The nurse can confirm with the patient whether this means he is ready to die. He may feel relief in having support that it is okay to die. Moreover, these statements signify it is time to discuss concerns with the patient about what he needs to do for end-of-life closure and offering support to the patient.

It may then be necessary for the nurse to coach families about the dying process. Often, family members recognize a patient's decline and understand death is near more easily than the patient. This comes from the necessity of providing more personal care or that the patient is eating less and sleeping more. Sometimes the family may be so overwhelmed they cannot see what is happening. It is then important for the nurse to gently explore how the patient's condition is changing and let the family come to an understanding that death is close.

Finally, the nurse may need to assist the family to allow and offer permission to the patient to let go. Families may need help with sample sentences such as "We will take care of Mom. It is okay to go," or " I will be okay. I don't want you to suffer. It is okay to go."

Depending on spiritual or religious tradition, the patient may ask for a spiritual counselor. Here the nurse can facilitate the presence of that person. If the family asks for this, the nurse must assess if it is for the patient or family. If it is clear the patient would not have wanted this, the nurse can discuss the use of ritual for the family outside of the patient's room.

Closer to Death

As the patient moves closer to death, the family may want to be in attendance. This is known as the vigil. It can be emotionally and physically draining. Permission should be given take care of themselves in this process. Support should be given to the family that they do not have to be there every minute. Encouragement should be given to take breaks to eat, drink, and sleep. Often the nurse can assist them in making a schedule of various family members for sharing in the vigil and taking breaks. See Case 3.3 for care of the family anticipating a loss.

The Death

Although nurses know when death has occurred, the family may need communication about the signs of death. Physical signs include absence of heart beat, absence of respirations, fixed pupils, pale and waxen skin color, and cool body temperature. There may be release of stool and urine and a relaxed jaw. The patient's eyes may remain opened or closed. When this occurs, the nurse should tell the family that death has occurred and allow quiet time. Then the nurse should prepare the family for the next steps of death notification and care of the body. More information and guidance is helpful at this time because families are emotional and may not retain details.

Often families ask about the timing of things in the initial post death period. They often want to know about timing of post mortem care of the body. The nurse can answer that death notification is first and care of the body second. Local statues may dictate timing. Nonetheless, body care should be explained and families should be offered the option and opportunity to participate. Some families find it healing and others find it morbid.

Death notification again should follow local jurisdiction. If the patient is enrolled in a hospice program, the nurse notifies the physician and hospice. Local authorities may need to be notified as appropriate.

If it is an expected home death with home health nursing services, there may be a different process. A death pronouncement may need to be completed for the authorities. Later, a death certificate will need to be completed. Additionally, the family may need assistance in notifying the funeral home for pick up of the body.

Finally, the nurse should wait with the family until the funeral home comes to take the body. Families may be afraid to be alone with the body. They may need time to do a life review. Or they may ask for help in notifying other relatives. This quiet time allows the nurse time for reflection of his involvement in the care and can help with caregiver stress of caring for the dying. Additionally during this time, the nurse performs a grief assessment to see how the family is doing. Safety for the family includes collecting the medications used by the patient in the dying process and destroying them. Various agencies may have policies on how this is done because it often needs to be witnessed.

BACK TO OUR CASE

Sundra became weaker and weaker. Her daughters stayed with her around the clock and provided meticulous personal care. They gave her an eye dropper of pain medications under her tongue before they provided any further care. They gently rubbed her skin with favorite lotions and oils. Even though she was thin, she had no bed sores. They cleaned her mouth with sponges and applied frequent applications of lip balm. As her weakness progressed, she could no longer eat or drink without coughing. They decided to stop food and fluids and all medications. Sundra talked quietly and told them she was comfortable and she appeared peaceful to the nurse. She said she was ready and asked her daughters if it was okay if she left. Her daughters tearfully told her they loved her and that it was time to go. Her vital signs decreased. The daughters knew she was close to death. The nurse told them what would happen, and reviewed the need for any other family to see her before she died or any religious rituals. Family gathered in the evening and Sundra died peacefully in the morning. Her daughters felt it was a gift to care for her at home.

TAKE AWAY POINTS

- The dying process includes some predictable signs and symptoms such as fatigue, weakness, loss of appetite, and less engagement of the patient.
- Information about the dying process may help families cope better.

REFERENCES

[1] Institute of Medicine. In: Field MJ, Behrman DE, et al., eds. *Approaching Death: Improving Care at the End of Life*. Washington, DC: Institute of Medicine, National Academy Press; 2003.

[2] American Nurses Association. *Nursing: Scope and Standard of Practice*. Washington, DC: American Nurses Association; 2010.

[3] Lynch M, Dahlin C. The National Consensus Project and National Quality Forum. Preferred practices in care of the imminently dying patient: Implications for nursing. *Journal of Hospice and Palliative Care Nursing*. 2007; 9(6):316–322.

[4] Lo K. Changes as Death Approaches. In: Panke J, Coyne P, eds. *Conversations in Palliative Care*, 2nd edition. Pittsburgh: Hospice and Palliative Nurses Association; 2006; 161–171.

[5] Callahan, M. *What is Normal for Dying Isn't Normal. Final Journey—A Practical Guide for Bringing Care and Comfort at the End of Life*. New York: Bantam Books-Random House; 2008.

Case 1.3 Accommodating Religiosity and Spirituality in Medical Decision-Making

Jennifer Gentry

HISTORY

Cynthia was a 50-year-old African-American woman admitted to the hospital with abdominal pain, nausea, and vomiting. Upon further evaluation, Cynthia was diagnosed with stage IV ovarian cancer. She underwent surgery for a suspected bowel obstruction, but the disease was too advanced for tumor de-bulking or placement of a gastrostomy tube. Post operatively, she was started on total parenteral nutrition as a bridge to receiving chemotherapy.

Cynthia's sister, Phoebe, was by her side throughout her hospital stay. Cynthia's only other family was an adult daughter and young grandchild, who lived in another state. Both Cynthia and Phoebe expressed the importance of their faith in tangible ways. Above the head of the bed was a banner that read, "Expect a miracle" and there were numerous outward expressions of faith visible in the hospital room including a Bible on the bedside table. Cynthia's sister met each staff person who entered the hospital room with one request: "If you don't have anything positive to say, stay out". The medical team believed that Cynthia would likely die from her illness within six months but attempts to discuss prognosis and goals of care were met with strong resistance from both Cynthia and her sister. Both the patient and her sister frequently referred to their belief in miracles and expressed the belief that God would miraculously heal Cynthia.

Case Studies in Palliative and End-of-Life Care, First Edition. Edited by Margaret L. Campbell.
© 2012 John Wiley & Sons, Inc. Published 2012 by John Wiley & Sons, Inc.

PHYSICAL EXAMINATION

Temperature: 37.4°C, Pulse: 112, respiratory rate: 22
Central nervous system: Alert, oriented, no focal deficits
Head, eyes, ears, nose, throat: Alopecia, temporal wasting, no other abnormalities
Cardiac: S1 S2 and tachycardia, no S3 or S4, no murmurs
Lungs: Clear lung sounds, diminished at bases, no accessory muscle use
Gastrointestinal: Firm, distended abdomen, occasional high-pitched bowel sounds, diffuse tenderness, midline incision with intact staple line
Genitourinary: Voiding
Extremities: 2+ bilateral lower extremity edema, no pressure ulcers or deformities

DIAGNOSTICS

Abdominal CT scan: Evidence of diffuse peritoneal carcinomatosis, small bowel obstruction
Chemistry and complete blood count: Unremarkable
Ca 125: 99.3 (normal range zero to 35)

CLINICAL QUESTION

How do providers accommodate religiosity when communicating a poor prognosis?

DISCUSSION

Defining Spirituality and Religiosity

Puchalski defines spirituality as that which gives people meaning and purpose in life, with religion being one expression of that spirituality. Mueller describes religion as something that "organizes the collective spiritual experiences of a group of people into a system of beliefs and practices" and goes on to define religiosity as "the degree of participation or adherence to the beliefs and practices of an organized religion".[1,2] Though some people consider spirituality important, they may do so without holding specific religious beliefs.

Religious beliefs can be the filter for how a serious illness is viewed and inform a person's response to it.[1]

Influence of Spirituality and Religiosity on Decision-Making

A divide exists between the public and the health care profession regarding the importance of religious beliefs in medical decision-making.[3] In one study, health care professionals considered religious beliefs less important in decision-making than the public at large.[3] Beliefs in divine intervention in situations deemed medically futile, such as recovery from a persistent vegetative state, are common.[3] The impact of these beliefs should not be underestimated by the health care team because they directly influence the type and aggressiveness of care provided, even when the patient's prognosis is poor. Despite the importance of religion in the lives of patients, spiritual needs frequently go unmet by the health care system.[4]

Balboni and colleagues studied the effect of serious illness on the need for spiritual support and how religiousness affects preferences for treatment.[4] African–Americans and Hispanics were more likely than Caucasians to consider religion very important.[4,5] Patients with higher degrees of religiousness have an association with preferences for more aggressive treatment and all measures to extend life.[4,5] Phelps and colleagues examined the influence of religious coping and aggressiveness of care in patients with end-stage cancer.[6] Religious coping referred to the use of religious beliefs and practices to understand and adapt to the stress of life-threatening illness. In this study, patients with a high degree of religious coping were significantly more likely to have preferences for aggressive, life-prolonging care such as mechanical ventilation, fewer advance directives, and fewer do not resuscitate (DNR) orders.[6] It is not difficult to imagine that strongly held religious beliefs may directly conflict with medical opinions regarding prognosis and course of treatment.

Care of seriously ill patients includes more than caring for the body but also caring for the human spirit. Acknowledging the multidimensional aspects of a person's being are essential to providing the type of care that both relieves suffering and supports coping at the most basic level. Spiritual beliefs become increasingly important as the end of life approaches,[7] and spiritual pain/existential suffering can exacerbate symptoms such as depression and anxiety.[8] Many patients would like their provider to inquire about their spiritual and religious beliefs if they become gravely ill, yet this is something with which many health care providers feel uncomfortable.[9] By first recognizing the importance of providing excellent spiritual care, the health care team can begin a respectful dialogue about spiritual/religious beliefs while keeping lines of communication open.

Spiritual Care Assessment

Engaging a patient and family in the discussion of their spiritual/religious beliefs can help to establish trust and understanding of the patient's approach to her illness. Health care professionals must consider spiritual assessment to be as important as a thorough medical history and physical examination. Several tools for spiritual assessment exist and one the best known, the FICA spiritual assessment tool, is an effective way for clinicians to integrate open-ended spiritual questions into the medical history:[10]

F: Faith, Meaning, Belief
- Religious/religiosity: Faith, including specific religious beliefs, rules of conduct, rituals, behaviors, values ("Do you consider yourself spiritual or religious?")
- Spirituality: Attitudes and beliefs in life, a higher-power, nature, value ("What gives your life meaning?")

I: Importance and Influence
- Importance of faith or belief
- How would you rate the importance of faith or belief in your life (0 to 5 point scale)?
- Do your beliefs help in handling stress?
- How do your beliefs affect making health care decisions?

C: Community
- "Are you part of a religious or spiritual community?"
- "How does this community offer support to you?"
- "Is there a group of people that are very important in your life?"

A: Address in Care
- "How can your health care team best support your spirituality?"
- "How would you like your health care team to use the information we have talked about in your care?"

Other clues that invite exploration of religious or spiritual beliefs are right in front our eyes and beg further investigation. Examples of helpful open-ended questions that can easily be included in conversation:[11]

Ask questions: "What has helped you get through this difficult time?", "Tell me more about how this has been helpful."

Listen for clues that patients and families give: "All I can do now is pray." "Miracles happen."

Look for clues such as religious/spiritual objects or books (Bible, Koran, inspirational books, religious objects/depictions).

Responding to Belief in Miracles

The use of the word "miracle" is common in health care settings and may be associated with religious beliefs.[12] Rushton describes miracles as "unexplainable events or actions that challenge the limits of humans, technology and apparently contradict known scientific laws".[12] When the word "miracle" is used by patients and families, professionals may assume that "denial" is present rather than an opportunity to explore. Using medical explanations to challenge a belief in miracles almost never works and may harm communication moving forward. Inviting further discussion with thoughtful questions and acknowledging the emotion of the situation can improve understanding. It is vital to involve spiritual care professionals when religious/spiritual beliefs, such as miracles, impact care. Rushton has identified strategies that can assist clinicians in working with families whose religious beliefs in miracles can affect decision-making:[12]

- Search for common ground: Acknowledge a mutual commitment to the patient's best interests
- Assess understanding: Ask "What do you understand about the situation" and provide accurate information and correct misunderstandings
- Understand the meaning of miracles, don't assume: "Tell me more about your belief in miracles"
- Honor one's faith: Faith traditions of both the patient and the professionals must be understood and honored
- Allow hope for a miracle: Acknowledge and respect another's beliefs, values, and faith

Respecting Professional and Personal Boundaries

Respecting the belief system and faith of a patient and family can be a challenge when the provider has personal spiritual or religious views that are very different. Though a spiritual assessment can provide information vital to the development of the plan of care, the patient's privacy should be respected if she does not wish to discuss her beliefs. Health care providers are in a position of authority and must guard against imposing personal perspectives on vulnerable patients.[13] Recognizing the value of professional chaplains and other spiritual care professionals in patient care is essential. There may be situations in which a patient has theological concerns and questions that require the expertise of a "spiritual care specialist" and making a referral can be very helpful.

Patients frequently ask their health care provider to disclose personal spiritual beliefs and opinions. In some situations, a patient may ask the provider to pray. Health care providers may feel uncomfortable with these conversations and struggle to find an appropriate response. Responding with "I am sorry but I can't do this" may inhibit future communication, convey a lack of empathy, or engender mistrust. Conversely, a provider offering: "Would you like for me to pray with you?" may lead to a vulnerable patient feeling obligated to comply.

Puchalski notes that it is seldom appropriate to share one's personal beliefs with patients unless one knows the patient and that sharing these beliefs would not influence or inhibit the sharing of these beliefs.[13] Answering the patient's request with a question such as "Tell me more about why you ask?" can further the conversation while conveying empathy and respect. A similar response, "I respect your beliefs. I would like to hear more about them and what they have meant to you," puts the focus back on the patient and off of the provider. Though some patients may not be satisfied with this response, the health care professional should not violate his own comfort level.[13]

BACK TO OUR CASE

Regrettably, Cynthia's condition deteriorated despite all efforts and she was transferred to the intensive care unit (ICU), where she was intubated and supported on vasopressors. Cynthia was unable to speak for herself and the medical team had a meeting with both her adult daughter and her sister. The grim prognosis was brought up by the team, who suggested discontinuing the life support, but the family remained steadfast in their desire that full resuscitative measures and aggressive care be in place. The family strongly expressed a belief that a miracle would happen and were upset that the team "wanted to give up." The patient remained on mechanical ventilation in the ICU for 12 weeks. Tension between the desires of the family and delivering what the team felt to be "futile" care remained constant.

Though chronically critically ill, Cynthia remained in the ICU for 12 weeks with her family by her side. During this time, discussions related to the goals for Cynthia's care became more focused on ways to manage symptoms, and to continue the course of treatment without initiating additional invasive treatments. During a care meeting, the family, ICU, and palliative care team were able to express a shared commitment to the goal of providing the best care for Cynthia: "Though we can continue to hope for a miracle, at the same time, there is much that can be done to improve her symptoms and avoid more discomfort."

Withdrawal of the ventilator was not open to discussion but a tracheostomy was placed to ease the discomfort caused by the endotracheal tube. Liberal visitation for family and friends was encouraged and faith-based rituals including prayer, singing, religious music, and "laying on of hands" were respected and accommodated as much as possible. The ICU staff took an approach that avoided confrontation and allowed for the open expression and practice of religious beliefs. It was this approach that facilitated trust between the patient, family, and health care team. At the end of her life, Cynthia was allowed to die without an attempt at resuscitation but remained on the ventilator.

! TAKE AWAY POINTS

- Spiritual needs have increasing significance at the end of life.
- Religious beliefs are important components of medical decision-making.
- High levels of religiosity are associated with increased use of aggressive care at the end of life.
- Spiritual assessment is an essential component of care for seriously ill patients.
- Open-ended, non-confrontational communication techniques are essential in exploring how religious beliefs affect decision-making.
- Providers should guard against imposing personal spiritual or religious beliefs on patients and their families.

REFERENCES

[1] Puchalski CM, Dorff E, Hendi Y. Spirituality, religion, and healing in palliative care. *Clinics in Geriatric Medicine.* 2004; 20:689–714.

[2] Mueller P, Plevak D, Rummans T. Religious involvement, spirituality, and medicine: Implications for clinical practice. *Mayo Clinic Proceedings.* 2001; 76:1225–1235.

[3] Jacobs L, Burns K, Jacobs B. Trauma death: Views of the public and trauma professionals on death and dying from injuries. *Archives of Surgery.* 2008; 143:730–735.

[4] Balboni TA, Wanderwerker LC, Block SD, Paulk E, Lathan CS, Peteet JR, Prigerson HG. Religiousness and spiritual support among advanced cancer patients and associations with end-of-life treatment preferences and quality of life. *Journal of Clinical Oncology.* 2007; 25:1140–1147.

[5] Johnson KS, Kuchibhatla M, Tulsky JA. What explains racial differences in the use of advance directives and attitudes toward hospice care? *Journal of the American Geriatric Society.* 2008; 56:1953–1958.

[6] Phelps AC, Maciejewski PK, Nilsson M, et al. Religious coping and use of intensive life-prolonging care near death, in patients with advanced cancer. *Journal of the American Medical Association.* 2009; 301:1140–1147.

[7] Steinhauser KE, Christakis NA, Clipp EC, McIntyre L, Tulsky JA. Factors considered important at the end of life by patients, family, physicians, and other care providers. *Journal of the American Medical Association.* 2000; 284:2476–2482.

[8] Delgado MO, Hui D, Parsons HA, et al. Spirituality, religiosity, and spiritual pain in advanced cancer patients. *Journal of Pain and Symptom Management.* March 2011; epub ahead of print.

[9] Ehman J, Ott B, Short T, Ciampa R, Hansen-Flaschen J. Do patients want physicians to inquire about their spiritual or religious beliefs if they become gravely ill? *Archives of Internal Medicine.* 1999; 159:1803–1806.

[10] Borneman T, Ferrell B, Puchalski CM. Evaluation of the FICA tool for spiritual assessment. *Journal of Pain and Symptom Management*. 2010; 40:163–173.

[11] Gentry JH, Galanos AN, Bryan L. Spiritual Warfare: Moral distress. Austin, Texas: Annual Assembly of the American Academy of Hospice and Palliative Medicine/Hospice and Palliative Nurses Association; 2009.

[12] Rushton CH, Russell K. The Language of miracles: Ethical challenges. *Pediatric Nursing*. 1996; 22:64.

[13] Braam A, Klinkenberg M, Deeg D. Religion and mood in the last week of life: An explorative approach based on after death proxy interviews. *Journal of Palliative Medicine*. 2011; 14:31–37.

Case 1.4 Discussing Cardiopulmonary Resuscitation When it May Be Useful

Kelli Gershon

HISTORY

Ed was a 67-year-old white man being evaluated at an acute care hospital after complaining of chest pain. He described the pain (eight out of 10) as stabbing in nature and it was associated with shortness of breath and "sweating." He also mentioned that he had been having shortness of breath at night and when he lays flat for weeks to months. He had driven himself to the emergency room because his family practitioner would not "call in something," because he had not been seen for three years.

Ed recently lost his wife to a long battle with breast cancer and the past three to five years he had been her primary caregiver. He was living alone in the house that they shared and he had three children that lived out of state. He stated his only past medical history included gastric esophageal reflux disease and arthritis. He treated both of these conditions with over-the-counter medications.

The emergency room physician asked Ed about resuscitation, specifically, "If you die do you want me to do anything?" Ed responded, "Are we talking about a DNR (do not rescusitate) order? If so I want to be DNR. All that stuff doesn't help anyway." With this information a palliative care consult was ordered.

Case Studies in Palliative and End-of-Life Care, First Edition. Edited by Margaret L. Campbell.
© 2012 John Wiley & Sons, Inc. Published 2012 by John Wiley & Sons, Inc.

PHYSICAL EXAMINATION

Temperature: 37.1°C, blood pressure: 180/100 mm Hg, heart rate: 32 bpm, respiratory rate 15
Central nervous system: Alert, oriented, diaphoretic
Head, eyes, ears, nose, throat: No defects or abnormalities
Cardiac: Bradycardic, III/VI midsystolic murmur, IV/VI systolic murmur, jugular vein distention 8 cm
Lungs: No wheezing or rales, good air movement, SpO_2 98% on room air
GI: Positive bowel sounds all four quadrants, non-tender/non-distended
GU: voiding
Ext: Lower extremities no pitting edema, 2+ dorsal pulse/pedal pulses

DIAGNOSTICS

Serum creatine: 1.0 mg/dl, hematocrit: 36%
Electrocardiogram (EKG): Sinus bradycardia with rate of 35 beats/minute, right bundle branch block with left anterior hemi-block, no acute ischemic changes
Echocardiogram: Ejection fraction 15%–20%, inferior wall hypokinesis, 3+ aortic insufficiency, 2+ mitral regurgitation, moderate left atrium enlargement, moderate dilation of thoracic aorta (over 5.5 cm)

CLINICAL QUESTION

How should cardiopulmonary resuscitation (CPR) be discussed when it may be beneficial?

DISCUSSION

History of CPR

Closed-chest cardiac massage or CPR was introduced in 1960 so that cardiac resuscitation could be done without open thoracotomy and direct cardiac massage. A monograph written in 1965 entitled *Fundamentals of Cardiopulmonary Resuscitation* declared:

"The first principal of CPR is the patient must be salvable: Cardiopulmonary resuscitation is indicated for the patient who, at the time of cardiopulmonary arrest, is not in a terminal stage of an incurable disease. Resuscitative measures on terminal patients will, at best, return them to the dying state. The physician should concentrate on resuscitating patients who were in good health preceding arrest, and who are likely to resume a normal existence. Resuscitation of the dying patient with irreparable damage to the heart, lungs, brain, or any other vital system of the body has no medical, ethical, or moral justification. The techniques described in this monograph are designed to resuscitate the victim of acute insult, whether it be from drowning, electrical shock, untoward side effects of drugs, anesthetic accident, heart block, acute myocardial infarction, or surgery."[1]

The American Heart Association has put out multiple standards over the years and all have emphasized that CPR is not indicated in all situations. In the early standards it clearly states, "CPR is the prevention of sudden, unexpected death, it is not indicated in certain situations, such as in cases of terminal irreversible illness where death is not unexpected."[2] In the more recent guidelines it encourages physicians not to offer CPR as an intervention if it is not going to be beneficial. Patients and surrogate decision makers have the right to choose from medically appropriate options but this does not imply that they have the right to demand care that is medically inappropriate and beyond accepted standards of care.[3]

Outcomes of CPR

The largest and most comprehensive source of in-hospital CPR outcomes is the National Registry of Cardiopulmonary Resuscitation (now called *Get With the Guidelines: Resuscitation*). Their most recent evaluation was done looking at 36,902 in-hospital adult resuscitation (2000–2004) from 10% of all U.S. hospitals.[4] The results are as follows:

- 45% to 67% of patients experienced return of spontaneous circulation.
- 38% to 62% of patients survived the event.
- 18% survived to discharge.
- 60% to 75% of survivors at discharge demonstrated ability to care for themselves.
- 18% of survivors were unable to care for themselves after discharge (functional level is unknown in the rest of the patients).
- Outcomes were better in ventricular fibrillation and pulseless ventricular tachycardia compared to pulseless electrical activity or aystole.

A meta-analysis of CPR hospital outcomes was reported in 1998; it included data from 49 research publications after 1980, totaling 9,838 patients.[5] The results are as follows:

- Immediate survival was 41%–44%.
- Survival to discharge was 13%–15%.

- Only five studies reviewed if patients discharged to home; 73 of 93 patients (78%) returned home.
- Factors that predicted a failure to survive to discharge included:
  - Sepsis prior to CPR
  - Serum creatine greater than 1.5 mg/dL
  - Metastatic cancer
  - Dementia
  - Dependent status

Outcomes of CPR in specific populations

Cancer

CPR in advanced cancer patients has been associated with a low (7%) success rate or failure to survive to discharge.[6] Factors that make this number lower include, metastatic disease, CPR in the critical care unit, and anticipated arrest.

Heart Failure

There are few studies that specifically look at survival rates in patients with heart failure who undergo CPR. A meta-analysis of studies reported that class III/IV heart failure was a weaker negative predictor of survival than cancer.[7] In one investigation, survival to discharge after CPR was only 19%.[8] Most (67%) heart failure patients undergoing an interventional procedure had a return of spontaneous circulation and 38% survived to hospital discharge, compared to patients without heart failure, with 80% return of spontaneous circulation and 61% survival to hospital discharge.[9] Fewer than 10% of patients survived a hospital cardiac arrest if the heart failure diagnosis was new.[10]

Chronic Obstructive Pulmonary Disease (COPD)

As with heart failure, there is limited data to educate us on how patients with COPD will do with CPR. Two studies are available that show:

- Of 42 patients who arrested, survival to discharge was 11.9% with diagnosis of COPD compared to 16.6% with no diagnosis of COPD.[8]
- COPD as a co-morbidity before hospitalization was not associated with low CPR survival (n=55); however, COPD as admitting diagnosis with subsequent arrest showed no survivors (n=5).[11]

Renal Failure

Outcomes during acute care hospitalization were reported:[12]

- 137 dialysis patient underwent CPR; survival to discharge was 14%
- Of 74 dialysis patients that had undergone CPR, only two (3%) survived six months compared to 9% of non-dialysis patients.

Talking with Patients about CPR and DNR

Even though the evidence regarding survival outcomes for patients receiving palliative care is limited, it is good to know which patients might be candidates for CPR and which ones will not benefit from CPR. The resuscitation discussion should be part of a larger discussion regarding advance care planning, a discussion that includes disease prognosis and mutually agreed upon goals of care. Meaningless "choices" such as CPR for imminently dying patients are to be avoided.[13]

Many patients and families have an unrealistic view of the outcomes associated with CPR; they get their information mostly from television, where almost everyone survives a "code." Lay people believe that CPR is successful in restoring a victim to prearrest status more than 50% of the time. Investigators have shown that if a patient or surrogate decision-maker is given a realistic probability about survival she is more likely to opt for DNR.[14,15]

An example of good communication when CPR is not warranted follows:[16] "I will provide you with maximal treatment for your pain or other symptoms you may experience; I do not recommend the use of breathing machines or other artificial means to prolong your life."

A recent development in advance directives discussion is the use of video to facilitate discussion about goals of care. Many times patients or their surrogates can appreciate a more realistic picture of advance disease or process of resuscitation if it is shown to them in videos. Videos are available that show patients with various chronic illness and how their lives are, therefore helping individuals better understand what their disease looks like.[17] Other videos are available that show different medical interventions including CPR and ventilators. El-Jawari and colleagues evaluated whether use of a video helped facilitate end-of-life discussion. Fifty participants were randomly assigned to either verbal narrative or video regarding their wishes of life-prolonging care, basic care, or comfort care. Their findings follow:[18]

Choice after discussion	Verbal	Video
Life-prolonging treatment	25.9%	None
Basic care	51.9%	4.4%
Comfort Care	22.2%	91.3%

BACK TO OUR CASE

During our palliative care consult, Ed was educated about his new diagnosis of heart failure (HF). On admission to the hospital Ed was by no means optimally treated for his HF; therefore, for him to make a decision about goals of care was not realistic. After a couple of days Ed's symptoms improved, as did his understanding of his new diagnosis. During the discussion about advance directives it became clear that he had decided to have a DNR designation based on information he was given by his wife's oncologist regarding her survival chances with CPR. Once Ed's case was discussed, he reversed his DNR and had a long discussion with his son regarding his goals of care. He decided if his quality of life was such that he could live alone and participate in his grandchildren's lives he wanted to continue to aggressively treat his heart failure. However, at any point he was unable to live alone or be active with his grandchildren he would not want to prolong his life.

Ed agreed with insertion of a pacemaker with automated implantable cardiovertor/defibrillator (AICD) due to his high risk of sudden cardiac death. In his goals of care discussion with his son he instructed his son that he would want his AICD turned off if he was not able to live the quality of life he wanted.

! TAKE AWAY POINTS

- There is limited research available to educate patients regarding outcomes of CPR in advanced illness, especially in relationship to quality of life.
- Outcomes of CPR vary by diagnosis. Do not offer CPR to a patient who will not benefit from the intervention.
- The DNR decision should be part of a larger advance care planning discussion including prognosis and mutually agreed upon goals.
- Consider using videos to help patients and families better understand their diagnosis and resuscitation.

REFERENCES

[1] Jude JR, Leam JO. *Fundamentals of Cardiopulmonary Resuscitation*. Philadelphia: F.A. Davis Company; 1965.
[2] National Conference on Cardiopulmonary Resuscitation and Emergency Cardiac Care. Standards and guidelines for cardiopulmonary resuscitation and emergency cardiac care, Part V: Medicolegal considerations and recommendations. *JAMA* 1974; 227:864–866.
[3] American Heart Associations. *Advance Cardiac Life Support*. Dallas: American Heart Association; 1994.
[4] Jacobs I, Nadkarni V. Cardiac arrest and cardiopulmonary resuscitation outcome reports. *Circulation*, 2004; 110:3385–3397.
[5] Ebell MH, Becker LA, Barry HC, Hagen M. Survival after in-hospital cardiopulmonary resuscitation: a meta analysis. *J Gen Intern Med* 1998; 13:805–816.

[6] Schneider, AP, Nelson DJ, Brown DD. In-hospital cardiopulmonary resuscitation: a 30-year review. *J Am Board Fam Pract.* 1993; 6(2):91–101.

[7] Cohn, EG, Lefevre F, Yarnold PR, et al. Predicting survival from in-hospital CPR: a meta–analysis and validation of a prediction model. *J Gen Intern Med.* 1993; 8(7):399–400.

[8] Ballew KA, Philbrick JT, Caven D, et al. Predictors of survival following in-hospital cardiopulmonary resuscitation: a moving target. *Arch Intern Med.* 1994; 154:1416–1432.

[9] Sprung J, Ritter M, Charanjit S. et al. Outcomes of cardiopulmonary resuscitation and predictors of survival in patients undergoing coronary angiography including percutaneous coronary interventions. *Anesth Analg.* 2006; 102:217–224.

[10] de Vos R, Koster R, Haan R, et al. In-hospital cardiopulmonary resuscitation: pre-arrest morbidity and outcome. *Arch Intern Med.* 1999; 159(8):845–850.

[11] DiBari M, Chiarlone M, Fumagalli S, et al. Cardiopulmonary resuscitation of older in-hospital patients: immediate efficacy and long-term outcome. *Crit Care Med.* 2000; 28(7):2320–2325.

[12] Hijazi F, Hossey JL. Cardiopulmonary resuscitation and dialysis: outcome and patients' views. *Semin Dialysis* 2003; 16:51–53.

[13] Gillick M. Decision making near life's end: A Prescription for change. *Journal of Palliative Medicine.* 2009; 12(2):121–125.

[14] American Heart Association in collaboration with the International Liaison Committee on Resuscitation. Guidelines 2000 for cardiopulmonary resuscitation and emergency cardiovascular care: An international consensus on science, Part 2: Ethical aspects of CPR and ECC. *Circulation* 2000; 102(Suppl I):I12-I-21.

[15] Agich GJ, Arroliga AC. Appropriate use of DNR orders: A practical approach. *Cleve Clin J Med* 2000; 67:392–400.

[16] Weissman, D. Do not resuscitate orders: A call for reform. *Journal of Palliative Medicine.* 1999; 2(2):152.

[17] Volandes A, Paasche-Orloff M, Gillick M, Shaykevich S, Abbo ED, Lehmann L: Health literacy not race predicts end of life care preferences. *J Palliative Med* 2008; 11:754–762.

[18] El-Jawahri A., Podgurski L, Volandes A. Use of video to facilitate end-of-life discussions with patients with cancer: A randomized controlled trial. *American Society of Clinical Oncology.* 2010; 28(2):305–310.

Case 1.5 Discussing CPR When it is a Non-Beneficial Intervention

Judy Passaglia

HISTORY

Valerie was a 48-year-old Asian woman who was admitted to the hospital following a visit to the outpatient neuro-oncology clinic, where she presented with significant functional decline. Valerie had a history of metastatic non-small cell lung cancer, diagnosed in 2007. She was status post resection and chemotherapy. In 2009, Valerie developed multiple metastases to the brain (parietal and frontal). On her last admission, the brain MRI revealed new areas of central nervous system (CNS) metastasis, hemorrhage, and a growing lung lesion. Valerie was non-verbal due to her CNS disease; therefore, the history was obtained from her husband, Conner, and her brother, Jim. Conner reported that Valerie was managing relatively well in a rehabilitation facility until two weeks prior to hospital admission. She could stand with one person assisting her and she could speak, although unintelligibly. Since then, there had been an overall decline in her speech, mobility, and level of alertness. Valerie did not have enough strength to sit up in her chair and spent more than 50% of her day in bed sleeping. She required assistance with feeding and had difficulty with swallowing, with occasional choking episodes. Valerie had been incontinent of urine and had constipation, requiring an enema every other day.

Valerie lived with her husband and 12-year-old daughter. They had an interracial marriage, as her husband, Conner, was Caucasian. Her parents lived next door and only spoke Mandarin. They spent much of

Case Studies in Palliative and End-of-Life Care, First Edition. Edited by Margaret L. Campbell.
© 2012 John Wiley & Sons, Inc. Published 2012 by John Wiley & Sons, Inc.

the day with her, at home and in the hospital. All family members were emotionally devastated with her overall decline and were very concerned about the effect her condition would have on the patient's daughter. Valerie was an architect who was functional until the disease progressed six months prior to hospitalization.

Valerie was referred to the palliative care consult service to review the goals of care; at referral, Valerie's orders included "full code." In other words, she would have received an advanced cardiac life support (ACLS) resuscitation attempt if she died while in the hospital. Based on the disease progression and functional decline, Valerie met criteria for a hospice referral. However, the patient's husband, parents, and brothers were searching for additional treatment options.

PHYSICAL EXAMINATION

Temperature: 36.2°C, blood pressure: 111/63, respiratory rate 17

Central nervous system: Eyes open, regards examiner, tracks, does not follow commands, non-verbal, unable to move right arm, spontaneous movement of left arm

Head, eyes, ears, nose, throat: within normal limits

Cardiac: Regular rate and rhythm

Lungs: Clear on auscultation bilaterally with no wheezes, rales, or rhonchi, SpO_2 96% on room air

Gastrointestinal: Abdomen soft and non-tender with active bowel sounds

Genitourinary: Incontinent of urine, diapered

Extremities: No edema or discoloration with palpable pulses

DIAGNOSTICS

Lumbar puncture: No malignant cells or intracellular micro organisms. Total protein elevated 125 (reference range < 45 mg/dl), glucose 66

CT chest abdomen pelvis: February 2007, 7-cm left lower lobe mass; CT-guided biopsy confirmed a non-small cell lung cancer favoring adeno carcinoma. PET/CT demonstrated a 7.7-cm left lower lobe lesion as well as two lymph nodes, one subcarinal lesion, the second a left hilar node.

MRI brain: September 2010, interval increase in the area of hemorrhage. Increased size of the large complex left thalamic metastatic lesion with both solid and hemorrhagic components. Increased mass effect causing ventricular obstruction likely at the level of the cerebral aqueduct with ventriculomegaly. Interval increase in bilateral, lateral, and third ventricular size concerning for worsening hydrocephalus.

?	**CLINICAL QUESTION**

How is the discussion regarding cardiopulmonary resuscitation (CPR) approached, in the setting of advanced illness, when it will not likely offer benefit?

✓	**DISCUSSION**

Performance status is a measure of the level of functional capacity, which is indicative of how well a person is able to carry on activities of daily living while living with cancer. Performance status is more important than cancer type in determining prognosis, because it is a predictor of survival.[1,2] When this is the situation, it is important to address resuscitation (see Table 1.5.1).

A patient with advanced illness and decreased performance status will not benefit from resuscitative efforts. Survival for hospital-based

TABLE 1.5.1. Steps toward resuscitation status clarification.

Preparation
Review the medical record to fully understand the disease status.
Assess frequency of emergency room or inpatient hospital admissions.
Review the advance directive.
Identify the agent for health care decision making.

Assess the patient
Conduct a physical examination.
Assess functional status.
Assess caregiving needs.

Family meeting (Include the patient if appropriate)
Assess patient/family understanding of the illness.
Provide an update of the disease status.
Ask what the patient/family are hoping for.
Establish the goals.
Discuss the prognosis.
Address cardiopulmonary resuscitation.
Reinforce that DNR/DNI does not exclude other treatment modalities.
Commit to follow up with the patient/family in a timely manner.
Provide contact information.

Strategies for success
Listen actively.
Provide strategic pauses in the dialogue.
Share empathy.
Explore questions and concerns.

CPR is 10% to 15% and is much lower for patients with metastatic cancer.[3] See Case 1.4 for an overview of CPR outcomes. The discussion regarding resuscitation status is best incorporated into the "goals of care" discussion, which involves an exploration of values, perception of illness, and hopes for the future.[4,5] When a patient is non-verbal and/or no longer has capacity, the discussions about advance care planning should be held with the patient's surrogate decision maker. If the patient has an advance directive, it is best to review the document before meeting with the surrogate decision maker and/or family because it may help facilitate a discussion about goals of care and treatment choices.[6]

It is important to perform a through physical, psychosocial, and spiritual assessment before approaching a discussion regarding advance care planning.[7]

Formal communication typically occurs in a family conference, which is the next step in the decision-making process. In this setting, the team can explore the values and goals of the patient and family.[8] It is important that cultural differences be acknowledged and respected to develop a trusting relationship with all participants.[9]

The discussion begins with a question relative to the patient's and family's understanding of the illness, which is a means of framing the goals of care discussion.[4,5] Whomever is leading the meeting should first introduce all participants, including the professional staff and services represented. It is essential that the team actively listen and express empathy.[10,11] The process of telling the story provides an opportunity for the family to acknowledge the patient's decline. Inability to recognize that a patient is nearing the end of her life is a barrier to a discussion of code status.[12]

Before asking the family to engage in a shared decision-making process, it is essential to review the anticipated course of illness and the probable outcome of the disease.[11,12] As a means of establishing the goals, it is helpful to ask an open-ended question such as "As you think about your wife's illness, what are you hoping for?"[13]

The discussion regarding cardiopulmonary resuscitation is addressed in the context of the advanced illness, patient's response to treatment, and overall performance status. Downar suggests the clinician start with asking the patient/family what they know about CPR before proceeding to describe an actual arrest (cardiopulmonary resuscitation, artificial respirations, and chest compressions).[4] It is important to reinforce that cardiac arrest is a natural consequence of the underlying disease. The team should express empathy in response to emotionally laden statements, which will ensure patients and families are heard and their emotions are validated.[10, 15]

If CPR does not achieve the goals expressed by the patient and family, it is not an appropriate intervention.[13] It is important that the discussion be framed in a way that addresses CPR survival benefit.[4,12,14]

The team should be prepared to make recommendations based on the clinical situation.[14] This serves to release the burden that is shouldered by the family in the decision-making process.[4, 11] It is important for the team to communicate that saying no to CPR does not mean they are saying no to all other interventions.[3, 16.]

The communication needs of the family remain a focus of the palliative care team throughout the process. Timely communication serves to reduce conflict and stress for all involved.[17] Through this process, trust is developed, decisions are made, and there is a gradual transition in the goals of care.

BACK TO OUR CASE

The patient had a Karnofsky performance status of 20/100 and was dependent upon others for all activities of daily living. She had many signs of decline including increased somnolence and anorexia. The patient was also non-ambulatory and non-verbal.

There was an advance directive in place that named her husband as her agent for health care decision-making. The advance directive was vague in that it did not specify what the patient would want if she were faced with an irreversible medical condition.

The palliative care team, attending physician, and advanced practice nurse examined the patient and met her parents. The patient was sitting up in the wheelchair. Occasionally, she shifted her eyes toward a voice and uttered a sound. She did not follow commands, but appeared to be relatively comfortable. Her mother massaged her hands and feet while her father sat quietly in a chair. Because the patient's parents spoke Mandarin, a hospital interpreter was present. Through the translator, the palliative care team learned that the family provided twenty-four hour care and that the patient was no longer eating and was somnolent. There were no resources in the home other than the durable medical equipment (hospital bed, commode, and wheelchair). The patient's parents were emotionally distraught as evidenced by their tears and worried expressions.

Following the physical assessment, the palliative care team met with the patient's husband and eldest brother. Although the patient's husband was the surrogate decision maker, the patient's family influenced him in the decision making process. The patient's husband embraced the "big picture," whereas the patient's brother and parents focused on life-sustaining therapies, including nutrition, intravenous fluids, and physical therapy. This may have represented cultural differences.

At the family meeting, the patient's husband reviewed the history of his wife's disease. He stated that she was diagnosed in 2007 and initially responded to treatment. He understood that the disease had recurred with multiple metastases to the brain. He articulated the recent changes including four weeks of profound weakness and increased somnolence. He stated that his wife was non-verbal, but he thought she could understand. The patient's brother nodded in agreement to everything that was shared. The palliative care team responded to the family with empathy by acknowledging their physical distress and sadness: "We are so sorry this is happening to your whole family; we understand you are all suffering."

The team proceeded to provide an update regarding the patient's medical condition: "We reviewed the medical record and spoke with the oncology team. The work-up revealed your wife has a new brain lesion and a growing lung lesion." This was followed by an interval of silence for the family to process the information.

In reviewing the disease status, the palliative care team explained the correlation between the tumor growth and the increase in intracranial pressure, which contributed to the decrease in level of alertness. The palliative care team asked, "What are you hoping for as you look to the days or weeks ahead?" The patient's husband responded, "We hope my wife will be strong enough to have additional chemotherapy, as we have a 12-year-old daughter, who needs her mother." The palliative care team replied, "The team appreciates you are hoping for cancer treatment, but, if your wife is not strong enough for chemotherapy, then what would be most important?" The family was told "Chemotherapy could cause harm and the patient may die sooner because of the side effects of treatment." This was followed by an interval of silence so the family could think about what was discussed and formulate questions.

The team explained that if the patient had a cardiac arrest, which means if she stopped breathing or her heart stopped beating, she would die. In this case, it would be a result of the advanced cancer. The palliative care team then tried to illicit what the patient would want if she could participate. They asked, "If the patient could speak to us right now, how might she guide us in our decision-making?" The patient's husband responded with certainty. "I think she would say she wants to continue to fight."

The team explained that the patient was currently "full resuscitation," which was described in the following manner: "Your wife would be on an artificial breathing machine. She would be in an intensive care setting. She would have a tube inserted down her throat and oxygen would be pushed into her lungs. It is not a comfortable intervention. Having a tube down one's throat is not natural; thus, the inclination is to pull it out. Therefore, most patients are restrained. I know this is a difficult conversation. I am sorry for that."

The palliative care team explained, "Resuscitation outcomes have been extensively studied in patients with metastatic cancer. If your wife was to stop breathing or her heart stopped, this would be her natural dying process, which is a result of her advanced illness. In this case, CPR is not a bridge to a good outcome and it is not recommended by the oncology or the palliative care team. This recommendation is based on a disease that is not reversible. The mechanics of resuscitation would cause more suffering for your wife and the family. What are your thoughts about letting your wife die peacefully, if she was to stop breathing or her heart stopped?"

The team reassured the family if they made the decision to proceed with do not resuscitate/do not intubate (DNR/DNI), their loved one would continue to get other therapeutic interventions. This decision is only applicable to CPR—chest compressions and intubation. If the patient's heart stopped beating, the focus would be to assure a peaceful and comfortable death.

In this case, the palliative care team met the husband and various family members on multiple occasions. Ultimately, the patient's resuscitation status was changed to DNR/DNI. The family was not ready for hospice. However, they hired a 24-hour caregiver and enrolled in a "bridge to hospice" program.

TAKE AWAY POINTS

- Performance status has been found to predict survival in cancer patients.
- Disease prognosis is a starting point for a discussion about CPR.
- A goals of care discussion includes an active exploration of patient/family values, perception of the illness, and hopes for the future.
- Resuscitation outcomes are extremely poor in the setting of serious malignant disease.
- A do-not-resuscitate (DNR) order does not mean a patient cannot obtain other life-sustaining treatments.

REFERENCES

[1] Yun YH, et al. Impact of awareness of terminal illness and use of palliative care or intensive care unit on the survival of terminally ill patients with cancer; prospective cohort study. *Journal of Clinical Oncology.* 2011; 29(18):2472–2480.

[2] Lamont EB, Christakis NA. Epidemiology and prognostication in advanced cancer. In: *Palliative Care and Supportive Oncology.* Philadelphia: Lippincott Williams & Wilkins. 2007; 471.

[3] Bass M. Should patients at the end of life be given the option of receiving CPR? *Nursing Times.* 2001; (105):26–29.

[4] Downar J, Hawryluck L. What should we say when discussing "code status" and life support with a patient? A Delphi analysis. *Journal of Palliative Medicine*. November 2010; (13):190–191.

[5] Kaldjian LC, et al. Code status discussions and goals of care among hospitalized adults. *Journal Medical Ethics*. 2009; 35:338–342.

[6] Tulsky J. Beyond advance directives. Importance of communication skills at the end of life. *JAMA*. 2005; 294(3):349.

[7] Engel G. The clinical application of the bio psychosocial model. *American qournal AMA of Psychiatry* 1980; 137(5):535–544.

[8] Curtis J, et al. The family conference to improve communication in the intensive care unit: opportunities for improvement. *Critical Care Medicine*. 2001; (29):26–33.

[9] Kagawa-Singer M, Blackhall LJ. Negotiating cross-cultural issues at the end of life. "You Got to Go Where He Lives". In: *Care at the Close of Life*. New York: McGraw Hill Professional. 2011; 417–418.

[10] Steinhauser J, et al. Factors considered important at the end of life by patients, families, physicians and other care providers. *JAMA*. 2000; 284(19):2476–2482.

[11] Levin T, Moreno B, et al. End of life communication in the intensive care unit. *General Hospital Psychiatry*. 2010; (32):433–442.

[12] Heyland D, Frank C, et al. Understanding cardiopulmonary resuscitation decision making. *Chest Journal*. August 2006; 130(2):419–427.

[13] Quill E, et al. Discussing treatment preferences with patients who want "everything." *Annals of Internal Medicine*. 2009; 151(5):345–349.

[14] Taylor R, et al. Improving do not resuscitate discussions: A framework for physicians. *Journal of Supportive Oncology*. 2010; 8:42–44.

[15] Quill T, et al. "I wish things were different": expressing wishes in response to loss, futility, and unrealistic hopes. *Annals Internal Medicine*. 2001; 135(7):551–555.

[16] Smith CB, Bunch-ONeill L. Do not resuscitate does not mean do not treat. How palliative care and other modalities can help facilitate communication about goals of care in advanced illness. Available at Wiley Inter Science (www.intersciencewiley.com). Accessed 2008; Mount Sinai Journal of Medicine.

[17] Norton S, et al. Life support withdrawal: communication and conflict. *American Journal of Critical Care* 2003; (12):548–555.

Case 1.6 Discussing Brain Death, Organ Donation, and Donation after Cardiac Death

Christine Westphal and Rebecca Williams

HISTORY: CASE 1

Kevin was a 28-year-old man who suffered a cardiac arrest due to a heroin overdose. He was admitted to the emergency department with resuscitation in progress after 14 minutes of anoxia. Upon transfer to the intensive care unit (ICU), he showed no spontaneous eye opening, no verbal response, and extension of extremities in response to pain. His Glasgow Coma Scale score was 4/15. Kevin met the clinical triggers established for potential organ donors so the nurse contacted the Organ Procurement Organization (OPO). The nurse informed the OPO of Kevin's past medical history, including the illicit drug use. An OPO representative visited the hospital and talked to the nurse about the case. Brain death testing was not yet initiated, thus the family was not approached about donation. The OPO representative directed the staff to call the OPO with changes.

Later that day, the nurse called the OPO staff to inform them that Kevin's condition deteriorated. The brain death examination protocol was planned for the morning. The next day a donation coordinator, an OPO "designated requestor," arrived to collaborate with the team about medical suitability for donation and family understanding of the prognosis. After the family was informed that the clinical examination was consistent with brain death the designated requestor talked to the family about donation.

Case Studies in Palliative and End-of-Life Care, First Edition. Edited by Margaret L. Campbell.
© 2012 John Wiley & Sons, Inc. Published 2012 by John Wiley & Sons, Inc.

How should organ donation be discussed with the organ donor's family?

The philosophy of palliative and hospice care nursing focuses on living well until the moment of death; however, the nurse can also be part of a team that helps the patient transcend death and live on through the gift of life. This unique opportunity requires specialized knowledge and skill.

History of Tissue and Organ Transplantation and Donation

The history of transplanting tissue can be traced in mythology, religious literature, and historic artifacts to ancient times. It has only been within the last 100 years, however, that human tissue and solid organ transplantation have been clinically successful. The earliest tissue transplants were blood, skin, and corneas. Now tissue transplants also include bone, tendons, marrow/stem cells, heart valves, veins, and arteries. Cadaveric kidney transplants were the first attempts at human organ transplant in 1962, followed by the lungs and liver in 1963 and heart in 1967. Unfortunately, early transplants often culminated in tissue rejection and/or recipient death in a very short time. The evolution of brain death criteria, advances in surgical techniques, and immunosuppressive therapy improved the success of non-related donor transplants, particularly related to organs. Organ transplants between living donors are more successful; however, the availability of living donors is relatively low. Thus, the majority of transplants occur from cadaver non-related donors.[1]

The number of people waiting for transplants continues to grow. Today there are more than 110,000 people in the United States waiting for organ transplants, and each day 18 people die waiting.[1,2] Although some tissue and organs can be donated by living donors, the majority of donations are realized from donors after death; in other words, from cadavers. Therefore, the legal definition of death and the opportunity to retrieve tissue/organs are intimately interwoven. Prior to the 1960s, cardiopulmonary criteria (absence of heart beat and breathing) were used to declare death and define the time at which tissues and organs could be donated. The development of brain death criteria shifted the donation paradigm.

Donation after Brain Death

In 1968 an ad hoc committee of the Harvard School of Medicine asserted that death can be determined if there is absence of whole brain function, even in the presence of heart beat.[3] This concept, supported by the President's Commission in 1981,[4] led to the passage of the Uniform Determination of Death Act which defined death as the cessation of cardiopulmonary function or cessation of entire brain and brain stem functions (neurologic criteria).[5] Virtually all states have adopted the Uniform Determination of Death Act, with two notable exceptions. For example, the New York statute requires hospitals to have procedures for reasonable accommodation of individuals with moral or religious objections.[6] In New Jersey a physician cannot apply neurologic criteria to declare death if this would violate the individuals' personal religious beliefs.[7]

Although the majority of religious and cultural groups do not oppose donation or transplant,[8] in some schools of thought within Islam, Orthodox Judaism, and Buddhism, the concept of brain death may be controversial and not accepted.[9] Cultural beliefs maybe interpreted to be opposed to brain death.[10] Clinical dilemmas may develop if the law related to declaration of death by neurologic criteria is in opposition to family's cultural and/or religious beliefs. Guidelines or policies may provide direction in these difficult situations; however, there is no single "right" approach to resolve this dilemma.

Evidence-based guidelines for clinically determining cessation of brain function in adults and children were originally published by the American Academy of Neurology (AAN) in 1995[11,12] and an ad hoc task force of pediatric specialties in 1987, respectively.[13] According to these guidelines three primary criteria must be met: (1) irreversibility of the neurologic condition, (2) the coexistence of coma and apnea after ruling out all other potential etiologies, and (3) absence of brain stem function as determined by cranial nerve testing. Various confirmatory tests, most commonly electroencephalograms, radionuclide flow studies, and cerebral flow studies, can be used in conjunction with the clinical examination, but are not mandatory. In 2010, the AAN Quality Standards Subcommittee researched the evidence and did not recommend any changes to the original guidelines.[14] Even with the guidelines, protocols for the actual determination of brain death vary across hospitals.[15,16] The declaration of death by neurologic criteria (brain death) has increased the number and success of transplants. However, as the transplant waiting list grows, and more families ask about organ donation, there is renewed interest in donation after cardiac death.

Obtaining Consent

Government and regulatory donation guidelines require that only those individuals who receive special training can become "designated requestors" due to the complex, sensitive nature of the request.[17]

Designated requestors must receive special training from the OPO and may be representatives from the OPO, the local tissue or eye bank, or the hospital. Conversations about donation require knowledge, interpersonal skills, and an interdisciplinary approach. Nurses can help by working closely with the designated requestor to provide the option of donation to the family or become designated requestors.

Although a nurse may be an OPO designated requestor, most often the nurse is part of the health care team collaborating with an OPO designated requestor. This collaboration includes sharing the patient's medical history, unique family dynamics, language barriers, and possible religious concerns, and evaluating the family's understanding of the prognosis before talking to the legal next of kin. Thus, the nurse must also be knowledgeable about key concepts related to donation in order to reinforce and support the information provided by the designated requestor. Ambiguity, inconsistent communication, and use of medical terminology can cause confusion, increase family anxiety, and impact consent.[18] The nurse helps validate the family's understanding, answer questions, and address concerns. For example the nurse can validate the family's understanding by asking them to repeat explanations in their own words or to ask open-ended questions that require them to provide a brief response. The nurse can also encourage the family to invite their religious/spiritual advisor to address concerns about donation after brain death (DBD) and donation after cardiac death (DCD). This collaborative approach will help the family make an informed choice in an emotional situation.

Care of the Donor and Donor's Family

The grieving donor family is a major focus of care for the nurse. Irrespective of the criteria used to declare death, the loss of a loved one is difficult to accept. It can be even more difficult when death is declared using brain death criteria because the use of mechanical ventilation and residual effects of medications make the body appear life-like. This can be very discordant and evoke ambivalent feelings for the family, as well as the nurse. The nurse has a responsibility for helping the family understand that death has occurred.

Modifying the environment to reflect the fact that the patient has died can be useful. Strategies include dimming lights, providing tissues, playing soft music, facilitating chaplain visits, arranging the body and linens, encouraging the family to perform end-of-life rituals significant for them, and, if part of hospital/hospice practice, placing signage on the door indicating that death has occurred. Nurses must also attend to ambivalent language that would suggest that the patient is still alive. For example, avoid saying "He looks comfortable" or "The vital signs are still stable." Instead, the nurse should offer condolences and support. Once death is declared comfort care measures for the patient should be stopped. Interventions to maintain and improve the organs for transplantation need to be explained to the family by the OPO coordinator, together with the nurse, so that the family understands that these measures are not for the patient but for the success of the donation.

BACK TO OUR CASE

The OPO coordinator talked to Kevin's family along with members of the critical care team and palliative care service. The family had decided to donate Kevin's organs if he was declared brain dead and knew several people on the national wait list, including a member of Kevin's family. Initial clinical examination supported a diagnosis of brain death. The family requested a confirmatory brain scan which showed no blood flow to Kevin's brain. The nurse, together with the physician, showed the family Kevin's blood flow scan alongside a normal blood flow scan and addressed their questions and concerns. Kevin was declared dead in accordance with hospital policy. Kevin's family signed the consent for donation and listed their potential directed donations if Kevin's organs were compatible.

The OPO coordinator evaluated Kevin for potential organ recovery and transplantation. Concurrently, offers were made to transplant centers, and donor management was initiated to optimize transplant potential. The palliative care nurse supported Kevin's family and called the family's church on their behalf. The family remained at the hospital until the recovery was completed early the next day. They found some comfort knowing that Kevin's heart, lungs, kidneys, and liver were transplanted to five waiting recipients, including Kevin's kidneys to his grandfather.

HISTORY: CASE 2

Jim suffered a witnessed cardiac arrest at home with 10 minutes of anoxia. He was admitted to the hospital's cardiac care unit with an anoxic brain injury. An EEG was done the next day, showing slowing brain activity. Clinical examination showed eye opening and withdrawal to pain and no verbal response, which indicated significant neurologic impairment. His Glasgow Coma Scale score was 7/15. Jim's family wanted full resuscitation and aggressive medical management at that time. Ten days later, the family realized that Jim was not recovering. They made a decision to change the goal to comfort and remove Jim from the ventilator. Marie, Jim's nurse, called the local OPO to inform them that the family was discussing possible ventilator removal. The OPO asked Marie questions about Jim's medical history, legal next of kin, current treatments, lab values, and likely survival time after removal from the ventilator. The OPO informed Marie that Jim was a potential organ donor and a designated requestor came to the hospital to meet with the family.

?   CLINICAL QUESTION

How should organ donation be discussed with the organ donor's family?

✓   DISCUSSION

Donation after Cardiac Death

The increasing gap between the need for and the availability of organs piqued a renewed interest in optimizing recovery of organs using cardiopulmonary death criteria, referred to as donation after cardiac death (DCD), previously known as "non-heart-beating donation." Although this was not a new concept, as the first organ donations historically occurred after cardiac death, new DCD protocols improve organ tissue viability by rapid recovery of organs after death. DCD is supported by the Institute of Medicine,[19,20] the Society for Critical Care Medicine,[21] the Joint Commission,[22,23] and the Association for Organ Procurement Organizations.[24]

Candidates for DCD are patients who suffer neurological devastation and are on life support therapies, but are not declared brain dead. Potential candidates may also include patients with a non-recoverable illness that require life support, such as amyotrophic lateral sclerosis or chronic obstructive pulmonary disease COPD. To be considered for DCD, it is necessary that the decision has been made to withdraw life support and subsequent cardiopulmonary arrest is expected within 60 to 90 minutes or less, depending on the organs to be recovered.[25] The United Network of Organ Sharing (UNOS) published guidelines for donor identification, consent, withdrawal, pronouncement, and organ recovery, which can include kidneys, pancreas, liver, lung, and intestines.[26] Kidney and liver transplant studies have shown no statistically significant difference between DBD and DCD transplant outcomes.[26,27] Thus, DCD provides another effective way to save lives through transplantation.

Hospital protocols may vary slightly, but should follow the UNOS guidelines. The OPO is called once the decision is made to remove life support, but prior *to* the actual withdrawal from the ventilator and/or extubation. If the OPO determines that the patient is a potential candidate for organ donation, a designated requestor from the OPO or hospital will discuss donation options with the legal decision maker(s). The hospital clinician follows the standard hospital protocol for termination of ventilator support and comfort care measures if donation consent is given.

Unlike patients who are declared brain dead, the potential DCD donor is not dead until cardiac and respiratory functions cease. Palliative care interventions must be used to ensure relief of symptoms and support of the family who is experiencing anticipatory grief. Comfort care must be ensured throughout the process until death is declared.[28]

Medication to maintain organ quality, such as heparin to minimize clotting, may be requested by the OPO to optimize organ function. Because it is important to recover the organs very soon after death is declared, the ventilator weaning and extubation needs to occur in a location near or in the operating room. All aspects of patient care before death, including comfort care medications, ventilator weaning, extubation, and declaration of death are done by the hospital team according to hospital policy. OPO coordinators are present to document the patient's vital signs, work with the family, and interact with the transplant teams. The transplant team(s) should be in a separate area and cannot be involved with the withdrawal of support. It is considered a conflict of interest and ethically inappropriate for the OPO and the transplant team to care for the patient before death is declared.[29]

If death occurs within the time frame necessary for donation there is also a wait time delineated by hospital policy, typically five minutes, before organ recovery can begin to ensure that the heart does not auto-resuscitate. If death does not occur within the established time frame, then the patient is no longer a DCD candidate. The patient is moved to a room appropriate for continued comfort care. Tissue donation may be a possibility after death occurs.

Care for the Donor and Donor's Family

Sometimes, despite the family's desire to honor a patient's wish to be a donor, the patient may not progress to donation. For example, the brain dead donor may suffer a cardiac arrest before organ recovery occurs. When this occurs, the family grieves the loss of their loved one as well as the loss of the opportunity to have their loved one live on through donation. In DCD the patient who is withdrawn from support may not die within a time frame to allow for donation. This family will continue to experience anticipatory grief and may grieve the lost opportunity to donate.

Typically, these patients die within a short time. Palliative care interventions may help with symptom control and end-of-life care and a referral to hospice should be considered. Although a brain dead patient would not be enrolled in hospice, the family can be referred for community based bereavement support provided by hospices and other agencies. The OPO will also refer families to community resources.

BACK TO OUR CASE

The OPO coordinator talked with the team to discuss Jim's potential for DCD, reviewed the medical record to determine the potential for donation, including estimated time until death after withdrawal, and discussed family dynamics with the team. It was agreed that the discussion would be led by the palliative care team and the OPO coordinator. The nurse asked Jim's wife, Susan, about her decisions to change goals and withdraw the ventilator. Susan tearfully stated that Jim would never have wanted to be maintained on life support, so withdrawal was her only option. The OPO coordinator explained that there may be an option that would allow Jim to save lives through organ donation and further explained the option of DCD. The nurse addressed Susan's concerns that her husband be comfortable. Susan signed the donation consent forms for both organ and tissue donation.

Jim's extubation was planned for the morning and took place in the operating room; however, a private room was reserved on a medical unit in the event Jim survived and was not a candidate for donation. The OPO coordinator evaluated potential organs to be recovered and concurrently made offers to transplant centers. Jim's nurse and physician managed the care for Jim and supported his wife, Susan. Their favorite music was played, and lights were dimmed. Jim was given scopolamine prior to extubation to reduce secretions and morphine sulfate to reduce his work of breathing. The extubation was uneventful and Jim was breathing comfortably. The OPO coordinator monitored vital signs and informed the transplant teams waiting in another room of Jim's status. After 90 minutes, Jim continued to have a heartbeat, blood pressure, and respirations, although agonal. The time allowing for donation had elapsed. The transplant teams left and Jim was moved to the private room with a referral to hospice. Seven hours later, Jim died with Susan at his side. While he was unable to donate organs, Susan also consented for tissue donation. Bone, skin, and corneas were recovered and helped 82 people. Hospice offered bereavement support to Susan and Jim's family.

SUMMARY

As for all donor families, the OPO contacted Kevin's and Jim's families to let them know how many lives were impacted by their gifts, to gain their perspective on the donation experience, and to invite them to become part of the community of donor families. The OPO may offer resources for bereavement support and may have a ceremony or other special way to honor donors celebrate their lives and thank their families for the generous gift.

Nurses can make significant contributions as part of the interdisciplinary team caring for potential organ/tissue donor patients and their families. Nurses provide education, support the decision-making process, provide symptom control until death, facilitate hospice transition, and support the family through their loss and grief. Through collaboration with the health care team and the OPO, patient and family needs are met and team members, as well as families, are gratified knowing that the patient's gift to others leaves a living legacy.

TAKE AWAY POINTS

- There are two types of organ donors: brain dead and donation after cardiac death.
- Per regulatory requirements, only "designated requestors" who receive special training from the OPO can discuss organ and tissue donation with families of potential donors.
- Nurses are integral members of the team throughout the processes associated with organ donation.

REFERENCES

[1] Linden PK. History of solid organ transplantation and organ donation. *Critical Care Clin.* 2009; 25:165–184.
[2] U.S. Government Information on Organ and Tissue Donation and Transplantation. *Waiting List Candidates as of 9/24/2010.* http://optn.transplant.hrsa.gov/. Accessed December 22, 2010.
[3] 2009 Annual Report of the U.S. Organ Procurement and Transplantation Network and the Scientific Registry of Transplant Recipients: Transplant Data 1999-2008. U.S. Department of Health and Human Services, Health Resources and Services Administration, Healthcare Systems Bureau, Division of Transplantation, Rockville, MD; 2009.

[4] Ad Hoc Committee of the Harvard Medical School. A definition of irreversible coma. Report of the Ad Hoc Committee of the Harvard Medical School to examine the definition of brain death. *JAMA*. 1968; 205:337–340.

[5] Guidelines for the determination of death. Report of the Medical Consultants on the Diagnosis of Death to the President's Commission for the Study of Ethical Problems in Medicine and Biomedical and Behavioral Research. *JAMA*. 1981; 246:2184–2186.

[6] National Conference of Commissioners of Uniform State Laws. Uniform Determination of Death 1981. Chicago, IL. http://www.law.upenn.edu/bll/archives/ulc/fnact99/1980s/udda80.htm. Accessed December 30, 2010.

[7] New York State Department of Health. Determination of Death. Regulation 10 NYCRR § 400.16; 1987.

[8] State of New Jersey. New Jersey Declaration of Death Act. 1991; NJSA Codified Title 26:Chapter 6A Section 5.

[9] U.S. Government Information on Organ and Tissue Donation. Religious views on donation. U.S. Department of Health and Human Services, Washington DC. http://www.organdonor.gov/aboutRelViews.asp. Accessed June 20, 2011.

[10] Bresnahan MJ, Mahler K. Ethical debate over organ donation in the context of brain death. *Bioethics*. 2008; 24(2):54–60.

[11] Bowman K, Richard S. Culture, brain death and transplantation. *Progress in Transplantation*, 2003; 13(3):211–215.

[12] Quality Standards Subcommittee of the American Academy of Neurology. Practice parameters for determining brain death in adults (Summary Statement). *Neurology*. 1995; 45:1012–1014.

[13] Wijdicks E. Determining brain death in adults. *Neurology*. 1995; 45:1003–1011.

[14] Task Force for the Determination of Brain Death in Children. Guidelines for the determination of brain death in children. *Archives in Neurology*. 1987; 44(6):587–588.

[15] Wijdicks E, Varelas P, Gronseth G, et al. Evidence-based guideline update: Determining brain death in adults: Report of the Quality Standards Subcommittee of the American Academy of Neurology. *Neurology*. 2010; 74:1911–1918.

[16] Greer DM, Varelas P, Haque S, et al. Variability of brain death determination guidelines in leading U.S. neurologic institutions. *Neurology*. 2008; 70:284–289.

[17] Powner D, Hernandez M, Rives T. Variability among hospital policies for determining brain death in adults. *Critical Care Medicine*. 2004; 32(6):1284–1288.

[18] Centers for Medicare and Medicaid Services Department of Health and Human Services. Chapter IV Conditions of Participation for Hospitals, Section 482.45. Organ, tissue and eye procurement. Washington DC, 2004. http://www.access.gpo.gov/nara/cfr/waisidx_04/42cfr482_04.html. Accessed June 22, 2011.

[19] Rassin M, Lowenthal M, Silner D. Fear, ambivalence and liminality: key concepts in refusal to donate an organ after brain death. *Journal of Nursing Administration Healthcare, Law, Ethics and Regulation*. 2005; 7(3):79–83.

[20] Institute of Medicine, National Academy of Sciences. *Non-Heartbeating Organ Transplantation: Medical and Ethical Issues in Procurement*. Washington, D.C.: National Academy Press. 1997.

[21] Institute of Medicine. *Non-Heart-Beating Organ Transplantation: Practice and Protocols*. Washington, D.C.: National Academy Press; 2000.

[22] Ethics Committee, American College of Critical Care Medicine. Recommendations for non-heart-beating organ donation. *Critical Care Medicine*. 2001; 29(9):1826–1831.

[23] Joint Commission on Accreditation of Healthcare Organizations. Health care at the crossroads: Strategies for narrowing the organ donation gap and protecting patients. Joint Commission, Chicago IL, 2004. http://www.jointcommission.org/assets/1/18/organ_donation_white_paper.pdf. Accessed March 16, 2011.

[24] Joint Commission. APPROVED: Revisions to Standard LD.3.110. Joint Commission, Chicago IL, June 2006. http://www.lopa.org/hospitals/JCAHO/Standard_LD_3_110.pdf. Accessed March 16, 2011.

[25] Eidbo E. Position on donation after cardiac death. Association of Organ Procurement Organizations. Personal communication, March 16, 2011.

[26] Bernat JL, D'Alessandro AM, Port FK, et al. Report of a national conference on donation after cardiac death. *American Journal of Transplantation*. 2006; 6:281–291.

[27] Steinbrook R. Organ donation after cardiac death. *New England Journal of Medicine*. 2007; 357(3):209–213.

[28] Fujita S, Mizuno S, Fujikawa T, et al. Liver transplantation from donation after cardiac death: A single center experience. *Transplantation*. 2007; 84(1):46–49.

[29] Hospice and Palliative Nurses Association. Role of palliative care nursing in organ and tissue donation. Pittsburgh, PA; 2008. www.HPNA.org. Accessed March 24, 2011.

Case 1.7 Discussing Physiological Futility

Judy C. Wheeler

HISTORY

David was a 48-year-old African-American male with a devastating medical history of hypertension and stroke. Approximately one year prior to hospital admission he was diagnosed with chronic obstructive pulmonary disease (COPD) after more than 20 pack/years as a cigarette smoker. He began to experience frequent trips to the emergency department for exacerbation of COPD, relieved with oral and inhaled steroids and bronchodilators.

Eight weeks prior to his death he was admitted to the hospital for exacerbation of COPD. On day two after admission he experienced an episode of pulseless electrical activity, with an anoxic interval of approximately ten minutes. He was resuscitated and transferred to the intensive care unit, where he failed to show any signs of neurologic improvement, with new onset of myoclonic seizures, sluggish pupillary reaction, no corneal reaction, and positive cough and gag reflexes. His family was informed of his grave prognosis but consented to tracheostomy and percutaneous endoscopic gastrostomy (PEG) tube for feeding, in hopes that with time he would improve. He was subsequently discharged to an extended care facility with no improvement in neurologic status.

David returned to the hospital ten days after hospital discharge with exacerbation of COPD and heart failure secondary to hypertension

Case Studies in Palliative and End-of-Life Care, First Edition. Edited by Margaret L. Campbell.
© 2012 John Wiley & Sons, Inc. Published 2012 by John Wiley & Sons, Inc.

and COPD. In spite of aggressive therapy, his condition continued to worsen, with labored respirations and copious secretions. His mother insisted that every possible measure, including intensive care unit (ICU) admission, ventilator support, and cardiopulmonary resuscitation/advanced cardiac life support (CPR/ACLS) interventions be ordered. He was admitted to the ICU and placed on ventilator support, but his mother was informed that in the event of a cardiac event resulting in death, he would not receive CPR/ACLS support, and that his code status would be do not resuscitate (DNR): clinical management with limitations. His mother continued to insist on full code status.

PHYSICAL EXAMINATION

Temperature: 38.6°C, blood pressure 102/68, apical rate 126, respirations 28

Lab values: White blood cell count 13.6, neutrophils 9.3; blood culture shows no growth after one day

Chest X-ray: Negative for consolidation or infiltrate

DIAGNOSTICS

No diagnostic studies were conducted during this visit.

CLINICAL QUESTION

How should physiological futility of aggressive life-sustaining treatment be discussed with patients or their surrogates?

DISCUSSION

Anyone who is a fan of the media—movies and television shows—about medicine has an opinion about the life-sustaining skills of medicine. Unfortunately, those expectations are often based on erroneous beliefs and unrealistic depictions of medical miracles. Investigators have shown that the more media people are exposed to, the more unrealistic are their expectations of what can be done for critically ill people.[1] Combine these erroneous beliefs with the cultural and religious convictions that many have about end-of-life care, and the relatively poor training and skills that clinicians have in communicating futility and the discussion of futile care can become fraught with opportunities for misunderstanding.

Futility: Conceptual Frameworks

Physiological futility refers to those conditions in which treatment is considered futile when it is unable to achieve the physiologic goal for which it is intended. For example, in the case of our clinical situation, ventilatory support might be considered appropriate for the patient with acute pneumonia, but might be considered futile for long-term management of end-stage COPD, because ventilatory support would not change the underlying physiologic cause of respiratory failure.

The American Medical Association's (AMA) Code of Medical Ethics[2] position statement on futility (Opinion 2.035, Medical Futility in End-of-Life Care) addresses the difficulties in attempting to define futility, and leaves it to individual practitioners and institutions to define the process by which futility will be determined. The AMA does identify several requirements for the resolution of disputes regarding medical futility, including joint decision-making between clinicians and responsible parties, negotiation of all disagreements regarding decisions, and offering patients and/or families the transfer of care to other physicians or other institutions in the event of disagreement. AMA standards in combination with state laws are used to guide decisions regarding medical futility, with the AMA position very firmly advocating that physicians are not morally or ethically required to provide treatment which they consider futile, but silent on the precise determination of futility.

State laws vary greatly, from defining very specific policies to be followed in cases in which medical futility is disputed to remaining silent on the process. For example, Texas addressed the problem of defining futility in its Advance Directives Act of 1999. While this law is also called the Texas Futile Care Law, it actually leaves the determination of futility up to the physicians caring for the patient.[3] Most states are silent regarding a specific definition of futility, and hospital ethics committees often become involved in making recommendations. In general, these decisions are based on ethical principles and are unbiased, but the makeup of an ethics committee can occasionally sway the direction in which decisions are made because most committees are comprised of clinicians who are likely to favor the medical opinion. It should be noted that these principles apply to American health care alone, and that standards of care in other nations may differ according to their ethical standards. Most notably, the Canadian health care system has recognized the right to refuse care, but is less clear on the right to withhold futile care.[4]

An argument can be made that determination of futility can be dominated by consideration of cost, and, although cost may be a consideration when futility is determined, it should never be a primary consideration when determining medical futility. Even the most inexpensive treatments can be withdrawn or denied if considered medically futile, while the most expensive treatments should be offered when there is a reasonable chance of a positive outcome, no matter the financial burden they may create to the institution, payer, or patient.

Kasman identified medical futility as "a clinical action serving no useful purpose in attaining a specified goal for a specific patient".[5] Kasman addresses three critical ethical concepts for the discussion of futility with patients and families. First, the physician is never obligated to provide care that is believed to be ineffective or harmful. Second, any requests for futile treatment should be met with education and discussion of alternatives rather than with a blanket denial. Finally, withdrawal of futile treatment does not mean withdrawal of medical care that is aimed at comfort and palliation. Kasman speaks to the need for humility and professional integrity in the communication of these difficult principles.

Reasons Patients or Families Request Futile Treatment

A survey regarding perceptions of futile care among staff in 16 intensive care units found that while physicians, nurses, and respiratory therapists were generally in agreement regarding how to define futile care, they felt that such care was provided for reasons other than patients' best interests.[7] These reasons included family demands, inadequate or untimely communication with families, and lack of consensus among the treatment team. Factors which made the transition to palliation more difficult included patient's age, family members' misunderstanding of the severity of the illness, family conflict about proposed medical treatment, and shifting medical treatment decisions. Younger age of patients was associated with increased discomfort with determination of futility, as were unrealistic expectations for positive outcomes from poorly informed family members. Family discord also resulted in nurse discomfort, especially when family members appeared to have ulterior motives, for example, financial gain, in decision making.

Finally, nurses were frustrated with inconsistent medical practices, especially when physicians appeared willing to continue to provide futile care in response to pressure from families. Nurses were most positively impacted by consensus amongst the medical staff, the patient's family, and the patient. They also reported that their comfort with palliative nursing practice was enhanced when treatment options had been exhausted, when the patient obviously failed to respond to aggressive treatment, and by their own desire to promote comfort.[6]

Some specific incidences which may complicate the discussion of medical futility are circumstances in which death occurs by trauma (unexpected), when death is of a child, or when cultural variables are present. For example, a study conducted among the general public and trauma professionals regarding preferences for palliative vs. aggressive critical care for a trauma victim described as "dead at the scene" found that the public is more likely to believe that they have the right to demand futile treatment (public 62.7% vs. professionals 51.9%) and overwhelmingly more likely to believe (public 57.4% vs. professionals 19.5%) that divine intervention could save a trauma victim once medical futility was determined.[7]

In the case of neonatal and pediatric patients, the American Academy of Pediatrics Committee on Bioethics is relatively silent on the issue of medical withdrawal of futile treatment while recognizing parental autonomy to refuse treatment, leading to potential conflicts for parents who are not prepared to come to grips with medical palliation.[8]

Westra, Willems, and Smith found that communicating a decision to withhold or withdraw life-sustaining treatment to Muslim parents was culturally incongruent with the ethical principles of autonomy and nonmaleficence.[9] In Islamic law, consent for withdrawal of treatment is not possible because only God is seen as able to make decisions regarding life and death. Similarly, nonmaleficence, or the action of doing no harm, can be used to justify withholding or withdrawing futile treatment from our cultural perspective, but is used in Islamic ethics to forbid any action which could harm life. The authors suggest that resolution of this religious and cultural dilemma can be achieved by exploring shared beliefs, clarifying the desire to allow natural death, and acknowledging both shared and unique values.

Treatment

In applying the AMA standards to cases in which physicians and health care providers have determined that treatment is futile, the patient or their advocate should be informed of the rationale and negotiations regarding the plan of care attempted. If the patient or family continues to demand treatment that is considered futile, they should be offered the opportunity to find a provider willing to undertake the desired treatment, and transfer to that provider should be expedited. If no other provider is willing to assume care, the physician and facility are not obligated to continue to provide futile care, but the patient and family must be informed of the decision to discontinue treatment and should continue to receive all comfort measures and support required during this difficult process.

Burns and Truog[10] have proposed a more refined approach to the identification of medical futility, focused on what they call "principled negotiation." This approach involves the evaluation of what they call qualitative futility based on quality of life judgments, quantitative futility which uses data about the probability of success of an intervention or treatment, and physiologic futility in which the goal is return to an accepted level of function. Their primary focus is the relationships between providers and families, with an emphasis on trust and communication. The principled negotiation approach includes four recommendations:

- Separate the people from the problem: Identify a few appropriate physicians/providers to communicate with a few appropriate family members.
- Focus on problem resolution rather than emotional responses: Allow time for emotional responses but emphasize the resolution of remaining problems.
- Generate a variety of possible options before coming to agreement: Identify all recommended treatment options from the care team and seek consensus before presenting to the family.
- Insist that agreements be based on objective criteria: Establish timelines and expected outcomes for treatment and reevaluate with each clinical change.

Not surprisingly, dispute regarding the clinical determination of futility continues.

Exactly how one communicates poor prognosis and the concept of medical futility has been the subject of some research. Curtis identifies some principles for communicating end-of-life care to patients and families in the ICU.[11] Some data conclude that communication with physicians and nurses is the most important determinant in family members' evaluation of end-of-life experiences in the ICU setting. A study of 51 family interviews found that family satisfaction with physician communication was inversely related to the amount of time that physicians spoke during these contacts.[12] In fact, the more opportunity the family was given to speak, the greater their satisfaction with the outcome of the conversation and the less likelihood there was for physician-family conflict throughout the relationship. By speaking too much, physicians missed opportunities to engage families in discussion about personal values and goals of care as well as to communicate comfort measures. In general, these discussions should occur early on, be repeated regularly, and involve the same primary decision makers and clinicians to avoid confusion and conflict. Because nurses are most often the clinician at the bedside with family, they should be included in discussions. In fact, nurses often recognized signs of medical futility sooner than physicians.

↰ BACK TO OUR CASE

With David's respiratory condition continuing to decline and the need for long-term ventilator support were he to survive, the intensive care team and the palliative care team were consulted, with both recommending a palliative approach to care due to the futility of further intervention. His mother and brother were identified as the appropriate contact people based on their continued presence at his bedside and their identification as contacts on previous medical records. They were called to a family conference at his bedside, and were informed that due to the medical futility of resuscitation, his resuscitation status would be prescribed as do not resuscitate. Discussion centered on the family's knowledge of David's values and past discussions he had about "what if" he were ever in this type of circumstance. They were certain that he would not wish to continue to be kept alive in his current condition without hope of recovery, with uncontrolled seizure activity and no meaningful interaction with others, and without hope of independence from the ventilator, but they were also suspicious that not enough time had passed to allow for improvement.

Information was shared regarding David's neurologic damage with repetitive reminders that his "brain could not be repaired," that his lung condition was irreversible, and that immobility would result in further complications. The spiritual care consultant was asked to join this discussion and she expressed her confidence in the integrity of the recommendations. David's mother and brother agreed that if there were truly no hope of David regaining independence or interaction with his environment that he would not wish to continue to live in his current condition. They elected to admit him to the palliative care service, where he was withdrawn from the ventilator and treated for comfort measures with seizure medications and morphine. He died less than 24 hours later with both his mother and brother at his bedside.

❗ TAKE AWAY POINTS

- Discussion of futility should be based on knowledge of hospital policy, state law, and the principles of medical ethics.
- The cultural and personal values of patients and families must be acknowledged and respected, even if they conflict with medical recommendations. However, patient and family wishes should not entice practitioners to provide care that is futile.

- Gentle negotiation of differences, along with reassurance that palliative withdrawal of treatment never means withdrawal of comfort, can result in outcomes that are ethical, medically appropriate, and supportive to those involved.

REFERENCES

[1] Van den Bulck J. The impact of television on public expectations of survival following inhospital cardiopulmonary resuscitation by medical professionals. *European Journal of Emergency Medicine.* 2002; 9(4):325–329.

[2] AMA Code of Medical Ethics. http://www.ama-assn.org/ama/pub/physician-resources/medical-ethics/code-medical-ethics/opinion2035.page. Retrieved on September 21, 2011.

[3] Fridman V. Ethical Dilemmas: Medical Futility the Texas Approach. http://www.clinicalcorrelations.org/?p=661 retrieved on September 21, 2011.

[4] Gedge E, Giacomini M, Cook D. Withholding and withdrawing life support in critical care settings: ethical issues concerning consent. *Journal of Medical Ethics.* 2007; 33:215–218.

[5] Kasman DL. When is medical treatment futile? *Journal of General Internal Medicine.* 2004; 19:1053–1056.

[6] Badger JM. Factors that enable or complicate end-of-life transitions in critical care. *American Journal of Critical Care.* 2005; 14(6):513–521.

[7] Jacobs L, Burns K, Jacobs B. Views of the public and trauma professional on death and dying from injuries. *Archives of Surgery.* 2008; 143:730–735.

[8] Fine R, Whitfield J, Carr B, Mayo T. Medical futility in the neonatal intensive care unit: hope for a resolution. *Pediatrics.* 2005; 116:1219–1222.

[9] Westra A, Willems D, Smit B. Communicating with Muslim parents: "The four principles" are not as culturally neutral as suggested. *European Journal of Pediatrics.* 2009; 168:1383–1387.

[10] Burns JP, Truog RD. Futility: a concept in evolution. *Chest.* 2007; 132:6.

[11] Curtis JR. Communicating about end-of-life care with patients and families in the intensive care unit. *Critical Care Clinician.* 2004; 20:363–380.

[12] McDonagh JR, Elliott TB, Engelberg RA, Treece PD, Shannon SE, Rubenfeld GD. Family satisfaction with family conference about end-of-life care in the ICU: increased proportion of family speech is associated with increased satisfaction. *Critical Care Medicine.* 2004; 32(7):1484–1488.

Case 1.8 Wounded Families: Decision-Making in the Setting of Stressed Coping and Maladaptive Behaviors in Health Crises

Kerstin McSteen

HISTORY

Jeff was 38 years old and a father of four children, ages 5, 7, 11, and 13, when he was diagnosed with non-Hodgkins lymphoma. His initial prognosis was good with expected cure; however, after several months of treatment, he began to develop respiratory problems, requiring a reduced dose of Bleomycin because of concerns about pulmonary toxicity. A few days after receiving chemotherapy, Jeff developed acute and severe dyspnea, called 911, and on arriving at the emergency room, had a full cardiac and pulmonary arrest. He had sepsis and quickly developed adult respiratory distress syndrome (ARDS).

As Jeff's large family gathered in the intensive care unit, the staff began to understand more of the dynamics at play. Jeff was married to Allie, but at the time he was diagnosed with cancer, the couple had been in the process of divorcing and were involved in other committed relationships. Because of health insurance, they decided to postpone the divorce until he was through the initial cancer treatment. However, they never explained this to their children or their extended family, allowing them to believe that they had officially divorced but were living in the same household for practical and financial reasons.

Both Jeff's and Allie's parents were divorced and remarried. Allie had no siblings; Jeff had eight step-siblings who were overtly hostile toward Allie and often took the staff aside to share derogatory stories of Allie's behavior in the marriage. Jeff's parents argued openly and

Case Studies in Palliative and End-of-Life Care, First Edition. Edited by Margaret L. Campbell.
© 2012 John Wiley & Sons, Inc. Published 2012 by John Wiley & Sons, Inc.

caustically at the bedside. Jeff's father was an imposing figure who believed he was the rightful primary decision maker, given the unstable marriage of Jeff and Allie. Additionally, Jeff's girlfriend would visit him frequently, holding his hand and crying at the bedside, causing some awkward discomfort for Allie, the children, and the nurses.

All of these issues came to a head when after two weeks in the intensive care unit (ICU), with ongoing complications and deterioration of Jeff's condition, the attending physician discussed resuscitation with Allie, recommending do not resuscitate (DNR). She agreed, but when this information "leaked" out to the rest of the family, the tension and confrontation rose to a level that disrupted the peace of the unit and the care of Jeff. A family care conference was convened and attended by Allie and her mother and Jeff's parents, stepparents, and a few siblings.

? CLINICAL QUESTION

How is decision-making in a family with intra-familial discord and maladaptive behaviors optimized?

✓ DISCUSSION

Any health care situation has the potential to escalate to a crisis, especially when the outcome of an illness or injury may be death. Serious illness is a primary developmental challenge for all families, but for families with maladaptive or distorted behavioral and emotional patterns, the potential for conflict between family members and care providers is high and can complicate the decision-making process regarding goals of care and treatment preferences. An understanding of family systems and relationship-centered care can provide insights into how the nurse can work collaboratively with families, especially when the family presents with less than optimal coping skills.

There has been a shift in the health care community's perspective of what traditionally have been labeled as "dysfunctional families." Instead of viewing them as "damaged," health care professionals now recognize the variations in the strength of family attachment bonds, the nature of family communication, and the degree of collaborative decision-making.[1] Common characteristics observed in families with maladaptive coping and distorted behaviors include the following:[2]

- Assume extreme all-or-none positions regarding change
- Alternate between feelings of hopelessness that any change can occur and unrealistic expectations for goals that are unlikely to be met

- Commonly fluctuate between extremes of enmeshed/disengaged and rigidity/chaos
- Enmeshed families resist any efforts to promote physical separation, fearing catastrophe and total cut-off if they leave
- Incongruence between verbal and nonverbal messages
- Little empathy or ability to listen attentively, often belittling others, or engaging in disrespectful communication

Hospice pioneered the idea of the patient and family as the unit of care but this approach has become the standard of many other health care fields that recognize the importance of extending the focus beyond that of the individual patient and recognizing the mutual influence of family functioning and physical illness.[3] Additionally, there are growing expectations on the part of patients and families that their care providers attend not only to the physical but also the psychosocial challenges of significant health issues.[1] Approaches to working with challenging families should focus less on controlling negative behaviors and more on understanding the importance of relationships between patients, families, and care providers, and finding collaborative ground on which to work together. Unfortunately, most care providers have not received specialized training or education in family-centered care.[1] The nature of palliative care demands that nurses understand the basics of family systems theory and are able to assess family functioning. At a minimum, the nurse should be able to identify critical issues with coping and when to refer to a specialist for appropriate support and intervention.

Rolland first developed the Family Systems Illness Model in 1984; since then it has been used widely to understand the developmental phases of an illness, the psychosocial demands the illness places on the family, the movement of the patient and family through their life cycles individually and collectively, and the influence and importance of family belief systems. Family belief systems include individual and multigenerational family experiences along with the families' cultural orientation. Cultural orientation includes historical context, ethnicity, medical understanding/perception, and religious and moral values and beliefs. Additionally, the societal context provides a level of meaning at a systems level that includes economic, political, and institutional forces.[4]

Rolland's Family Systems Illness Model emphasizes the importance of collaboration between the health care providers and the patient and family as an evolutionary process involving relationship and connectivity. The provider who strives to understand the belief systems, or in other words, the "story" of the patient and family, can protect against the disconnection that can develop when the health care team is focused on the disease and the family is focused on what the illness means to them personally. If families feel neglected or not respected in their beliefs, it can lead to further marginalization, separation, withdrawal, and misunderstanding.[4]

Along with the Family Systems Illness Model, Rolland applies a Family Resilience Framework, with resilience defined as "the ability to withstand and rebound from serious crises and persistent life challenges."[1] In practice, stressed families have often been viewed through a "deficit-based lens" and are seen as damaged or dysfunctional. The intent of a resilience-oriented approach shifts the providers' perspective to a collaborative and relationship-based approach, recognizing the strengths that families bring to the crisis, and assisting them in their coping, adaptation, and growth, even in the face of terminal illness.[1]

As the importance of relationships in health care began to emerge in full a few decades ago, in 1992 the Pew Health Professions Commission and the Fetzer Institute formed a partnership to examine ways to promote an integrated approach to health care that would affirm the interaction of the biomedical and psychosocial factors in health. The work of this task force was published in 1994 and produced the model of relationship-centered care (RCC), identifying it as "the vehicle for putting into action a paradigm of health that is focused on caring, healing, and community."[5] As the prerequisite to effective care and healing, RCC is founded on four principles: (1) relationships in health care should include the personhood of the participants, (2) affect and emotion are important components of these relationships, (3) all health care relationships occur in the context of reciprocal influence, and (4) the formation and maintenance of genuine relationships in health care is morally valuable. In RCC, relationships between patients and clinicians remain central, although the relationships of clinicians with themselves, each other, and the community are also emphasized.[6] RCC is becoming accepted in the rapidly changing health care culture as the standard of care.

While in practice nurses are able to quickly identify when family dynamics are impacting the care of the patient, valid and reliable tools to assist care providers in assessing family functioning have been lacking in the field of palliative care.[7] The Checklist of Family Relational Abilities was developed and revised to provide clinicians with an efficient method to assess families.[8] The tool is based on Wynne's epigenetic model of family relational functioning and the attachment/affection bonds between the individual members.[9] The checklist rates three separate categories: the strength of family attachment bonds, the nature of family communication, and the degree of collaborative decision making. The overall rating can then guide a plan of care that considers what level of intervention should be directed to the family. The capabilities and needs of the family are categorized into four levels (see Table 1.8.1).

Practical Management of Intra-Familial Conflicts

Working with "wounded" families is stressful and difficult. No matter the setting—hospital, home, skilled nursing facility—maladaptive

TABLE 1.8.1. Rating of family relational abilities.

4 Naturally resilient	Strong bonds, clear and open communication, effective and collaborative decision-making	Little if any intervention indicated
3 Overwhelmed	Generally strong relationships but temporarily stressed by the intensity and complexity of the situation	Brief and focused family support to assist in accessing inherent family strengths
2 Closed or fixed	Significant difficulty in communication and/or decision-making	Targeted intervention of family consultation indicated
1 Wounded	Damaged bonds of attachment, intensely negative or conflictual communication and decision-making	Family therapy indicated to address longstanding grievances

coping and disruptive behaviors in families can have a negative impact on the optimal functioning of the care providers and on the patient. Providing therapy for families with severe maladaptive behavior patterns is beyond the scope of practice of the nurse and requires the expertise of psychology, social work, and spiritual care to address the needs of these patients and families. However, for the nurse at the bedside who has sustained and repeated contact with these high-need families, it requires the ability to maintain focus and boundaries while providing appropriate emotional support. Besides acquiring knowledge of family systems theory and relationship-centered care, the following are strategies for the nurse to keep in mind in these challenging situations; they will aid in supporting families in making difficult treatment decisions:

- Be transparent. Explain what you are doing and why. Explain unit and facility routines and rules and the rationale for having them. Encourage families to ask questions and to ask for clarification.
- Be professional. When emotions are high, it is easy to slip into defensive postures and assert one's authority unnecessarily. If a situation is causing you to feel angry and stressed, call on management to assist, if only to take a break to leave the setting for a few minutes and compose yourself.
- Avoid labeling and stereotyping. Demonizing certain family members is not uncommon, but can impede optimal care of the family. Rolland found that staff tends to ally with the family member who best supports the unit's purpose, priorities, and mission; these members also tend to be less disruptive and thus easier to work with. This can develop into a labeling process of who is normal and who is sick in the family system, which can shut down communication and increase tensions.[4]

- Beware of triangulation. Nurses may unwittingly be drawn into the middle of the family drama, taking sides and identifying victims and perpetrators. This triangulation can split team members and increase conflict among staff. Maintain neutrality and do not try to fix generations of discord and dysfunction.
- Establish communication. Because information may need to be repeated frequently in less cohesive family systems, it is important to clearly identify a primary contact person in the family and clarify a chain of communication for information sharing with the family. Nurses can find themselves being constantly pulled away from the care of the patients to talk with family at the bedside and on the phone. Place some responsibility for dispersing pertinent medical information on the family in an agreed upon plan. Family conferences are important in supporting and promoting family decision-making but have been found to be more effective when families are cohesive and collaborative. However, it is still an important intervention with less cohesive families in order to get everyone around the table, hearing the same information, and having a safe place to talk.
- Maintain safety. Involve security, patient representatives, and risk management early on to assist in setting necessary limits. This may include written contracts, if needed, to specify expected behaviors of family, as well as consequences if their behavior falls outside the contract. Staff safety is a top priority and may require a more visible presence of security on the unit. Do not hesitate to call for security escorts for disruptive family members.
- Practice self reflection. The nurse will be more effective if he has reflected on his own belief system. Think about your own family history, multigenerational attitudes, health practices, stories, secrets, unresolved losses. What do you bring to the bedside?[4]

BACK TO OUR CASE

The pertinent details to consider from our case include:

- Four children at different stages of development and ability to understand illness, loss, and death
- Reconfigured/blended families: Each parent had divorced and remarried and relationships remained acrimonious
- Dormant family conflicts that resurfaced in a crisis
- Secrets
- Confusion and disagreement in the family and in providers about who was the legal and rightful health care decision maker for Jeff
- Suspicions in the family and some care providers about Allie as being the rightful primary and legal decision maker, with

concerns about conflict of interest, and whether she had his best interest at heart

- No written health care directive
- Potential for triangulation of the treatment team members

Prior to the family care conference, all providers met beforehand to review what the team was aware of in terms of relationships and the current conflicts that would be present, whether or not the family would choose to speak about them openly. At the introduction of the conference, the palliative care clinician identified how incredibly stressful and frightening this situation was for the family. She communicated that the team was aware of the many conflicts within the family and assured them that the team did not come to them from a place of judgment, but rather from a place of wanting to support them as a family and in their individual relationships with Jeff. It was also noted that one of the goals of the conference was to clearly identify a primary decision maker and a communication plan for the family. It was explained that boundaries would be established if family behaviors were having a negative effect on Jeff or impeded the nurses and staff in being able to care for him.

At the point in the conference when the resuscitation issue was addressed, Jeff's father angrily and tearfully accused Allie of making Jeff DNR so that he would die and she could "move on." Security was called because of uncontrolled language (content and volume) and fears that behaviors had the potential to become physically threatening.

Though the discussion during the family care conference became very heated and emotionally charged, requiring a call to security to be present outside the conference room, Jeff's family was able to find safety in the nonjudgmental approach of the team and see the team as unbiased facilitators who had their loved one's best interest at the center. They were assured that the team would always be honest with them about Jeff's condition and would make medical recommendations based on expected outcomes and potential benefit. Given how critically ill Jeff was, the team stressed that there may be acute changes in his condition requiring urgent decisions, and the family was able to agree that Allie was the most appropriate primary decision maker in a crisis. The family also discussed their fears and emotions behind the idea of DNR, essentially that Jeff may die, but they agreed that it was the correct treatment choice at the moment. A plan was made to schedule weekly care conferences to maintain healthy communication between family and the care team.

Jeff died in the ICU several weeks later, surrounded by his family. Though they continued to struggle with their longstanding issues, they were receptive and appreciative of psychosocial and spiritual interventions, especially to support the children.

! TAKE AWAY POINTS

- Patients and families expect their care providers to attend to psychosocial issues in addition to the physical challenges of health crises.
- The nurse who has an understanding of family systems and relationship-centered care is able to work more collaboratively with families, especially when the family presents with less than optimal coping skills.
- When the providers' perspective shifts to a collaborative and relationship-based approach, the strengths that families bring to the crisis can be recognized and supported, which can then assist them in their coping, adaptation, and growth, even in the face of terminal illness.
- Remember the importance of transparency, professionalism, avoiding labeling and triangulation, maintaining safety, and self reflection when working with challenging families.

REFERENCES

[1] Rolland JS, Walsh F. Systemic training for healthcare professionals: The Chicago center for family health approach. *Family Process.* 2005; 44(3):283–301.

[2] Olson DH, Gorall DM. Circumplex model of marital and family systems. In: Walsh F, ed. *Normal Family Processes.* New York: Guilford; 2003:514–547.

[3] Weihs K, Fisher L, Baird M. Families, health and behavior. *Family Systems and Health.* 2002; 20:7–47.

[4] Rolland JS. Beliefs and collaboration in illness: Evolution over time. *Families, Systems, & Health,* 1998; 16(1–2):7–25. doi: 10.1037/h0089839.

[5] Tresolini CP, and the Pew-Fetzer Task Force. Health professions education and relationship-centered care. San Francisco: Pew Health Professionals Commission 1994; reprinted 2000.

[6] Beach MC, Inui T. Relationship-Centered Care Research Network. Relationship-centered care: A constructive reframing. *J of Gen Int Med.* 2006; 21 (S1):S3–S8. doi: 10.1111/j.1525–1497.2006.00302.x

[7] Payne S, Hudson P. Assessing the family and caregivers. In: Walsh TD, et al., eds. *Palliative Medicine.* Philadelphia: Saunders Elsevier. 2009; 320–325.

[8] Wilkins VM, Quill TE, King DA. Assessing families in palliative care: A pilot study of the checklist of family relational abilities. *J Palliat Med.* 2009; 12(6):517–519. doi:10.1089/jpm.2009.0021.

[9] Wynne LC. The epigensis of relational systems: a model for understanding family development. *Fam Process.* 1984; 23:297–318.

Case 1.9 Notification of an Expected Death

Peg Nelson

HISTORY

Eve had advanced pancreatic cancer; she was 53 years old. She had been diagnosed six months earlier and had been taking palliative chemotherapy up until three weeks prior to hospital admission, when she became so weak she could no longer get out of bed without assistance. She was admitted to the hospital with dyspnea, severe pain, and nausea. Her symptoms were controlled, but her overall condition remained grave with progressive renal failure, debility, malnutrition, and pneumonia. Her oncologist asked the palliative care team to assist her to tell Eve and her family that she was dying with prognosis only days. Eve was not surprised but was sad and verbalized regret not to see her children grow older. Her family also understood death was close and were openly grieving. Eve's husband Joe and her three children, two boys and a girl, spent the last two days at her side. Eve remained in the hospital under care of the palliative care team as her death appeared imminent and required titration of high doses of intravenous opioids. At the time of death Eve's family called the nurse into the room because they thought Eve had stopped breathing.

CLINICAL QUESTION

How should a family be notified that an expected death has occurred?

Case Studies in Palliative and End-of-Life Care, First Edition. Edited by Margaret L. Campbell.
© 2012 John Wiley & Sons, Inc. Published 2012 by John Wiley & Sons, Inc.

☑ **DISCUSSION**

Preparation

Preparation for notification of a death—whether expected or not—involves understanding the dying experience from the family's perspective. Those involved in the care of the dying patient need to understand that if the patient is not managed properly, needless suffering for the family as well as the patient occurs, and the distress to the family will likely continue long after the patient dies.[1] Bereaved families have reported high rates of unmet needs for symptom management for their loved one, concerns regarding physician communication, lack of emotional support for themselves and their other family members, and the belief that often their loved one was not treated with respect. Furthermore, the concerns expressed by family regarding the poor quality of care for their loved one is reported to be higher if the patient dies in a hospital or nursing home.[2]

Understanding these findings when combined with the specific knowledge of how the patient died and the suffering that has been occurring with the patient and family before death are important for the clinician to know as she prepares herself to notify family about the death and determine how best to support them in their grief. Determining if the family was well prepared/coached for the death in the last days of life builds a foundation that supports trust, mutual understanding and communication.[3] Meeting with the family to notify them of a death is an important part of the care experience. The process requires sensitivity, compassion, and thoughtful communication. Too often it is relegated to a junior clinician who has little or no training.[4] Different states, as well as hospital policies, differ as to what type of medical professional may make a death pronouncement.

Notification Process

1. Before entering the room, confer with nursing and review the medical record; be prepared to answer questions regarding the patient's death and/or illness.
2. Determine if family has previously requested an autopsy or if the death occurred in a manner such that an autopsy is appropriate. Refer to hospital or community policies regarding autopsy procedures and contact the medical examiner before talking with the family if an autopsy is necessary to understand the procedure in order to best explain the next steps to the family.
3. Understand the procedures that are practiced regarding request for organ, tissue, and bone or eye donation before meeting with the family.

4. Have the nurse or the chaplain accompany the pronouncing clinician, especially if the clinician is not known to the family.
5. Introduce yourself to the family and explain why you are there and tell them they are welcome to stay during the exam or leave, whatever is most comfortable for them.
6. Observe the patient and look for signs of life. Gently touch the patient, and examine for respirations, pulse, and heartbeat. There is no need to perform common practices such as checking a pupillary response or doing a sternal rub; these actions are unnecessary and strongly discouraged.[5]
7. If family is present, state clearly that the patient is dead and offer sympathy for their loss. "Mr. Smith has died. I am so sorry for your loss."
8. Ask about and allow for any cultural or special rituals that family may request.
9. Ask the family if they have any questions and/or if they would like to talk.
10. If yes, offer to go to a private area. Sit down during the conversation. If it is necessary to discuss organ donation or autopsy, allow the family some time for their questions before bringing up these subjects. See Case 1.6 for a discussion of organ donation. Even though the death was expected, many families are surprised and/or have questions and it is an opportunity for you to share your condolences and, if you knew the patient, your respect for the person.
11. Affirm the family's care and love for the patient. Many families have regrets or feel inadequate in some of their care for or relationship with their loved one and find solace in words from the clinician. "Family and friends who are present at the time of death look to the physician for information, reassurance, and direction regarding the weeks and months ahead. The lasting impression and memories that family members have regarding the manner in which they received word that their loved one died may affect the grief process and eventual integration of the loss within the survivors' world. Research has demonstrated that the skills of compassion and sensitivity can be learned and must be incorporated into the practice of all physicians."[6]
12. Give the family a contact number that they can use if they have further questions or concerns.
13. Document the date and time of the death in the medical record, and whether an autopsy was offered or requested. Also document the family members who were present and notification of the attending physician as appropriate.

Supporting the Bereaved

Even an expected death may evoke significant grief reaction and the clinician can help begin the healing process for a family member. See Case

3.3 for a comprehensive discussion of acute grief after an expected death. There is not one best way to support a recently bereaved person, but the EASE tool provides a simple guide for assisting families with acute loss:[7]

Educate family about normal variations in grief responses, support and validate their expressions of loss, and affirm that different people will have different ways to grieve.

Assess health—mental and physical—as well as loss history and grief responses.

Support by listening to the feelings of loss, sharing information about and encouraging family to participate in support groups or counseling, and sending a sympathy card and/or attending memorials or funerals.

Explore what works best for each individual.

BACK TO OUR CASE

After being called by the nurse, the palliative care nurse practitioner went into the room; she found the family all lying on the bed surrounding the patient, quietly crying. She waited until the family had time to be with the patient. She introduced herself and told them that she needed to do a brief examination. She assessed the pulse, respirations, and heartbeat. She said, "As you suspected, she has died. My condolences to you, I knew her for the last few days and could tell she was a special person. I am so glad you were here with her when she died. I know your presence comforted her." She then sat down at their request and answered their questions and listened to their stories about the patient.

TAKE AWAY POINTS

- The pronouncement of death is a solemn privilege and the clinician must prepare by understanding the general and specific needs of the bereaved.
- Although the steps are simple, if the family is present, the process of examination and communication involved must be done in a sensitive and compassionate manner.
- Although death may be expected, the family will continue to require support as they cope with this highly emotional event.

REFERENCES

[1] LeGrand SB, VonGunten CF, Emanuel LL. Competency in end-of-life care: last hours of life. *Journal of Palliative Medicine.* 2003; 6:605–613.

[2] Teno JM, Clarridge BR, Casey V, et al. Family perspectives on end-of-life care at the last place of care. In: Meier DE, Isaacs SL, Hughes, RG, eds. *Palliative Care: Transforming the care of serious illness.* San Francisco: Jossey-Bass. 2010; 235–245.

[3] Andershed B. Relatives in end-of-life care—part 1: a systematic review of the literature the five last years, January 1999-February 2004. *Journal of Clinical Nursing.* 2006; 15(9):1158–1169.

[4] Bailey FA, Williams BR. Preparation of residents for death pronouncement: a sensitive and supportive method. *Palliative Supportive Care.* 2005; 3(2): 107–114.

[5] Hallenbeck J. Palliative care in the final days of life. In: McPhee SJ, Winker MA, Rabow, MW, et al., eds. *JAMA Evidence Care at the Close of Life.* New York: McGraw-Hill Company, Inc. 2011; 301–309.

[6] Midland D. Informing significant others of a patient's death, 2nd edition. *Fast Facts and Concepts.* Milwaukee, WI: End of Life/Palliative Education Resource Center; month year. Available at: http//www.eperc.mcw.edu/fastFact/ff_64. tm. Accessed July 17, 2011.

[7] Carrington N, Bogetz J. Normal grief and bereavement: letters from home. *Journal of Palliative Medicine.* 2004; 7(2):309–323.

Case 1.10 Death Notification after Unexpected Death

Garrett K. Chan

HISTORY

Paramedics brought in a 25-year-old woman with a chief complaint of shortness of breath. The patient's mother activated the Emergency Medical System because the patient had been having progressive shortness of breath and abdominal pain. The patient had stage IV ovarian cancer that had metastasized to the lung and liver. The patient was undergoing experimental chemotherapy treatment and just had an infusion three days prior to arrival to the emergency department (ED).

On arrival to the ED, the patient was obtunded with abdominal retractions with bradypnea. After being brought in to the ED for five minutes, the patient went into a pulseless electrical activity (PEA) rhythm. Because no advance directive accompanied the patient, the ED team began chest compressions and endotracheally intubated the patient. Given the severity and advanced stage of her cancer, the decision was made to stop resuscitative efforts after 15 minutes. The mother had still not arrived at the ED.

The mother arrived at the ED approximately 50 minutes after the ambulance left the home. The social worker greeted the mother at the ED entrance and brought her back to the family room and gathered the ED team to disclose the death.

Case Studies in Palliative and End-of-Life Care, First Edition. Edited by Margaret L. Campbell.
© 2012 John Wiley & Sons, Inc. Published 2012 by John Wiley & Sons, Inc.

| ? | **CLINICAL QUESTION** |

How should the ED team handle disclosing the death to the family?

| ✓ | **DISCUSSION** |

Approximately 10% of all deaths in the United States are a result of a sudden event.[1] In the pre-hospital setting, cardiopulmonary arrest and trauma are common causes of death. In the acute care setting, death can come without warning due to a sudden change in severity of illness or due to the nature of invasive interventions. Sudden death can occur across the life span from fetal/neonatal death to death of an elderly person. The age of the decedent as well as the ages of the survivors has an effect on how the survivors are affected by the death.[2] Death from medical error can have a distressing effect on the clinicians as well as the survivors.

Death notification and bereavement support to survivors of patients who die from sudden death is an essential skill for nurses and physicians. However, personal fears of death, fear of being blamed for the death, and difficulty in dealing with survivors' grief reactions are potential barriers to delivering the death notification well.[3] Poorly conducted death notification and bereavement care can contribute to the development of traumatic stress, post-traumatic stress disorder, complicated grieving, or depression.[4, 5] Early morbidity and mortality from cardiac pathology, suicide, and cirrhosis of the liver can develop after sudden death of a loved one.[5] Delivering death disclosure in a direct and compassionate way improves the survivors' abilities to plan and cope and gives emotional support during the devastating news.[6]

In a study by Jurkovich and colleagues, the most important elements of giving bad news in trauma settings include the perceived attitude of the news-giver, clarity of the message, privacy of the conversation, and adequate knowledge on the part of the news-giver to answer family questions.[7] Respondents in the same study were mixed in their desire to have clergy present, the amount of detail of the event vs. general information that preceded the event, and touching. Negative aspects of the death notification included complaints about parking, long waits, and frightening hospital scenes. These results help give context about how to deliver bad news in a sensitive way.

Strategies for Death Notification

Core elements should be included to promote empathic death notification such as (1) appearing calm and speaking directly to the

TABLE 1.10.1. GRIEV_ING acronym.

Gather	Gather the family; ensure that all members are present.
Resources	Call for support resources available to assist the family with their grief, i.e., chaplain services, ministers, family, and friends.
Identify	Identify yourself, identify the deceased or injured patient by name, and identify the state of knowledge of the family relative to the events of the day.
Educate	Briefly educate the family as to the events that have occurred in the emergency department; educate them about the current state of their loved one.
Verify	Verify that their family member has died. Be clear! Use the words "dead" or "died."
_Space	Give the family personal space and time for an emotional moment; allow the family time to absorb the information.
Inquire	Ask if there are any questions, and answer them all.
Nuts and bolts	Inquire about organ donation, funeral services, and personal belongings. Offer the family the opportunity to view the body.
Give	Give them your card and access information. Offer to answer any questions that may arise later. Always return their call.

Reprinted from Hobgood C, Harward D, Newton K, Davis W. The educational intervention "GRIEV_ING" improves the death notification skills of residents. *Academic Emergency Medicine*. Apr 2005;12(4):296–301 with permission from John Wiley & Sons, Inc.

survivors, (2) comforting the survivors, (3) allowing adequate time for questions, (4) disclosing the news of death in a timely fashion, and (5) explaining the events that surrounded the death.[6] Clinicians should also prepare the environment for the death disclosure by ensuring privacy, allowing for people to sit down, making sure that the patient is correctly identified, and ensuring that the patient's body is ready for viewing provided there are no relative contraindications (e.g., coroner's/medical examiner's case). Additionally, clinicians should give a warning phrase that sets the tone of the discussion. Often, this is called a "warning shot," meaning that bad or serious news is coming. Phrases such as "I'm afraid I have bad news" or "I have some very serious news to discuss with you" allow the recipient of the serious news a chance to adjust or begin to cope with the news and to minimize the surprise.

To improve the delivery of death notification and to help reduce clinician anxiety, Hobgood and colleagues found that structuring the steps to death notification improved a sense of confidence and competent delivery.[8] The authors created an acronym, GRIEV_ING (Table 1.10.1), to address the important aspects of death notification in sudden death situations.

Quest and colleagues created a structured educational program to teach and evaluate the subtle affective aspects of sensitive death disclosure called the Affective Competency Score (ACS) (Table 1.10.2).[9] The ACS is designed to help learners practice death disclosure before it is actually needed. Learners are evaluated giving death notification during a standardized patient or a role-play scenario. Feedback is shared with the learner and the scenario is played again until competence is achieved.

Interventions and Considerations

The following interventions and considerations should be made when preparing for a sudden death disclosure, depending on the situation. Being prepared and thinking about these issues will help promote an empathic death disclosure. In addition, including members of an interdisciplinary team such as chaplaincy and social work is vital to support the bereaved and clinicians. Cultural considerations of the patient and survivors should be assessed and honored before delivering the death notification.

Organ/Tissue Donation

Organs and tissues can be procured after cardiac death or brain death. Federal law (Public Law 99-5-9; section 9318), Centers for Medicare and Medicaid Services, and the Joint Commission require hospitals to have written protocols regarding organ and tissue donation and allow the surviving family members the chance to authorize donation of their family member's tissues and organs. Evidence suggests that having in-house organ transplant coordinators who are not part of the hospital staff and who are trained specifically to inquire about organ donation increases the rates of organ donation and procurement.[10] In the absence of in-house coordinators, health care organizations should work closely with their local organ procurement organization (OPO) to create procedures for approaching families. See Case 1.6 for a comprehensive discussion of communication around organ donation.

Family Presence During Resuscitation

Family presence during resuscitation is a hotly debated topic. Commonly cited fears of clinicians include fear of litigation, performance anxiety, and concern that families may interfere with resuscitation efforts or the family may become distressed and then need care.[11] However, family presence during resuscitation supports family- and patient-centered care principles that are consistent with the philosophy of palliative care.

There are two important characteristics of successful family presence programs. First, there must be a formal program and

TABLE 1.10.2. Affective Competency Score.

Checklist		
Check one		Criteria (evaluation of physician)
Yes	No	
		Introduced self/role
		Sat down
		Assumed comfortable communication distance
		Tone/rate of speech acceptable
		Made eye contact
		Maintained open posture
		Gave advanced warning of bad news
		Said "dead"/"died"
		Tolerated survivor's reaction
		Used no medical jargon, used language that was clear and easily understood
		Offered viewing of deceased
		Offered to be available to survivor
		Concluded appropriately

Affective evaluation					
	Check ONE only				
	1 Unsatisfactory	2 Below average	3 Average	4 Above average	5 Superior
Confident					
Comfortable					
Empathetic/ sensitive					
Respectful/ professional					
Informative					
Comforting					

Global assessment ratings			
	Check ONE only		
	Needs basic instruction before further survivor encounters	Perform with faculty supervision only	Able to perform independently
Notification of survivor of sudden death			

Reprinted from Quest TE, Ander DS, Ratcliff JJ. The validity and reliability of the affective competency score to evaluate death disclosure using standardized patients. *J Palliat Med.* Apr 2006; 9(2):361–370 with permission from Mary Ann Liebert, Inc.

procedure in place to support the family and the clinicians during this time of crisis. If the opportunity is hastily coordinated, many things can go terribly wrong such as surprising or angering the resuscitation team or abandoning the family who is witnessing the resuscitation, among others. A formal program with education and preparation of the clinicians is vital for the success of the program. An essential component of this formal program is to ensure there is a hospital employee who is assigned to the family at all times to assess their interest and capacity to witness the event, explain the action being witnessed, re-assess the family members during the resuscitation to evaluate whether they need to be escorted from the room, and debrief after the code has been stopped if the patient survives the resuscitation.

Second, the program should be optional for both resuscitation team and families alike. Resuscitation teams need to have the ability to judge a particular situation and deem it unsuitable for family presence. Alternatively, families should be offered the option and not forced to witness an event that could be damaging to them. The Emergency Nurses Association has a toolkit available for institutions to implement family presence.[12]

Medicolegal Investigation of Death

In the United States, we have three systems of medicolegal investigation of death: the coroner system, the medical examiner system, or a hybrid of both.[13] The purpose of medicolegal investigation is to determine whether the death was from natural or unnatural causes by employing forensic pathology principles. Examples of deaths that are investigated include violent deaths, sudden deaths not caused by readily recognizable disease, deaths under suspicious circumstances, or deaths related to disease which might constitute a threat to public health.[13] In these cases, it is important for the resuscitation clinicians to preserve the body as evidence. Access to the deceased should be restricted. This can potentially complicate the bereavement of survivors. One recommendation is to allow the survivors to see the body through a window. This facilitates the grieving while preserving the evidence.[14]

Considerations for Children During Death Disclosure

Sudden death disclosure should be carefully considered when children are present. Loud or demonstrative grieving can frighten young children. Adolescents, depending on the level of maturity, may be able to hear the news. It is less than ideal to have children hear the news at the same time as the adults.[6] Support should be given to the adults on how to disclose the news to children.

"Sign-Out" Death Disclosure

Ideally, the primary team who took care of the patient and who declared the death is the team that delivers the death disclosure. However, in cases where the death happens during a change in shift, having clinicians stay and wait for families to come to the hospital may be impractical.[6] When the care team must leave, it is important to "sign out" or "give report" to the oncoming shift, giving details of the resuscitation event and the follow-up needs including potential coroner/medical examiner investigation, organ or tissue donation, and bereavement support.

Death Disclosure over the Telephone

Telephone death disclosure should be used as a last resort. Reasons for not disclosing the news over the phone include concern that the survivors may get into an accident trying to rush to the hospital and not being able to assess the psychological adaptation of the survivors to the news.[15] However, if barriers exist to disclosing the death in person such as distance or physical frailty of the survivors, clinicians may need to disclose the news over the phone.

Iserson has an excellent telephone notification protocol in his book *Grave Words: Notifying survivors about sudden, unexpected death*.[15] The protocol is divided into three parts: before making the call, making the call, and phrases that help with questions the survivors may ask. A central theme to this protocol is to do everything possible to avoid giving the death notification over the telephone, and trying to convey to the survivors the seriousness of the situation and to get them to the hospital so the death notification can be delivered in person.

If the death notification must be done over the telephone, it is best to have someone with the survivor when they receive the news.[15] This may be difficult to arrange; however, the survivor should get a relative, friend, neighbor, or clergy member to come to their home and then call the hospital back. In some cases, hospital personnel can arrange for local police to do a welfare check on the person and be there when the news is delivered. Hospital staff should contact support services in the survivor's local area to be available to the survivor after the death notification.

BACK TO OUR CASE

The mother was brought into the ED family room. She waited with the social worker and ED charge nurse, who elicited additional history of the patient's illness trajectory. The patient had been receiving intensive chemotherapy and had a surgical resection of her tumors over the past year. The patient had not been feeling well during the 12 hours prior to EMS transport; she had increasing abdominal pain and shortness of breath. The patient was supposed to have an appointment with the medical oncologist that afternoon. The social worker asked the mother if there should be any other people called to be with her and the mother said no. The ED charge nurse took all the information back to the emergency physician and primary nurse to prepare for the death notification while the social worker stayed with the mother.

The emergency physician, primary nurse, and charge nurse approached the mother, sat in a circle, and each introduced themselves by name, title, and role in the ED. The charge nurse started the conversation by asking the mother what happened after she activated the Emergency Medical System. The mother said that she was worried about her daughter because she had been having increasing abdominal pain and shortness of breath. The emergency physician then described the chain of events and started delivering the death notification. "I'm sorry but we have some bad news. When the paramedics picked up your daughter, she was not doing well. She had very low oxygen levels that we believe were from her extensive cancer. The paramedics tried to give her very high doses of oxygen to help her body. When she came into the emergency department, your daughter continued to have very low oxygen levels despite our most aggressive treatments. After being in the emergency department for about five minutes, your daughter's heart and breathing stopped. We immediately started our resuscitation efforts to try and re-start the heart and lungs. Unfortunately, those interventions did not work. I'm so sorry to tell you that your daughter died."

After delivering the death notification, the ED team allowed time for the mother to absorb the information. The team sat with the mother for about three minutes in silence. Tissues were offered to the mother and to the ED team. The primary nurse broke the silence by telling the mother that this was a lot of information and devastating news. The primary nurse and charge nurse said that they would be available until 7 pm to answer any questions. The social worker offered to stay with the mother and contact other family members who should come to the hospital. The charge nurse said that she would come back to ask about funeral services and offered to have the mother see her daughter in the emergency department to view the body. The mother said yes, she wanted to see her daughter and the charge nurse prepared the mother for what she would see. The emergency physician told the mother how sorry he was about the mother's loss of her child and left the family room. The charge nurse, primary nurse, and social worker accompanied the mother to the resuscitation room after it had been tidied by the ED technician.

Additional family members arrived to the ED and were given the opportunity to view the body. With the additional social support with the mother, the charge nurse called the coroner and obtained clearance to release the body to the funeral home. The charge nurse inquired whether the mother thought of any funeral home she might want to contact and then made arrangements for that funeral home to come after the family had left.

As the family was getting ready to leave, the social worker gave the mother her business card and some resources for local bereavement groups in the area and encouraged the mother to call her if she had any questions. The social worker walked the mother out to the parking lot to go home in the care of her family. The emergency physician called the medical oncologist to let her know that the patient had died in the ED.

TAKE AWAY POINTS

- Sudden death notification is challenging and is given during a time of crisis for survivors.
- Be prepared, use a structured approach, and rehearse the death notification before you actually deliver the news.
- Create protocols and resources for the bereaved survivors that address critical issues such as organ donation, medical examiner/ coroner processes, and special populations.

REFERENCES

[1] Lunney JR, Lynn J, Hogan C. Profiles of older Medicare decedents. *JAGS.* 2002; 50:1108–1112.

[2] Roesler R, Ward D, Short M. Supporting staff recovery and reintegration after a critical incident resulting in infant death. *Adv Neonatal Care.* Aug. 2009; 9(4):163–171; quiz 172–163.

[3] Knopp R, Rosenzweig S, Bernstein E, Totten V. Physician-patient communication in the emergency department, part 1. *Academic Emergency Medicine.* Nov. 1996; 3(11):1065–1069.

[4] Boelen PA, van de Schoot R, van den Hout MA, de Keijser J, van den Bout J. Prolonged Grief Disorder, depression, and posttraumatic stress disorder are distinguishable syndromes. *J Affect Disord.* Sep. 2010; 125 (1–3):374–378.

[5] Zalenski R, Gillum RF, Quest TE, Griffith JL. Care for the adult family members of victims of unexpected cardiac death. *Academic Emergency Medicine.* Dec. 2006; 13(12):1333–1338.

[6] Emanuel L, Quest T, eds. *The education in palliative and end-of-life care for emergency medicine.* Chicago: The EPEC™ Project; 2007.

[7] Jurkovich GJ, Pierce B, Pananen L, Rivara FP. Giving bad news: the family perspective. *J Trauma.* May 2000; 48(5):865–870; discussion 870–863.

[8] Hobgood C, Harward D, Newton K, Davis W. The educational intervention "GRIEV_ING" improves the death notification skills of residents. *Academic Emergency Medicine.* Apr 2005; 12(4):296–301.

[9] Quest TE, Ander DS, Ratcliff JJ. The validity and reliability of the affective competency score to evaluate death disclosure using standardized patients. *J Palliat Med.* Apr 2006; 9(2):361–370.

[10] Salim A, Berry C, Ley EJ, et al. In-house coordinator programs improve conversion rates for organ donation. *J Trauma.* Mar. 10 2011.

[11] Dougal RL, Anderson JH, Reavy K, Shirazi CC. Family presence during resuscitation and/or invasive procedures in the Emergency Department: one size does not fit all. *Journal of Emergency Nursing.* Mar. 2011; 37(2): 152–157.

[12] Emergency Nurses Association. *Presenting the option for family presence,* 3rd ed. Des Plaines, IL: Author; 2007.

[13] Godwin TA. End of life: natural or unnatural death investigation and certification. *Dis Mon.* Apr. 2005; 51(4):218–277.

[14] Chan GK. Trajectories of approaching death in the emergency department: Clinician narratives of patient transitions to the end of life. *J Pain Symptom Manage.* May 28 2011.

[15] Iserson KV. Grave Words: *Notifying Survivors About Sudden, Unexpected Deaths.* Tuscon, AZ: Galen Press; 1999.

Section 2

Symptom Management Case Studies

Case 2.1	**Pain: Cancer in the Home**	87
	Constance Dahlin	
Case 2.2	**Treating an Acute, Severe, Cancer Pain Exacerbation**	98
	Patrick J. Coyne	
Case 2.3	**Pain and Advanced Heart Failure**	104
	Margaret L. Campbell	
Case 2.4	**Dyspnea and Advanced COPD**	110
	Margaret L. Campbell	
Case 2.5	**Dyspnea and Heart Failure**	117
	Garrett K. Chan	
Case 2.6	**Treating Dyspnea during Ventilator Withdrawal**	128
	Margaret L. Campbell	
Case 2.7	**Cough Associated with COPD and Lung Cancer**	138
	Peg Nelson	
Case 2.8	**Hiccups and Advanced Illness**	145
	Marian Grant	
Case 2.9	**Treating Nausea Associated with Advanced Cancer**	152
	Judy C. Wheeler	
Case 2.10	**Nausea Associated with Bowel Obstruction**	161
	Terri L. Maxwell	
Case 2.11	**Nausea Related to Uremia, Dialysis Cessation**	168
	Linda M. Gorman	
Case 2.12	**Opioid-Induced Pruritus**	176
	Richelle Nugent Hooper	
Case 2.13	**Pruritus in End-Stage Renal Disease**	183
	Linda M. Gorman	
Case 2.14	**Opioid-Induced Constipation**	190
	Grace Cullen Oligario	
Case 2.15	**Depression in Advanced Disease**	198
	Todd Hultman	
Case 2.16	**Treating Anxiety**	205
	Darrell Owens	
Case 2.17	**Terminal Secretions**	213
	Terri L. Maxwell	
Case 2.18	**Fungating Wounds and the Palliative Care Patient**	220
	Laura C. Harmon	
Case 2.19	**Pressure Ulcer Care in Palliative Care**	229
	Laura C. Harmon	
Case 2.20	**Treating Ascites**	239
	Darrell Owens	
Case 2.21	**Delirium Management in Palliative Care**	247
	Kerstin McSteen	

Overview

No one should suffer while dying. Patients with unrelieved symptoms are unable to fully attend to activities of daily living, work, and engagement with others. Patients with terminal illnesses often fear "dying" more than death because of concerns about comfort and suffering.

Symptom prevalence varies by diagnosis and illness trajectory. Pain, dyspnea, nausea, constipation, and delirium are common across diagnoses. More is known about the symptom experience of patients with cancer than with other conditions. Pain is more common among patients with cancer, while dyspnea is more common among cardio-pulmonary diseases.[1] The interventions for each symptom vary by etiology; hence, the next section has more than one case for the more prevalent symptoms. For example, cancer pain interventions may not be appropriate for treating pain associated with heart disease. Similarly, treating dyspnea associated with heart failure entails different interventions than managing dyspnea from chronic obstructive pulmonary disease (COPD).

In each of the subsequent cases in this section the authors take an evidence-based approach to describing the symptom etiology, assessment, and treatment. Treatment entails both pharmacological and non-pharmacological along with complementary and alternative methods that are supported by evidence.

Pain is an unpleasant sensory or emotional experience associated with actual or potential tissue damage or described in terms of such damage.[2] Pain management is discussed in cases 2.1 through 2.3. A comprehensive description of pain assessment and treatment can be found in Case 2.1 (cancer pain) with application of the generic principles in Case 2.2 (cancer pain exacerbation) and Case 2.3 (pain in heart failure).

Pulmonary symptoms entail several cases. Dyspnea is a subjective experience of breathing discomfort that consists of qualitatively distinct sensations that vary in intensity.[3] Dyspnea treatment under three different conditions is described in Case 2.4 (COPD), Case 2.5 (heart failure), and Case 2.6 (ventilator withdrawal), along with cough (Case 2.7). Retained secretions, conventionally referred to as "death rattle," are discussed (Case 2.17).

Gastrointestinal symptoms are addressed, including hiccups (Case 2.8), nausea (Cases 2.9 through 2.11), opioid-induced constipation (Case 2.14), and ascites (Case 2.20). Psychological symptoms such as depression (Case 2.15), anxiety (Case 2.16), and delirium (Case 2.21) are discussed. Skin and wound problems include pruritis (cases 2.12 and 2.13), fungating wounds (Case 2.18), and pressure ulcers (Case 2.19).

Fatigue is a common complaint across diagnoses and trajectories. The evidence base for a palliative approach to fatigue is so limited that the topic has not been included.[4]

! TAKE AWAY POINTS

- Unrelieved symptoms diminish patient and family quality of life.
- Effective interventions exist for most symptoms that produce distress.

REFERENCES

[1] Solano JP, Gomes B, Higginson IJ. A comparison of symptom prevalence in far advanced cancer, AIDS, heart disease, chronic obstructive pulmonary disease and renal disease. *Journal of Pain and Symptom Management.* Jan 2006; 31(1):58–69.

[2] IASP Subcommittee on Taxonomy. Pain terms: a list with definitions and notes on usage. *Pain.* 1980; 8:249–252.

[3] American Thoracic Society. Dyspnea. Mechanisms, assessment, and management: a consensus statement. *Am J Respir Crit Care Med.* Jan 1999; 159(1):321–340.

[4] Campbell ML, Happ MB, Hultman T, et al. The HPNA research agenda for 2009-2012. *Journal of Hospice and Palliative Nursing.* 2009; 11(1):10–18.

Case 2.1 Pain: Cancer in the Home

Constance Dahlin

HISTORY

Terry was a 50-year-old woman who presented with severe abdominal pain and was subsequently diagnosed with advanced pancreatic cancer. After her diagnosis she moved closer to her parental home for support. After several months, Terry was referred to a home palliative care program for pain and symptom management after being unable to eat or drink; she stated she felt pressure or fullness at her abdomen.

Terry reported 10/10 pain in her right upper quadrant of her abdomen, which radiated through her abdomen. She also complained of banding bilaterally from her umbilicus around to her spine. She had been on oxycodone 30 mg q three hours, but with little relief. She stated she was desperate to have her pain managed. She also had constipation from the medications and was quite fearful of worsening pain.

Terry was the youngest of five children. She was a binge drinker from age 17 to 35. She lived out of state and was a house cleaner until her diagnosis. After her diagnosis she lived with her elderly parents with siblings nearby. She had difficulty understanding the gravity of her prognosis. Her two sisters were nurses and helped with her care.

Case Studies in Palliative and End-of-Life Care, First Edition. Edited by Margaret L. Campbell.
© 2012 John Wiley & Sons, Inc. Published 2012 by John Wiley & Sons, Inc.

PHYSICAL EXAMINATION

Temperature 38.2°C, blood pressure 125/70, heart rate 100, respiratory
rate 16

General: Disheveled, in fetal position on bed, severe pain

Head, eyes, ears, nose, throat: Normocephalic; pupils equal, round, and
reactive to light; extra-ocular movement intact; no scleral icterus; dry
mucosa; no thrush

Chest: Bilateral clear breath sounds, no accessory muscle use

Heart: Regular rate rhythm, S1, S2, no murmur or rub

Abdomen: Positive bowel sounds, firm, tender to palpation in right
upper quadrant and epigastric area

Extremities: Warm, well-perfused, no edema, no deformities

Neurologic: Alert and oriented in three domains, cranial nerves II-XII
grossly intact

Hematological: No bruising

Skin: Multiple bruises on arms and legs

DIAGNOSTICS

Laboratory

White blood count: 3.0, red blood count: 2.97, hemoglobin: 9.2, hematocrit:
27.2, mean corpuscular volume: 92, mean corpuscular hemoglobin:
31.0, sodium: 134, potassium: 4.1, chloride: 98, carbon dioxide: 28.3,
blood urea nitrogen: 10, creatinine: 0.37, epidermal growth factor
receptor: > 60, glucose: 106

Cancer antigen 19-9: 148, carcinoembryonic antigen: 5.4

Calcium 8.1, phosphate: 4.7, magnesium: 1.5

Alanine transaminase/serum glutamic pyruvic transaminase: 12, aspartate aminotransferase and alanine aminotransferase: 10, alkaline
phosphatase: 88, total bilirubin: 0.4, direct bilirubin: 0.1

Prothrombin time: 14.8, prothrombin time and international normalized
ratio: 1.2, partial thromboplastin time: 28.0

Radiology

CT scan of abdomen and pelvis: Locally advanced pancreatic adenocarci-
noma involving the head and uncinate process with circumferential
encasement of the superior mesenteric vein, superior mesenteric artery,
and gastroduodenal artery. The superior mesentery vein is obstructed
with multiple venous collaterals in the upper abdomen. Metastatic
lymphadenopathy in the peripancreatic space and porta hepaticus. Suspicious tumor invasion in the second/third portion of the duodenum.

CT scan of chest: No evidence of intrathoracic metastasis.

| ? | **CLINICAL QUESTION** |

How do you assess and manage cancer pain for a patient at home?

| ✓ | **DISCUSSION** |

Cancer Pain

Pain was described by McCaffrey as "whatever the experiencing person says it is, existing whenever the experiencing person says it does".[1] The International Association for the Study of Pain defines pain as "an unpleasant or emotional experience associated with tissue damage."[2] There are two types of pain: acute and chronic. Acute pain lasts a brief time and is usually caused by a specific incident such as tissue damage, inflammation, a brief disease process, or surgery. Chronic pain lasts past the normal time of healing, usually longer than three months. It is persistent and may worsen over time. Chronic pain is categorized into malignant and non-malignant pain.[3,4] Chronic pain may be caused by cancer or cancer therapy such as chemotherapy and radiation. Cancer pain is chronic in nature because it usually persists for longer than three months.[3]

Etiologies of Cancer Pain

Organic

Different types of pain may occur in cancer: nociceptive and neuro-pathic pain. Nociceptive pain includes visceral or tumor pain and bone pain. Visceral pain is caused by the tumor or metastatic sites. Somatic or bone pain is caused by cancer invasion into the bones. Neuropathic pain may be caused by the tumor irritating the nerve by metastases, tumor swelling which puts pressure on the nerve, nerve irritation from a procedure such as chest tubes, hand and arm swelling from breast or chest surgery, or hand and foot numbness from chemotherapy.

Different types of cancer have various pain syndromes. In pancreatic cancer, it is common to have abdominal pain from the tumor. Additionally, a patient may experience neuropathic pain from the tumor swelling, causing hepatic stretch and innervating nerves along the way. Lung cancer patients may not have pain in their lung, but rather referred pain in the chest wall or back area. Patients with colorectal cancers may have abdominal pain, fullness, and back pain. Breast cancer patients usually have painless breast lumps, but as the disease progresses, bone metastases develop, which cause pain.

TABLE 2.1.1. Guidelines for the management of cancer pain.

National Comprehensive Cancer Network. *NCCN Clinical Practice Guidelines in Oncology. Adult Cancer Pain.* Vol 1: 2011; http://www.nccn.org/professionals/physician_gls/f_guidelines.asp. Accessed May 1, 2011.

American Pain Society. *Principles of Analgesic Use in the Treatment of Acute Pain and Cancer Pain,* 6th edition. Glenview, IL: Author. 2008.

National Cancer Institute. *Pain PDQ. Management with Drugs.* http://www.cancer.gov/cancertopics/pdq/supportivecare/pain/Patient/page4. Accessed July 24, 2011.

World Health Organization Pain and Palliative Care Communication Program. *Two Decades of Clinical Practice Guidelines for the Management of Cancer Pain.* http://www.whocancerpain.wisc.edu/?q=node/99. Accessed July 24, 2011.

Idiopathic

A patient with cancer pain may have a psychologic component. This may include guilt around developing cancer. Or the patient may feel they deserve cancer because of events that have occurred in their life of which they are ashamed. They may also have anxiety about having pain, which may increase the intensity of the pain. Finally, cancer represents death and for some people the psychological distress of this alone can affect cancer pain.[5]

Pain Assessment at End of Life

Assessment

As part of an initial evaluation, it is essential to discuss the patient's experience and description of their pain. In asking about pain, the nurse normalizes the fact that people experience pain. There are many guides for managing cancer pain available from many profession organizations (see Table 2.1.1). The important thing is to chose one guide and use it consistently. Initial assessment of pain includes reviewing the multifactorial aspects of pain. This includes a detailed review of the pain.[4,5]

Description: The clinician must have the patient describe the pain. This will assist in determining whether the pain is from bone, nerve, or tumor. The descriptions help delineate the type of pain such as nocioceptive pain, which includes visceral or tumor pain and bone pain, or neuropathic pain. Nocioceptive pain is well localized and can be constant or intermittent. It can be located in skin, muscle, soft tissue, or bone. It is often describes as constant, a dull ache, or cramping. Somatic pain is usually bone pain and patients describe this as throbbing or aching. Neuropathic pain is caused by damage to nerve fibers.

Intensity: Common tools to assess pain intensity include numeric scales anchored from 0 to 10 or 0 to 100. Other patients may need to use a color scheme with white representing no pain and red signifying worst pain. For some patients, the use of a visual analogue is helpful, such as happy faces evolving to sad faces. Another useful scale is a pain thermometer. The challenge is to ensure that culturally, a patient is allowed to express pain.[4]

Location: Having patients localize pain helps to determine a plan. It also requires that each site be assessed. Sometimes the location can give clues to the coping of the patient. For instance, when a patient says it hurts all over, there may be a psychological aspect that needs attention.

Onset: Onset is helpful to determine if a particular condition or activity initiated the pain.

Duration: Duration establishes whether the pain is constant or intermittent. Asking the patient if it lasts for minutes, hours, or days is helpful in considering causes.

Aggravating and alleviating factors: Reviewing the factors that increase or reduce pain is important to determine if activity is a factor. There also may be a pattern to the pain.

Affective

The patient may have emotional responses to pain. Such responses may include anger, depression, or anxiety; when pain begins, she may moan or cry. These conditions may also need to be treated to reduce pain. After getting a patient's perception of the pain, it is important to have a patient describe how the pain is affecting her quality of life. This includes exploration into the four domains of physical well being (including function), psychological well being (including coping), spiritual well being (including the meaning of the pain), and social well being (including the changes in their roles and relationships from the pain).[5]

Sociocultural

A number of sociocultural considerations follow: What is the age of the patient? If he is older, he may be resigned to pain. If she is younger, the pain may be preventing interaction with family. What are the norms for dealing with pain for this patient within her culture or religion? Is he supposed to be quiet and bear the pain? Is she supposed to be more verbal? What is the patient's support system? What roles has the patient given up?

Treatment

Using the assessment, the nurse can recommend an appropriate regimen. The treatment of cancer pain usually requires a multidrug approach of opioids and adjuvant medications.[6] At home, the focus is on the simplest, least invasive, and least expensive regimen. Moreover, consideration should be given to the dosing in older adults due to slower gastrointestinal absorption, altered kidney function, and sensitivity to anticholinergic side effects.[7]

Opioids

At home, opioids are the primary medication of choice because they are inexpensive, effective, and safe. Additionally, they can be given by many routes including orally, sublingually, rectally, transdermally, intravenously, and subcutaneously. Many hospices have medications compounded in various forms. It is important to consider a medication's properties as to whether certain forms of compounding will be effective.[8] The adage is if a patient can tolerate oral medications, it is best to start with the oral route. In determining a dose, it is important to consider maximizing the use of long-acting medications to reduce the numbers or times a patient needs medications. A patient should be on a long-acting medication to maintain pain, and a short-acting medication for breakthrough dosing. The National Comprehensive Cancer Network (NCCN) guidelines and the American Pain Society (APS) guidelines are all good sources to review for dosing.[9,10] Pasero and McCaffrey and Arnstein also offer step-by-step coaching.[6,11] The general rule is to add the total amount of medication and calculate a divided dose for long-acting agents. The short acting dose should be about 10% to 20% of the 24-hour total. Patients may need a chart or pill box to remind them of medication schedules because that will help keep blood levels more consistent.

Patients react differently to different medications. This may be evident by pain rating, decreased function, and/or adverse side effects from medications. The etiology may be due to inadequate dosing, disease progression, or intolerance to certain medications.[12] Often, it may take some creativity to find an effective regimen.

Morphine, a hydrophilic opioid, is the gold standard for severe and cancer pain. It is the best understood, least expensive medication available in a variety of routes.[5,8] Extended-release tablets, short-acting tablets, and liquid solutions in concentrated forms are available by the oral route. Suppositories can be compounded to high concentrations. For difficult pain syndromes, morphine may be administered by intravenous and subcutaneous routes, but this is less common with all the options of oral medications. Intramuscular injections should be avoided because of discomfort and inconsistent absorption when the patient is hemodynamically unstable, as may characterize the dying patient. It should be noted that compounded gels, creams, or patches are for local treatment of a specific tissue; they are not absorbed systemically. For opioid naïve patients, it is best to start at 5 to 10 mg of an immediate release formulation every four hours as needed. This may need to be adjusted for older adults with renal insufficiency.

Oxycodone, a synthetic hydrophilic opioid, is effective as well. It is about one-third stronger than morphine and available in long-acting pills, short-acting pills, or liquid.[5,8,13] However, access can be an issue for patients who are prescribed oxycodone. Many hospices that use various national pharmacies deny access to oxycodone by not including it as part of the hospice plan of care, or their formularies, making patients pay for it out of pocket. It is best to use simple oxycodone rather than mixed oxycodone/acetaminophen preparation so titration can be done without the risk of acetaminophen toxicity.

Fentanyl transdermal, a highly lipid-soluble anesthetic, is an option for patients who cannot take pills or need more constant delivery.[5,8] The lowest patch preparation is 12 mcg/hour. It is not a first line opioid to initiate because the peak effect is 12 to 18 hours after application and the patient's effective dose is unknown. Patients should have their pain stabilized using immediate-release oral or parenteral formulations, then have the parenteral morphine equivalents converted to an equi-analgesic dose of fentanyl. Fentanyl is not recommended for cancer patients with cachexia or wasting because there is not enough fat for full absorption. It is more expensive than morphine or oxycodone. It is also available as oral lozenges and quick-acting buccal tablets for break-through use. These are often not covered by private insurance.

Hydromorphone, another synthetic lipophilic opioid, is also very strong, with many formulations and a short half life. Hydromorphone is recommended for patients with altered kidney function who may become delirious from the metabolites from morphine. It is a good choice for patients with hepatic or renal impairment.[5,8,13]

Methadone is a synthetic lipophilic opioid that can be used if other opioids are ineffective. It is a very strong medication that can be used for both visceral and neuropathic pain. Methadone is inexpensive and was the only long-acting medication used before long-acting morphine and oxycodone were developed. Methadone has complex properties that can cause a long half life ranging from five to 130 hours.[13] It should be used with caution in older adults because of the long half life and potential for confusion. This medication carries the stigma of being used in the maintenance programs of people with substance abuse; patients require counseling about methadone's use for severe or cancer pain.

The cost of and the access to prescription medications should be a consideration in treatment. Insurance coverage varies considerably among commercial insurance and for Medicare Part D coverage. Patients enrolled in hospice may have more access to pain medications not normally carried by commercial pharmacies. Large chain pharmacies may make it more difficult to access medications with three-day ordering requirements. Other pharmacies may not carry newer, more expensive medications. It is unknown how health care reform measures will change prescription coverage in the future.

Opioid-Induced Side Effects

It is important to remember that while opioids help pain, they also induce constipation, which does not abate over time. It is therefore essential to initiate a bowel regimen when initiating opioids. This should include a softener and stimulant. For many patients this can be as simple as senna and docusate once a day to three times a day. However, some patients may need more aggressive regimens including lactulose, miralax, or enemas. If those are ineffective, other agents may be considered, such as oral naxalone or methylnatraxone, both of which are expensive.

Adjuvants

Adjuvant medications include nonsteroidal anti-inflammatory drugs (NSAIDS), steroids, tricyclic antidepressants, and anti-convulsants. Nocioceptive pain or tumor pain may be responsive to acetaminophen, NSAIDS, bisphosphonates, and radiation or chemotherapy. Acetaminophen, which comes in pills or liquids, may be used with opioids to reduce pain; however it does not reduce swelling like NSAIDS does. Furthermore, care must be taken to monitor dosing so as to reduce the risk of liver toxicity. Patients should receive no more than 3,000 mg of acetaminophen each day. NSAIDs include aspirin, ibuprofen, naproxen, and celecoxib.[5,8] These come in pills, liquids, and patches. They may affect the kidneys so care must be taken for older patients or patients with kidney impairment. They may also affect platelet aggregation; therefore, previous clotting issues should be considered.

Bisphosphonates can relieve bony cancer pain. They are usually administered intravenously on a monthly basis. Some patients experience flu-like symptoms. Patients who have side effects from NSAIDs may benefit from this. Because gastrointestinal protection is necessary for NSAIDS, a cost analysis of the use of bisphosphonates may be helpful.[5,8]

Neuropathic pain responds to antidepressants and anticonvulsants.[14] Antidepressants, including nortriptyline, desipramine, duloxetine, and vanlafaxine, are the most commonly used.[5,8] Cost and age may be considerations. Nortriptyline and desipramine are tricyclic antidepressants. They may be helpful if patients have sleep issues as well as nerve pain. However, because of their cholinergic side effects, they may not be tolerated by older adults. Duloxetine and vanlafaxine may be useful with patients with depression and pain. They have fewer side effects; however, some insurances and hospices do not cover the cost of these newer medications.

Anticonvulsants include gabapentin and pregabalin. Gabapentin is effective for chemotherapy-related neuropathic pain as well as cancer-related pain. It may make patients lethargic until they get used to the medication. If gabapentin fails, pregabalin may be used. For specific nerve pain caused by procedures, transdermal lidocaine may be helpful.

Both nerve pain and nocioceptive pain respond to steroids, which include dexamethasone and prednisilone. They help reduce swelling of a tumor or an impinged nerve. Their secondary effects are also helpful because they offer a sense of well being, alleviate fatigue, promote appetite, and reduce nausea and vomiting.[15] A low dose initially is helpful because often a small amount goes a long way. Consideration should be given to age of patient because older adults may have concurrent illnesses adding to pain syndromes and have a greater potential to experience side effects.

Nonpharmacological Treatments

Nonpharmacological strategies for patients at home with cancer pain are as important as pharmacological interventions.[11] Physical modalities include positioning when patients are no longer able to lie flat. They may need pillows, bolsters to help them sleep upright, easy chairs to elevate legs, or home hospital beds to ease the change of position.

Pacing of activities is also important. Cancer in itself causes fatigue, but often cancer treatments such as chemotherapy and radiation intensify fatigue. When patients are tired, their pain may worsen. Patients may need assistance in understanding the limits of daily activity that do not worsen their pain. They may also need assistance in reviewing the energy necessary for various activities.

The use of heat and cold can help. Patients may find that heating pads help in diminishing pain or they may find warm baths soothing. Ice packs may be helpful at times as well. The use of small bags of frozen vegetables or commercial formed frozen pea-size granules can conform better to awkward areas in the back, feet, and groin. Sometimes patients may alternate between heat and cold.

Psychosocial strategies include distraction such as reading, watching television, or listening to music. This helps refocus away from symptoms. Relaxation techniques such as deep breathing can also help. Hypnosis, acupuncture, and massage may also facilitate pain relief if there are specially trained practitioners who visit the home.

BACK TO OUR CASE

Terry needed a long-acting agent. Ideally, because she had been on oxycodone, she could be on a long-acting preparation of the same medication. Given that she was taking 30 mg every six hours, she was taking 180 mg a day but with little relief. Therefore, it was reasonable to increase the dose by 2% to 50% to 240 mg to 360 mg a day. It was dosed every eight hours or every 12 hours, which would make it 80 to 120 mg PO TID, or 120 to 180 PO BID using the tablets that come in doses of 60 mg, 80 mg, and 100 mg. The PRN breakthrough dose was 25 to 50 mg every three to four hours, which was 5% to 20% of the total 24-hour dose. Additionally, given that pancreatic cancer has a neuropathic component, it was reasonable to start gabapentin 100 mg PO TID. A bowel regimen included a senna/doucosate product with the Oxycontin dose. If Terry was unable or afraid to take pills, it would have been reasonable to use fentanyl patches. One could start at 75 to 100 mcg and see how she felt. Reassessment took place on each home visit.

! TAKE AWAY POINTS

- Assessment should review intensity, quality, and severity of pain to elicit whether it is nociceptive, bone, or neuropathic pain.
- Treatment of cancer pain at home includes both pharmacological agents including opioids, adjuvants, and non-pharmacological interventions.
- Opioid therapy should include a long-acting and short acting regimen.
- Constipation must be managed concurrently with opioids.

REFERENCES

[1] McCaffrey M. *Nursing Practice Theories Related to Cognition, Bodily Pain, and Man-Environment Interactions*. Los Angeles: UCLA Press. 1968; 95.

[2] Merseky H, Bogduk N., eds. *Classification of Chronic Pain, 2nd edition.* International Association for the Study of Pain, Task Force on Taxonomy. Seattle, WA: IASP Press. 1994; 209–214.

[3] Fishman S, Ballantyne J, Rathmell J, eds. *Bonica's Management of Pain.* Philadelphia: Lippincott, Williams & Wilkins. 2010; 78.

[4] Fink R, Gates R. Pain assessment. In: Ferrell BR, Coyle N, eds. *Oxford Textbook of Palliative Nursing, 3rd edition.* New York: Oxford University Press. 2010; 137–160.

[5] Coyle N, Goldstein-Layman M. In: Matzo M, Sherman D, eds. *Palliative Care Nursing—Quality Care to the End of Life.* New York: Springer Pub Co. 2010; 357–410.

[6] Pasaro C, McCaffrey M. *Pain Assessment and Pharmacologic Management.* St Louis: Mosby Elsevier. 2010.

[7] American Geriatrics Society. *Pharmacological Management of Persistent Pain in Older Adults.* 2009; 57:1331–1346.

[8] Paice J. Pain at the end of life. In Ferrell BR, Coyle N, eds. *Oxford Textbook of Palliative Nursing, 3rd edition.* New York: Oxford University Press. 2010; 161–185.

[9] National Comprehensive Cancer Network. NCCN Clinical Practice Guidelines in Oncology. Adult Cancer Pain. 2011:1. http://www.nccn.org/professionals/physician_gls/f_guidelines.asp. Accessed May 1, 2011.

[10] American Pain Society. *Principles of analgesic use in the treatment of acute pain and cancer pain,* 6th edition Glenview, IL. 2008.

[11] Arnstein P. Nondrug, complementary and alternative approaches to pain relief. *Clinical Coach for Effective Pain Management.* Philadelphia: FA Davis. 2010; 151–177.

[12] McPherson ML. *Demystifying Opioid Conversion Calculations—A Guide for Effective Dosing*. Bethesda, MD: American Society of Health System Pharmacists. 2010.

[13] Brant J. Practical approaches to pharmacologic management of pain in older adults with cancer. *Oncology Nursing Forum*. 2010; 37(5): Suppl; 17–25.

[14] Dworkin R, O'Connor A, Miroslay B, Farrar J, Finnerup N, et al. Pharmacologic management of neuropathic pain: Evidenced based recommendations. *Pain*. 2007; 132:237–251.

[15] Emanual L, Librach SL. In: Thai V, Fansinger R, eds. *Palliative Care: Core skills and Clinical Competencies*. Philadelphia: Saunders Elsevier. 2007; 96–114.

Case 2.2 Treating an Acute, Severe, Cancer Pain Exacerbation

Patrick J. Coyne

HISTORY

John was a 56-year-old man with metastatic non-small cell lung cancer. His cancer was diagnosed four months prior to hospital admission after he complained of generalized aching, fatigue, and dyspnea on exertion. He had received three rounds of palliative chemotherapy and several fractions of radiation therapy for pain and symptom management. His cancer was previously deemed inoperable. There were multiple bone and suspected liver metastases. He arrived in the emergency room with moaning, grimacing, and altered mental status.

His wife of 18 years and 15-year-old daughter accompanied him. They called 911 after having difficulty arousing him. According to his wife, he had been taking six to 10 tablets of oxycodone/acetaminophen daily and 45 mg of extended-release morphine every 12 hours for the last two weeks. This was a conservative equilanalgesic conversion equaling 120 mg of oral morphine equivalent every 24 hours, or 40 mg of parenteral morphine in 24 hours, or 1.7 mg of parenteral morphine per hour. John's wife reported that this pain regimen had not kept her husband comfortable, and his use of breakthrough oxycodone/acetaminophen had increased. Constipation was becoming more of an issue, per the family report. John was allergic to no medications, drank occasional alcohol, and continued to smoke approximately one pack of cigarettes daily. He was on disability; he had previously worked as a carpenter.

Case Studies in Palliative and End-of-Life Care, First Edition. Edited by Margaret L. Campbell.
© 2012 John Wiley & Sons, Inc. Published 2012 by John Wiley & Sons, Inc.

PHYSICAL EXAMINATION

Constitutional: Cachectic

Neurological: Lethargic, opened his eyes to verbal and light physical stimuli, followed some commands but did not respond to questions. He intermittently fell asleep. Moved all extremities without difficulty

Blood pressure: 160/92, pulse: 110, respiratory rate: 23, temperature 99°C

Pain: Reported pain as 7/10, using a nonverbal adult pain scale; guarded his left ribs on palpation.

Heart: Regular, tachycardic

Lungs: Diminished left lower lung sounds, SpO_2 91% on room air.

Lab results: Normal with the exception of a calcium level of 13.1 mg/dL, and hemoglobin of 9.6 g/dL.

DIAGNOSTICS

Chest X-ray: Confirmed metastatic lung cancer; of note, part of the sixth left rib was no longer visible and widespread spinal metastases were noted

CT scan of the head: Negative for metastatic cancer or hemorrhage

? CLINICAL QUESTION

How should an acute, severe, pain exacerbation be treated in advanced stage cancer?

✓ DISCUSSION

The estimate of death from lung cancer in 2010 in the United States is over 150,000, and it is the leading cause of cancer-related mortality in this country.[1] The leading cause of cancer remains smoking.

The five-year relative survival rate for patients with lung cancer is 15.7%. The five-year relative survival rate varies markedly depending on the stage at diagnosis, from 49% to 16% to 2% for patients with local, regional, and distant stage disease, respectively.[2] However, individuals with advanced metastatic disease may achieve improved survival and palliation of symptoms with chemotherapy, as well as with aggressive palliative care.[3]

Presentation in the emergency department (ED) because of acute pain exacerbation and other adverse effects is common in advanced cancer. Patients who are opioid tolerant rarely have altered mentation from their analgesics.

Hypercalcemia is common in patients with bone metastases. Often when cancer patients appear somnolent, altered, or constipated, opioids are blamed as the etiology of these symptoms. Therefore, it is important to remember that in opioid- tolerant patients in which minimal opioid titration has been done for a week prior to such symptoms, one must consider renal and hepatic function, electrolyte levels, especially calcium, infection of the urinary and respiratory tracts, and metastatic spread to the brain. Pain management should always be continued during this evaluation. See Case 2.1 for a comprehensive discussion of cancer pain etiologies and assessment.

Principles of Rapid Titration of Analgesia for Acute Pain Exacerbation

It is not unusual for patients having cancer pain to be admitted to a hospital for aggressive opiate titration when their pain is poorly managed or they have intractable symptoms from the analgesic regimen. Because cancer may produce rapid changes in the patient's comfort, clinicians must consider titrating opioids rapidly.

For severe pain, intravenous (IV) titration is indicated because pain control may be achieved more quickly than through an oral regimen or transdermal or subcutaneous routes. IV titration of opioids can be administered and increased every 20 minutes using short-acting opioids such as fentanyl, hydromorphone, and morphine. Rapid opioid titration is indicated for severe pain, increasing hourly doses by 50% to 100%.[4] Monitoring for changes in level of sedation and side effects is imperative as opioids are increased. When the patient is opioid tolerant there is low risk for respiratory sedation but with an opioid naïve individual there is a moderate risk and frequency of reassessment should be established based on the clinical circumstances. If a rapid opioid titration has been attempted and pain relief has not been achieved or the side effects become too problematic, then an opioid rotation is indicated.

Opioid rotation entails changing the patient from the opioid regimen that is no longer effective to another opioid. Individuals may respond better to one opioid than another. When opioids are rotated in a stable pain scenario the equianalgesic dose is often decreased by 25% to account for cross tolerance. However, with severe intractable pain many clinicians may choose to match the equianalgesic dose of the previous opioid.

When pain becomes stable patients should be converted to a long-acting opioid to maintain comfort. For example, 300 mg of IV morphine in 24 hours is equivalent to 900 mg of oral morphine which is divided into 3 doses at 300 mg of sustained-release morphine every eight hours. The morphine parenteral to oral conversion is 1:3.

Even when patients with stable pain are on long-acting opioids, breakthrough pain will occur so short-acting opioids must be available to treat this pain. Typically 10% to 20% of the 24-hour opioid dose is used to treat breakthrough pain. Therefore, with 300 mg of sustained-release morphine equaling 900 mg of PO morphine daily, the indicated breakthrough morphine dose is 90 mg of immediate release morphine every two or three hours as needed.

Other options that can be considered include epidural analgesia which is a relatively safe and uncomplicated procedure in experienced hands, but the care of the catheter and medication administration may be quite burdensome to some patients and their families.[5] In addition to opioids, some patients benefit from nonsteroidal anti-inflammatories (NSAIDS), lidocaine infusion, and the use of ketamine as an opioid-sparing agent. Invasive analgesic options include neurolytic blocks of the rib cage or a neurosurgical intervention to disrupt nerve transmission.

Complementary and/or alternative treatments such as acupressure and/or acupuncture might offer some comfort as well. The interventions used are dictated by the institutional resources and expertise of providers.

BACK TO OUR CASE

John required admission to the hospital for evaluation and treatment of severe pain, dyspnea, constipation, and altered mental status. On ED evaluation John's oxygen levels and respiratory effort were adequate. In reviewing his labs, the most likely cause of his drowsiness was the elevated calcium level. John had chest tenderness to movement and palpation; therefore, the likely etiology of his discomfort was from his bone metastases. Per radiology findings no impending fractures exist.

John's wife described initially good relief from morphine in the emergency room, so this medication was continued. As noted, 1.7 mg of parenteral morphine equivalent was being received by the patient with minimal benefit. Therefore, the emergency staff chose to increase John's morphine dose to 3 mg intravenously every 30 minute as bolus until relief while awaiting admission. After hospital admission John was started on 60 mg of long-acting morphine every 12 hours and 4 mg of IV morphine every hour as needed for pain. Morphine was continued as the primary opioid because his wife reported it had been providing good relief until prior to hospital admission. Should John never have received pain relief from morphine or failed to provide adequate analgesia with appropriate titration, opioid rotation would have been considered. John was also started on dexamethasone 8 mg as an adjunct treatment for bone pain, along with a proton pump inhibitor.

John had been taking oxycodone/acetaminophen combination but this was rotated to morphine to avoid excessive doses of acetaminophen. Within the first 24 hours he received 24 mg of IV morphine with reported good relief of his discomfort. This 24 mg of IV morphine in 24 hours was equivalent to 72 mg of oral morphine during this time frame. John was noted to be more alert and aware and able to respond to questions. He reported his pain as adequate, rating it as four out of 10 on the pain scale. He was able to participate in activities of daily living. Noting his opioid requirements, he was converted to 90 mg of long-acting morphine every 12 hours with 15 mg of immediate release morphine available every two hours as needed. His bowel regimen was increased to prevent future complications from opioid-induced constipation.

NSAIDS were not considered, given John was on corticosteroids and these agents in combination may increase the risk of gastrointestinal bleeding. No neuropathic pain was noted on the pain assessment; therefore, further adjunctive analgesics for neuropathy were not needed at this time. However, neuropathic pain is a common occurrence in patients with cancer and John may need them in the future. Radiation therapy offers analgesia in approximately 70% of patients receiving this intervention, usually within seven to 14 days, so a consult for radiation therapy was initiated.

Over the next 24 hours John was noted to be increasing his activity while his pain scores remained consistently between three and five. The team started at a slightly lower dose of extended-release morphine in hopes the radiation therapy would continue to decrease his pain and therefore opioid requirements. If it did not, he would still have the immediate release to use as needed. The corticosteroids were titrated over the 14 days. John did well on this regimen, with ongoing improvement in function and pain, and required infrequent break-through doses of immediate-release morphine. He was discharged home in the care of his family with hospice.

! TAKE AWAY POINTS

- Cancer pain is an evolving target. It may be chronic, acute, or both at any given time, requiring a complete pain reassessment with each change in the quality, intensity, or location in pain.
- There are a wide range of evidence-based safe, effective interventions for the treatment of cancer pain.

- Cancer pain may often be exceedingly complicated. Although its etiology often begins in a physical source, it is critical to assess the psychosocial and spiritual components of the pain, and to evaluate the patient physically, psychosocially, and spiritually, including support systems.
- There are many ways to treat cancer pain and one should never accept intractable pain without exploring all potential interventions.

REFERENCES

[1] American Cancer Society. Cancer facts and figures 2010.
[2] Ries LAG, Eisner MP, Kosary CL, et al. *SEER cancer statistics review, 1975–2002.*
[3] Temel JS, Greer JA, Muzikansky A, et al. Early palliative care for patients with metastatic non-small-cell lung cancer. *N Engl J Med.* 2010; 363:733–742.
[4] Miaskowski C, Cleary J, Burney R, Coyne P, Finley R, Foster R, Grossman S, Janjan N, Ray J, Syrjala K, Weisman S, Zahrbock C. Guidelines for the Management of Cancer Pain in Adults and Children, APS Clinical Practice Guidelines Series, No.3, Glenville, IL : American Pain Society. 2005.
[5] Brogan S, Junkins S. Interventional therapies for the management of cancer pain. *J Support Oncol.* 2010; 8:52–59.

Case 2.3 Pain and Advanced Heart Failure

Margaret L. Campbell

HISTORY

George was a 76-year-old white man who was admitted to the hospital via the emergency department (ED) with a report of severe chest pain complicating New York Heart Association (NYHA) stage IV heart failure; his ejection fraction was 28%. George reported severe pain at 10 of 10 on a numeric rating system. He was compliant with his heart failure medication regimen, monitored his weight daily, and reported rare dyspnea, particularly during exertion. He had an implantable cardioverter/defibrillator that had never fired.

George lived with his wife and they had three adult children that lived in the local area. He was independent with limited activities of daily living (eating, bathing, toileting) as long as he balanced rest with activity; he used a walker with seat when mobile outside their home.

PHYSICAL EXAMINATION

Temperature: 37.2°C, blood pressure: 100/60, heart rate: 86, respiratory rate: 14
Central nervous system: Alert, oriented, no focal deficits
Head, eyes, ears, nose, throat: No defects or abnormalities
Cardiac: S1 S2, no S3 or S4, no murmurs

Case Studies in Palliative and End-of-Life Care, First Edition. Edited by Margaret L. Campbell.
© 2012 John Wiley & Sons, Inc. Published 2012 by John Wiley & Sons, Inc.

Lungs: Clear to auscultation, SpO$_2$ 92% on room air

Gastrointestinal: Scaphoid abdomen, normal bowel sounds, no tenderness

Genitourinary: Voiding

Extremities: Cachectic, no pressure ulcers or deformities

DIAGNOSTICS

Chest X-ray: Cardiac hypertrophy

EKG: Normal sinus rhythm with occasional premature ventricular contractions, old anterior and lateral myocardial infarctions

Labs: Complete blood count within normal limits, sodium: 145, potassium: 3.2, chloride: 104, blood urea nitrogen: 30, creatinine: 1.6

? CLINICAL QUESTION

What treatments may reduce pain associated with advanced heart failure?

✓ DISCUSSION

Natural History of Heart Failure

Heart failure continues to be the leading cause of death in the United States, accounting for 616,067 deaths in 2009. It is worth noting that because deaths from heart disease have tended to decrease between 1980 and 2009, it is likely that at some point in the near future heart disease will no longer be the leading cause of death in the United States.[1]

There are two commonly used approaches to the classification of heart failure (HF). The American Heart Association/American College of Cardiologists (AHA/ACC) developed a classification that emphasizes the progression of HF.[2] The New York Heart Association classification categorizes patients according to their functional capacity.[3] The classification systems complement one another and are illustrated in Table 2.3.1.

Progression varies by patient. The strongest, validated prognostic tool is the Seattle Heart Failure Score (SHFS) with a number of variables and adjustments for medications and devices. The SHFS provides data at 1, 2, and 5 years.[4] Variables include:

- Age
- Gender
- NYHA class

TABLE 2.3.1. Classification of heart failure.

ACC/AHA stage		NYHA functional class	
Stage	Description	Class	Description
A	Patients at high risk of developing HF because of the presence of conditions that are strongly associated with the development of HF. Such patients have no identifiable structural or functional abnormalities of the pericardium, myocardium, or cardiac valves and have never shown signs or symptoms of HF.		
B	Patients who have developed structural heart disease that is strongly associated with the development of HF but who have never shown signs or symptoms of HF.	I	No limitation of physical activity. Ordinary physical activity does not cause undue fatigue, palpitation, or dyspnea.
C	Patients who have current or prior symptoms of HF associated with underlying structural heart disease.	II	Slight limitation of physical activity. Comfortable at rest, but ordinary physical activity results in fatigue, palpitation, or dyspnea.
		III	Marked limitation of physical activity. Comfortable at rest, but less than ordinary activity causes fatigue, palpitation, or dyspnea.
D	Patients with advanced structural heart disease and marked symptoms of HF at rest despite maximal medical therapy and who require specialized interventions.	IV	Unable to carry out any physical activity without discomfort. Symptoms of cardiac insufficiency at rest. If any physical activity is undertaken, discomfort is increased.

From the AHA/ACC in Hunt et al. (2001) and the NYHA in the Criteria Committee of the NYHA (1994).

- Weight
- Ejection fraction
- Systolic blood pressure
- Cause of heart failure
- Medication use
- Diuretic dose
- Anemia
- % Lymphocytes
- Uric acid
- Total cholesterol
- Serum sodium
- Intraventricular conduction delay
- Use of devices

Treatment

Heart failure regimens include diuretics, angiotensin-converting-enzyme (ACE) inhibitors, and beta blockers. Inotropes are indicated for class III to IV patients who have a left ventricular ejection fraction less than 35%. Implantable cardioverter-defibrillator is appropriate to prevent sudden cardiac death. At stage IV the patient should be evaluated for heart transplant and/or a left ventricular assist device.[5] In addition, at stage IV patients should have their preferences about life-sustaining therapies and cardiopulmonary resuscitation (CPR) reviewed and documented.[5]

The highly variable prognosis for heart failure limits hospice referral. Non-hospice palliative care, however, is appropriate in this condition that is fraught with complex symptoms and challenges to quality of life.[6] The most common symptoms that typify advanced heart failure include: dyspnea, pain, depression, fatigue, and edema. Pain in heart failure is the focus of this case.

Pain Etiology

The etiology of pain in heart failure is not fully understood.[7] Older patients may experience pain from sources other than cardiac such as osteoarthritis, but also have cardiac-associated pain such as angina.

NSAIDS

Nonsteroidal anti-inflammatory drugs (NSAIDS) are the mainstay for treating joint and muscle pain but are contraindicated in heart failure because of adverse effects on renal function leading to sodium and fluid retention that worsens heart failure.[8] Alternative analgesia should be applied including topical modalities such as cold or heat or joint injections.

Opioids

Opioids are safe, effective agents in the context of heart failure. Close monitoring for adverse effects is indicated as with any other opioid regimen. Morphine and codeine are safe but must be used cautiously in renal dysfunction.

BACK TO OUR CASE

George was compliant with his heart failure regimen at home and although he was frail he was largely free of the common complaint of dyspnea. His predicted survival with the SHFS was 3.7 years. He was not a candidate for transplant or re-vascularization or stenting. A palliative approach to treating George's pain was indicated.

George did not have continuous pain, it waxed and waned. In the face of mild renal insufficiency an "as needed" regimen of immediate release morphine was planned. George reported relief of pain with 15 mg of oral morphine with a decrease in his numeric pain score from 10 to three. A bowel regimen was initiated. George was discharged with a prescription for morphine, immediate release, 15 mg every two hours as needed for pain. Follow up in a palliative medicine clinic was recommended.

TAKE AWAY POINTS

- Heart failure is a progressive, irreversible leading cause of death; treatment is supportive and palliative.
- Dyspnea, pain, depression, fatigue, and edema are the most prevalent symptoms that produce patient distress.
- Opioids can be safely given in the context of heart failure; NSAIDS are contraindicated secondary to adverse renal effects and worsening heart failure.

REFERENCES

[1] Centers for Disease Control. *National Center for Health Statistics*. Hyattsville, MD. 2009.
[2] Hunt SA, Baker DW, Chin MH, et al. ACC/AHA Guidelines for the Evaluation and Management of Chronic Heart Failure in the Adult: Executive Summary. A Report of the American College of Cardiology/ American Heart Association Task Force on Practice Guidelines (Committee to Revise the 1995 Guidelines for the Evaluation and Management of Heart Failure): Developed in Collaboration With the International Society for Heart and Lung Transplantation; Endorsed by the Heart Failure Society of America. *Circulation*. Dec 11 2001; 104(24):2996–3007.

[3] The Criteria Committee of the New York Heart Association. *Nomenclature and Criteria for Diagnosis of Diseases of the Heart and Great Vessels*, 9th edition. Boston: Little, Brown & Co. 1994; 253–256.

[4] Levy WC, Mozaffarian D, Linker DT, et al. The Seattle Heart Failure Model: prediction of survival in heart failure. *Circulation.* 2006; 113:1424–1433.

[5] Goodlin SJ. Palliative care in congestive heart failure. *Journal of the American College of Cardiology.* 2009; 54(5):386–396.

[6] Adler ED, Goldfinger JZ, Kalman J, Park ME, Meier DE. Palliative care in the treatment of advanced heart failure. *Circulation.* 2009; 120:2597–2606.

[7] Goodlin SJ, Wingate S, Pressler SJ, Teerlink JR, Storey CP. Investigating pain in heart failure patients: rationale and design of the Pain Assessment, Incidence and Nature in Heart Failure (PAIN-HF) study. *J Card Fail.* May 2008; 14(4):276–282.

[8] Page J, Henry D. Consumption of NSAIDs and the development of congestive heart failure in elderly patients: an underrecognized public health problem. *Arch Intern Med.* Mar. 27, 2000; 160(6):777–784.

Case 2.4 Dyspnea and Advanced COPD

Margaret L. Campbell

HISTORY

Marjorie was a 72-year-old white woman who was admitted to the hospital via the emergency department (ED) with an acute exacerbation of advanced chronic obstructive pulmonary disease (COPD; forced expiratory volume – 1 second < 35%) secondary to a 50 pack/years history of cigarette smoking. This was her third admission in two months. On the last admission she spent two weeks in the medical intensive care unit (MICU), requiring intubation and mechanical ventilation. At her last discharge she indicated a preference for no future intubation/ventilation. However, although she met enrollment criteria, she was not referred to hospice; a palliative care consult was requested by the admitting physician.

Marjorie reported severe dyspnea using 10 of 10 on a numeric rating system. She validated a preference for no mechanical ventilation of any type (invasive or non-invasive). She confirmed a decision for no resuscitation and would accept any treatment to relieve her dyspnea except for the limitations previously stated.

Marjorie lived alone in a senior's apartment but had a housekeeper who came into the home three times a week to shop, clean, assist Marjorie with bathing, prepare meals, and do laundry. Marjorie was on home oxygen at 2l which she wore for most of the day and night. Marjorie was mobile in her apartment and occasionally went to

---

Case Studies in Palliative and End-of-Life Care, First Edition. Edited by Margaret L. Campbell.

a common room to socialize with other residents. She had no children and was a widow.

PHYSICAL EXAMINATION

Temperature: 37.2°C, blood pressure: 120/60, heart rate: 128, respiratory rate: 39

Central nervous system: Alert, oriented, no focal deficits

Head, eyes, ears, nose, throat: No defects or abnormalities

Cardiac: S1, S2 and tachycardia, no S3 or S4, no murmurs

Lungs: Large A-P diameter, distant lung sounds, diminished at bases, expiratory wheeze, tachypneic, accessory muscle use, SpO_2 83% on 4l humidified nasal cannula

Gastrointestinal: Scaphoid abdomen, normal bowel sounds, no tenderness

Genitourinary: Voiding

Extremities: Cachectic, no pressure ulcers or deformities

DIAGNOSTICS

Chest X-ray: Hyperinflation and bullae throughout bilaterally; no infiltrates or effusions

CLINICAL QUESTION

What treatments may reduce dyspnea associated with advanced COPD?

DISCUSSION

Natural History of COPD

COPD is characterized by the progressive development of airflow limitation that is not reversible and is inclusive of chronic obstructive bronchitis, emphysema, and mucus plugging. Most patients with COPD have all three conditions.[1] Chronic pulmonary diseases are the third leading cause of death for all people who die each year in the United States.[2] The resulting dyspnea, respiratory distress, cough, and secretions burden the patient and are the emphases of palliative care for terminal pulmonary disease.

Cigarette smoking is the leading cause of COPD in industrialized countries; environmental pollutants are important causes in developing countries. Irritants deposited in the lower respiratory tract from cigarette smoke or pollutants and the resulting histopathological responses produce alveolar wall destruction (emphysema) and mucus hypersecretion (chronic bronchitis). Quitting smoking slows but does not appear to halt the inflammatory process in the airways, suggesting that there are perpetuating mechanisms once inflammation has become established.[3]

Over time the person with COPD develops a chronic cough; experiences changes in the volume, tenacity, and purulence of sputum; and declines in pulmonary function. Weight loss and fatigue are typical because appetite is reduced and it is difficult to eat when dyspneic. The lungs become hyperinflated, producing an increased anterior-posterior thoracic diameter (barrel-chest), increased retrosternal airspace, bullae, and hilar vascular prominence. Hypoxemia, hypercarbia, and reduced peak expiratory flow rate develop.

The terminal stage is characterized by a continued decline in respiratory status, decreased ability to complete activities of daily living, and frequent emergency department visits or hospital admissions with acute exacerbations. At present there are no reliable tools to predict survival interval of less than six months.[4]

Assessment

The gold standard for measuring symptom distress is the patient's report. The numeric rating scale (NRS) anchored with "0" for no breathlessness to "10" for the most severe breathlessness may be helpful to measure the trend of the patient's response to treatment. Dyspnea is a multi-dimensional symptom and the NRS can be applied to measure any of the domains such as intensity, distress, impact on activities of daily living, and others.

Cognitive impairment typifies the period during an acute exacerbation, particularly if the pressure of arterial oxygen (PaO_2) is less than 50 mm Hg[5] and hypercarbia produces a narcotic effect at $PaCO_2$ levels greater than 70 mm Hg.[6] Patients with COPD who experience chronic blood gas alterations are likely to have mild cognitive impairment, even when their oxygenation is stable, with declines from baseline occurring when they are hypoxemic.[7] During an episode of cognitive impairment the NRS may be too difficult for the patient to comprehend. A simple query "Are you short of breath?" may yield a yes or no response and be a sufficient assessment until cognition is restored.

Cognitive impairment and decreased consciousness typifies the active dying stage and the patient may not be able to provide a simple yes or no response.[8] The Respiratory Distress Observation Scale (RDOS) is the only known tool for assessing respiratory distress when the adult patient cannot self-report dyspnea. The RDOS has undergone rigorous clinical testing to establish scale reliability, inter-rater reliability, convergent validity, construct validity, and discriminant validity.[9-12] The RDOS is an eight-item ordinal tool to measure the presence and intensity of respiratory distress; each item is scored from zero to two points and the points are summed. Higher scores suggest higher intensity respiratory distress. The instrument is not valid for use in children or when the patient is undergoing neuromuscular blockade or has amyotrophic lateral sclerosis.[12]

Treatment

Optimize COPD Regimen

COPD has no cure and treatment is largely supportive and palliative, directed at delaying progression, optimizing lung function, and minimizing symptom distress. Smoking cessation is the only measure that will slow the progression of COPD and is aided by nicotine-replacement therapies.[13]

Inhaled bronchodilators are the mainstay of current drug therapy for COPD. They are given on a scheduled and as-needed basis to prevent or reduce symptoms. The principal bronchodilator treatments are short and long-acting β_2-agonists (albuterol, sameterol), anticholinergics (ipratropium), and theophylline, usually used in combination.[13]

Antibiotics are important during acute exacerbations only if a bacterial infection is detected.[1] Long-term oxygen therapy (more than 15 hours/daily) reduces mortality and improves the quality of life in patients with severe COPD who have chronic hypoxemia (PaO_2 less than 55 mm Hg).[14]

An acute exacerbation of COPD is characterized by some combination of three clinical findings: worsening dyspnea, increase in sputum purulence, and increase in sputum volume. Acute exacerbations are treated by maximizing the patient's regimen of bronchodilators, anticholinergics, and oxygen. A brief course of intravenous corticosteroids followed by oral prednisone tapered over days has been successful in stabilizing patients with acute exacerbations. Mechanical ventilation is indicated when patient fatigue or respiratory failure are present, unless the patient refuses this level of support. Non-invasive mechanical ventilation, such as continuous positive airway pressure (CPAP), is less burdensome than intubation and ventilation and is employed if the patient is alert, cooperative, hemodynamically stable, able to maintain her own airway and secretions, and able to tolerate the mask.[15] The patient's goals determine whether mechanical ventilation is used.

Refractory dyspnea in the face of an optimized COPD regimen warrants a dyspnea treatment plan while the COPD regimen continues. An array of palliative interventions for dyspnea include positioning, balancing rest with activity, oxygen if hypoxemic, opioids, and benzodiazepines.

Positioning

A tripod position with the arms supported by pillows or on an over-bed table and the patient leaning forward may reduce dyspnea. Upright positioning with arms elevated and supported optimizes lung capacity.[16,17]

Oxygen

Oxygen is more effective than air in hypoxemic patients with terminal stage COPD.[18,19] However, little benefit in reducing dyspnea is achieved with oxygen when the patient is normally oxygenated.[20] Nasal cannulae are better tolerated than face masks; face masks can worsen the sensation of suffocation. High flow oxygen by nasal cannula leads to drying of the nasal mucosa and occasionally nosebleed; humidification of the flow reduces the adverse effects.

Increased air flow, fans, and cold air have also been therapeutic to reduce dyspnea.[21–24] The mechanism is not well understood; however, these simple interventions may be useful when oxygen is not indicated.

Opioids

Oral or parenteral opioids, most commonly morphine or fentanyl, are the mainstay of pharmacological management of terminal dyspnea, and effectiveness has been demonstrated in numerous clinical trials.[25] Doses for treating dyspnea are patient-specific, generally lower than those needed to relieve pain, and as with opioid use in managing pain no ceiling should be placed on dosage. Close bedside evaluation to assess the efficacy of the medication is essential.

Benzodiazepines

Fear and anxiety may be components of the respiratory distress experienced by the dying patient. The addition of a benzodiazepine to the opioid regimen has been successful in patients with advanced COPD.[26] As with opioids, these agents should be titrated to effect.

BACK TO OUR CASE

Marjorie was compliant with her COPD regimen at home; Salmeterol and ipratropium metered dose inhalers were continued every six hours. She received oxygen at 4l nasal cannula. No potentially reversible sequelae such as pleural effusion, infection, or pneumothorax were identified on chest X-ray.

An opioid regimen of morphine 10 mg by mouth every four hours with 10 mg every hour as needed for breakthrough dyspnea was initiated. Marjorie reported satisfaction with this regimen and her NRS decreased from 10 to 4. Plans for return home with a hospice referral were made. At discharge Marjorie's opioid regimen had been converted to morphine sustained-release 15 mg every eight hours with morphine immediate-release at 10 mg every hour as needed. She continued to use her inhalers and nasal oxygen at 3 l/minute.

! TAKE AWAY POINTS

- COPD is a progressive, irreversible leading cause of death; treatment is supportive and palliative.
- Frequent hospitalizations for acute exacerbation and dyspnea typify late stage disease.
- Mechanical ventilation is a reliable treatment for respiratory failure but the burdens often outweigh the benefits; patients with COPD may forgo this treatment.
- A continued COPD regimen with the addition of opioids may relieve refractory dyspnea in terminal stage disease.

REFERENCES

[1] Barnes PJ. Chronic obstructive pulmonary disease. *New England Journal of Medicine*. 2000; 343:269–280.
[2] Centers for Disease Control. *National Center for Health Statistics*. Hyattsville, MD. 2007.
[3] Rutgers SR, Postma DS, ten Hacken NHT, et al. Ongoing airway inflammation in patients with COPD who do not currently smoke. *Thorax*. 2000; 55:12–18.
[4] Fox E, Landrum-McNiff K, Zhong Z, Dawson NV, Wu AW, Lynn J. Evaluation of prognostic criteria for determining hospice eligibility in patients with advanced lung, heart, or liver disease. *JAMA*. 1999; 282:1638–1645.
[5] Moosavi SH, Golestanian E, Binks AP, Lansing RW, Brown R, Banzett RB. Hypoxic and hypercapnic drives to breathe generate equivalent levels of air hunger in humans. *Journal of Applied Physiology*. 2003; 94:141–154.
[6] Dean JB, Mulkey DK, Garcia AJ, Putnam RW, Henderson RA. Neuronal sensitivity to hyperoxia, hypercapnia, and inert gases at hyperbaric pressures. *Journal of Applied Physiology*. 2003; 95:883–909.
[7] Hung WW, Wisnivesky JP, Siu AL, Ross JS. Cognitive decline among patients with chronic obstructive pulmonary disease. *Am J Respir Crit Care Med*. July 15 2009; 180(2):134–137.
[8] Campbell ML, Templin T, Walch J. Patients who are near death are frequently unable to self-report dyspnea. *J Palliat Med*. Oct. 2009; 12(10):881–884.
[9] Campbell ML. Fear and pulmonary stress behaviors to an asphyxial threat across cognitive states. *Res Nurs Health*. Dec. 2007; 30(6):572–583.

[10] Campbell ML. Psychometric testing of a respiratory distress observation scale. *J Palliat Med*. Jan.-Feb. 2008; 11(1):44–50.

[11] Campbell ML. Respiratory distress: a model of responses and behaviors to an asphyxial threat for patients who are unable to self-report. *Heart Lung*. Jan.-Feb. 2008; 37(1):54–60.

[12] Campbell ML, Templin T, Walch J. A respiratory distress observation scale for patients unable to self-report dyspnea. *J Palliat Med*. Mar. 2010; 13(3): 285–290.

[13] GOLD Expert Panel. Global Initiative for Chronic Obstructive Lung Disease. 2005; www.goldcopd.org.

[14] Tarpy SP, Celli BR. Long-term oxygen therapy. *New England Journal of Medicine*. 1995; 333:710–714.

[15] Apostolakos MJ. COPD exacerbation. In: Kruse JA, Fink MP, Carlson RW, eds. *Saunders Manual of Critical Care*. Philadelphia: Saunders. 2003; 46–47.

[16] Barach AL. Chronic obstructive lung disease: postural relief of dyspnea. *Archives of Physical Medicine and Rehabilitation*. 1974; 55:494–504.

[17] Sharp JT, Drutz WS, Moisan T, Foster J, Machnach W. Postural relief of dyspnea in severe chronic obstructive lung disease. *American Review of Respiratory Disease*. 1980; 122:201–211.

[18] Guyatt GH, McKim DA, Austin P, et al. Appropriateness of domiciliary oxygen delivery. *Chest*. Nov. 2000; 118(5):1303–1308.

[19] Cranston JM, Crockett A, Currow D. Oxygen therapy for dyspnoea in adults. *Cochrane Database Syst Rev*. 2008; (3):CD004769.

[20] Abernethy AP, McDonald CF, Frith PA, et al. Effect of palliative oxygen versus room air in relief of breathlessness in patients with refractory dyspnoea: a double-blind, randomised controlled trial. *Lancet*. Sep. 4 2010; 376(9743):784–793.

[21] Burgess KR, Whitelaw WA. Reducing ventilatory response to carbon dioxide by breathing cold air. *American Review of Respiratory Disease*. 1984; 129:687–690.

[22] Burgess KR, Whitelaw WA. Effects of nasal cold receptors on pattern of breathing. *Journal of Applied Physiology*. 1988; 64:371–376.

[23] Liss HP, Grant BJB. The effect of nasal flow on breathlessness in patients with chronic obstructive pulmonary disease. *American Review of Respiratory Disease*. 1988; 137:1285–1288.

[24] Schwartzstein RM, Lahive K, Pope A, Weinberger SE, Weiss JW. Cold facial stimulation reduces breathlessness induced in normal subjects. *American Review of Respiratory Disease*. 1987; 136:58–61.

[25] Jennings AL, Davies AN, Higgins JP, Gibbs JS, Broadley KE. A systematic review of the use of opioids in the management of dyspnoea. *Thorax*. Nov. 2002; 57(11):939–944.

[26] Light RW, Stansbury DW, Webster JS. Effect of 30 mg of morphine alone or with promethazine or prochlorperazine on the exercise capacity of patients with COPD. *Chest*. 1996; 109:975–981.

Case 2.5 Dyspnea and Heart Failure

Garrett K. Chan

HISTORY

Jane was a 74-year-old woman with systolic dysfunction and heart failure, status post mitral valve repair (MVR) complicated by methicillin resistant *s. aureus* (MRSA) endocarditis, coronary artery disease (CAD) with three vessel coronary artery bypass graft (CABG) in 2002, diabetes mellitus Type 2 with sequela of neuropathy and retinopathy, and pulmonary hypertension. She was admitted from the clinic for shortness of breath. The patient reported that she did well until 2006 when she was admitted for fluid volume overload/pulmonary edema.

In May 2008, she was admitted for a non-ST segment elevation myocardial infarction (NSTEMI) with flash pulmonary edema. The patient underwent a cardiac catheterization, which demonstrated that the left anterior descending artery had an 80% proximal and 100% mid vessel occlusion. Jane was admitted three times from June to August 2008 with congestive heart failure (CHF) exacerbations. During each hospitalization, she would receive diuretics and be sent home. In May 2009, the patient decided to have surgical repair and underwent a mitral valve replacement. She had a 63-day hospital course due to complications of pulmonary edema, vancomycin-resistant enterococcus urinary tract infection, and acute renal injury. From June to November 2010, the patient was admitted three times for NSTEMI and pulmonary edema. Jane was admitted in December 2010 for volume overload and was subsequently found to have MRSA bacteremia and endocarditis. She became anuric in the setting of this infection

Case Studies in Palliative and End-of-Life Care, First Edition. Edited by Margaret L. Campbell.
© 2012 John Wiley & Sons, Inc. Published 2012 by John Wiley & Sons, Inc.

and was started on hemodialysis. Her daughter, Ella, reported that she stopped making urine in January 2011. She was treated with a four-and-a-half-week course of vancomycin and rifampin, but could not complete the full six-week course because of thrombocytopenia.

In the last hospitalization, the patient was doing well until she developed shortness of breath. She had a syncopal episode at home and was found down by her daughter. She quickly recovered consciousness and the paramedics brought her to the hospital. Her daughter reported that she was treated for pneumonia (vancomycin and levaquin). She was admitted for dyspnea. On admission, her weight was 67.35 kg and a brain natriuretic peptide of 21,060. In the intensive care unit (ICU), the patient had severe shortness of breath with persistent hypotension with systolic blood pressures in the 70s to 80s. She was placed on dopamine to increase her blood pressure and to attempt continuous veno-veno hemofiltration with dialysis (CVVHD) because she was hyponatremic and hyperkalemic, and her creatinine was 4.0 (previously 2.4). On day four in the hospital, the patient experienced day/night reversal (i.e., ICU psychosis) but could report that her dyspnea was a seven on a 0-10 numeric rating scale. Palliative care was consulted for symptom management and to clarify the goals of care of the patient.

PHYSICAL EXAMINATION

Temperature: 36.7°C (98.1°F), pulse: 75, blood pressure: 103/68 mm Hg, respiratory rate: 20
General: Pleasantly confused woman who can follow very simple commands
Eyes: Extraocular movements intact, no icterus
Neck: Jugular vein distention elevated at 12 cm, neck supple
Chest: Coarse lung sounds in bilateral bases, regular rate and rhythm, S1, S2, SpO$_2$: 97%
Abdomen: Soft, non-tender, non-distended, positive abdominojugular test, no hepatosplenomegaly
Extremities: 2+ pitting edema in bilateral lower extremities, chronic venostasis changes, no rash

DIAGNOSTICS

Transthoracic echocardiogram (March 2011):

- Normal left ventricular size with moderately reduced systolic function; segmental wall motion abnormalities are noted, estimated ejection fraction: 30%

- Severe tricuspid regurgitation with estimated right ventricular systolic pressure: 35 mm Hg; status post mitral valve repair with a mean gradient of 7 mm Hg (78 beats per minute)
- Compared to the prior transthoracic echocardiogram images on January 3, 2011, mitral valve mean gradient has decreased from 10 mm Hg, but heart rate is lower

Chest X-ray: Stable right internal jugular dialysis catheter, sternal wires, mediastinal clips and valve prosthesis. Overall, little change with stable prominent cardiac silhouette and signs of mild-to-moderate fluid overload.

?   CLINICAL QUESTION

What interventions will reduce dyspnea associated with advanced heart failure?

✓   DISCUSSION

Natural history of Heart Failure

Heart failure (HF) is a complex phenomenon that can be classified in many ways. Often, heart failure is a result of structural (e.g., valvular disease) or functional (i.e., atrial fibrillation with rapid ventricular response) abnormalities that impair the ventricle to fill or eject blood.[1] Heart failure is a clinical diagnosis made on the symptoms (e.g., fatigue or dyspnea) in the setting of physical exam findings (e.g., edema or rales), and there is no single diagnostic test for HF.[1] There are many palliative care interventions that should be included with disease management strategies to relieve the physical, psychosocial, and spiritual distress of patients with heart failure.[2]

It is common to first distinguish whether the left or right side of the heart is failing. Right-sided heart failure occurs when the right ventricle cannot pump effectively. The most common reasons for right-sided heart failure include left-sided HF or pulmonary artery hypertension due to either pulmonary disease or from a pulmonary embolus.

Left-sided HF occurs when the left ventricle cannot fill or empty properly. This leads to a back-up of blood that increases pressures in the left ventricle and atrium and causes congestion in the pulmonary vascular system. Left-sided HF is further classified into two categories: systolic dysfunction and diastolic dysfunction.

Systolic dysfunction is determined by measuring the ejection fraction. Ejection fraction (EF) is the percentage of the left ventricular

TABLE 2.5.1. New York Heart Association Functional Classification.

Class 1	No limitation of physical activity. Ordinary physical activity does not cause undue fatigue or dyspnea.
Class 2	Slight limitation of physical activity. Comfortable at rest, but ordinary physical activity results in fatigue or dyspnea.
Class 3	Marked limitation of physical activity without symptoms. Symptoms are present even at rest. If any physical activity is undertaken, symptoms are increased.
Class 4	Unable to carry on any physical activity without symptoms. Symptoms are present even at rest. If any physical activity is undertaken, symptoms are increased.

Created from information found in Criteria Committee of the New York Heart Association. *Nomenclature and criteria for diagnosis of diseases of the heart and great vessels,* 9th edition. Boston: Little, Brown, 1994.

end-diastolic volume (LVEDV) that is ejected out of the ventricle in one cycle. The volume of blood ejected is known as the stroke volume. For example, if the LVEDV is 100 mL and the stroke volume is 70 mL, the EF is 70%. Normal ejection fractions can range from 50% to 70%. Systolic dysfunction is defined as an EF of less than 40% due to a decrease in myocardial contractility. When the ventricle does not contract efficiently, the ventricle cannot eject a sufficient amount of blood and the end result is a decreased cardiac output.

Diastolic dysfunction is a complex physiological phenomenon that is not well understood. In diastole, the ventricular myocardium is supposed to relax to allow for filling. The filling of the ventricle occurs with passive filling as well as atrial contraction (i.e., atrial kick) that forces blood into the ventricle. If the ventricular myocardium is stiff or non-compliant, the relaxation of the myocardium is slow or incomplete.[3] There are many etiologies that contribute to diastolic dysfunction such as a short diastolic phase in tachycardia, atrial fibrillation with the loss of the atrial kick, or ventricular hypertrophy due to uncontrolled hypertension.

There are two classification systems that help categorize the severity of HF. The New York Heart Association (NYHA) Functional Classification[4] provides a framework to assess the severity of HF based on the functional ability of the patient (Table 2.5.1). The American College of Cardiology (ACC)/American Heart Association (AHA) Guidelines for Stages of Heart Failure[1] provides another method to classify the severity of the HF (Table 2.5.2). The ACC/AHA guidelines are meant to supplement and not replace the NYHA Functional Classification. ACC/AHA stages A and B describe those patients who are at risk of developing HF. Patients in stages C or D should have the NYHA Functional Classification applied to determine severity of symptoms.

TABLE 2.5.2. ACC/AHA Guidelines for Stages of Heart Failure.

A	Patients at high risk for heart failure because of the presence of conditions that are strongly associated with the development of heart failure. Such patients have no identified structural or functional abnormalities of the pericardium, myocardium, or cardiac valves and have never shown signs or symptoms of heart failure.
B	Patients who have structural heart disease that is strongly associated with the development of heart failure but who have never shown signs or symptoms of heart failure.
C	Patients who have current or prior symptoms of heart failure associated with underlying structural heart disease.
D	Patients with advanced structural heart disease and marked symptoms of heart failure at rest despite maximal medical therapy and who require specialized interventions.

Hunt SA, Abraham WT, Chin MH, et al. Focused update incorporated into the ACC/AHA 2005 Guidelines for the Diagnosis and Management of Heart Failure in Adults. A Report of the American College of Cardiology Foundation/American Heart Association Task Force on Practice Guidelines Developed in Collaboration With the International Society for Heart and Lung Transplantation. *J Am Coll Cardiol.* Apr. 14, 2009; 53(15):e1–e90. Reprinted with permission from Elsevier Ltd.

There are four mortality risk-stratification models available for HF: Seattle Heart Failure Model; Acute Decompensated Heart Failure National Registry Regression Model; American Heart Association Get With the Guidelines—Heart Failure Score; and the Association of Health Aging and Body Composition Heart Failure Score. The Seattle Heart Failure Model[5] has been shown to be the most accurate in estimating the mean, one-year, two-year, and five-year survival of patients with HF.[6]

Etiologies of Dyspnea in Heart Failure

Dyspnea is one of the defining symptoms in the clinical diagnosis of HF. Fluid overload, hypoxemia, fatigue, and ejection abnormalities can contribute to the sensation of dyspnea in HF.[7]

Assessment

Patient Report

Dyspnea can be triggered by pathology intrinsic or extrinsic to heart failure. For example, an intrinsic factor of HF that can exacerbate dyspnea is pulmonary edema. An extrinsic factor could be pneumonia that causes an exacerbation of dyspnea. Both intrinsic and extrinsic factors should be assessed to determine and ameliorate the underlying etiology of the dyspnea. Clinicians should assess the effects of body positioning and amount of exertion and the level of dyspnea. To assess the level of dyspnea while supine, clinicians should ask about orthopnea and paroxysmal nocturnal dyspnea (PND). Orthopnea is measured by the number of pillows the patient must use to breathe comfortably at rest. PND is measured by the average number of times per night or per week a patient has to sit up suddenly to catch his breath. Other questions to ask when assessing PND are "How much time passes before you can breathe normally?" and "Do you need to do anything besides sit up to relieve the shortness of breath?"[3]

To assess the level of dyspnea with exertion, clinicians should consider the following questions: "How many blocks and flights of stairs can you walk without stopping to rest or catch your breath?", "Do you stop because you cannot go farther or because you want to avoid getting short of breath?", "How many times must you rest while doing activities of daily living such as toileting or minor housework?"[3]

Other self-report assessment tools to determine the symptom severity of heart failure patients include the Memorial Symptom Assessment Scale (MSAS)[8] and the Edmonton Symptom Assessment Scale—Heart Failure (ESAS-HF).[9]

Common Tools

The physical exam is an important method to assess the contributing factors that lead to dyspnea in HF. Common signs of ACC/AHA Class D HF include cachexia, fatigued posture, jugular venous distension, an S_3 heart sound, rales/coarse lung sounds, abdominojugular reflux, and lower extremity edema.[3] Other diagnostic studies that help identify the underlying etiology of the dyspnea include the electrocardiogram (ECG), echocardiography, radionuclide ventriculography, chest radiography, and hemodynamic monitoring.

The ECG is used to assess the rate and rhythm that could lead to an exacerbation of HF. Structural changes can be detected such as atrial enlargement or ventricular hypertrophy. Dysrhythmias such as atrial fibrillation with a rapid ventricular rate or other tachydysrhythmias can reduce the time of systole or diastole and decrease the cardiac output and cause congestion of the pulmonary or systemic vascular systems.

Echocardiography can assess the structure and function of the heart and large vessels using ultrasound. Doppler technology can be used to assess the volume and direction of the blood flow through the heart and great vessels. Transesophageal echocardiography (TEE) is superior to transthoracic echocardiography (TTE) because the left ventricle sits more posteriorly in the chest and is close to the esophagus. Transesophageal echocardiography requires procedural sedation and is, therefore, more difficult to obtain.

Radionuclide ventriculography or multigated acquisition (MUGA) scans are used to accurately determine the EF using a radioactive isotope and are considered the "gold standard" for determining the EF because they do not rely on subjective interpretation like other diagnostic modalities.[3] In addition, a MUGA scan can describe wall motion abnormalities, dilation, and wall thickness. However, MUGA cannot determine valve function or blood flow direction (i.e., regurgitation). Chest radiography is used as a simple screening tool that allows clinicians to rule in or out infection, masses, pulmonary edema, pleural effusions, or other gross abnormalities.

Hemodynamic monitoring is an invasive method of monitoring HF in critical care units. There are three types of patients that benefit from hemodynamic monitoring via a pulmonary artery catheter (PAC).[3] The first type of patient that can benefit from invasive monitoring is the patient that has been empirically started on inotropes and IV diuretics but has not responded appropriately either through diuresis or in symptoms. The second type of patient that can benefit from a PAC is the patient with both chronic obstructive pulmonary disease (COPD) and HF. The PAC can help differentiate the underlying etiology of the decompensation. The third type of patient is the patient who continues to have ascites or peripheral edema and continues to have renal function results suggestive of worsening pre-renal azotemia. The PAC can help clinicians understand the fluid balance and status of the patient. Despite having hemodynamic monitoring values, evidence suggests that there has been no improvement in hospital mortality in patients with acute heart failure.[10]

To assess and measure the severity of breathlessness and the impact of the symptom on patients, Johnson and collagues[11] recommend combining a uni-dimensional measure such as the numeric rating scale (NRS) or visual analog scale (VAS) with a multi-dimensional measure such as the Chronic Heart Failure Questionnaire—dyspnea subscale.[12]

Treatment

Optimize HF Regimen

In 2009, the American College of Cardiology Foundation (ACCF)/ American Heart Association (AHA) revised their 2005 guidelines for the diagnosis and management of heart failure.[10] Identification and treatment of both structural and functional cardiac abnormalities are the cornerstones of medical and interventional treatment of HF. Health behavior modification such as tobacco cessation, exercise, lipid control, and nutrition are central to the management of HF. Additional medical therapies such as angiotensin-converting enzyme inhibitors (ACEI)/ angiotensin II receptor blockers (ARB), diuretics, and beta-blockers are core drug categories for management of advanced stages of HF. Bi-ventricular pacemakers or implantable defibrillators can be considered in selected patients to maximize heart functioning. In extraordinary cases, heart transplant, chronic inotropes, experimental surgery or devices, or permanent mechanical support such as the ventricular assist device (VAD) can be considered.

In hospitalized patients, IV loop diuretics should be titrated to relief of symptoms while monitoring renal function because loop diuretics can worsen renal function.[10] If patients suffer from anemia of chronic disease, blood transfusions should be considered to palliate dyspnea with furosemide IV between units to prevent fluid overload. Co-morbidities of anxiety or depression can exacerbate dyspnea and should be recognized and treated.[7] See Cases 2.15 and 2.16 for discussions of depression and anxiety.

Oxygen

The use of oxygen for patients with hypoxemia or who experience sleep apnea is well established[13] and recommended,[10] but in patients without hypoxemia, the literature is sparse. One Cochrane review by Cranston and colleagues[14] analyzed data from eight studies that included a total of 144 subjects with cancer (n=97), heart failure (n=35), and kyphoscoliosis (n=12) to determine whether oxygen therapy administered in non-acute care settings provided relief of dyspnea in the end stages of disease over breathing room air oxygen or placebo as controls. All subjects had breathlessness at rest or on minimal exertion and could be normoxemic or hypoxemic. The review could not demonstrate a benefit to the subjects with end-stage heart failure, although the sample size was very small.

Park and colleagues investigated the effects of oxygen on forearm hemodynamics in patients who were normoxemic with mild-to-moderate heart failure (NYHA class I and II) with left ventricular systolic dysfunction in 13 men.[15] Park et al. found that there was an increase in heart rate, systemic vascular resistance, and blood flow in the forearm hemodynamics when given a fraction of inspired oxygen (FiO_2) of 0.40. There was, however, no change in the natriuretic peptides (A-type [ANP], or pro-B type [BNP]) before or after oxygen administration. ANP and BNP are laboratory indicators of heart strain. The authors conclude that in the absence of hypoxemia, supplemental oxygen may have a negative impact on the workload of the failing heart. The results of this study should be taken with caution given the small sample size, single gender, and relatively healthier population than the population of advanced disease patients seen in palliative care.

Opioids

In palliative care, opioids serve as a cornerstone of medical management for dyspnea regardless of etiology,[16] yet commonly patients with HF do not receive opioids.[17] However, there are some instances when opioids may not be appropriate in acute HF. When a patient experiences pulmonary edema in the setting of an acute decompensation of HF (ADHF), Peacock and colleagues found an association between IV morphine and a greater frequency of mechanical ventilation, prolonged hospitalization (mean = 5.6 days vs. mean 4.2 days), more ICU admissions (38.7% vs. 14.4%), and a higher mortality (adjusted odds ratio 4.83, 95% CI 4.51, 5.18, p < 0.001).[18] However, caution must be used when interpreting these results. This was a retrospective observational study of a registry database. The only data available were whether a patient received IV morphine and the outcomes listed above. No data such as dose, indication for IV morphine, timing of morphine, or precise temporal relationships to adverse events were available for analysis in this study. Caution should be used when considering administering IV morphine to relieve dyspnea and balancing disease-modifying treatments in ADHF.

In the outpatient setting, investigators have demonstrated an equivocal effect of opioids on dyspnea without any reported negative sequelae.[19,20] Therefore, a time-limited trial to investigate whether opioids will have the intended effect of dyspnea reduction without exacerbating the underlying pathology is warranted in the outpatient setting. However, in a study by Oxberry and colleagues, patients who have chronic, stable CHF, oral short-acting opioids did not demonstrate a decrease of dyspnea against placebo.[20] The researchers used a crossover randomized design and enrolled 39 patients to three interventions of oral morphine 5 mg four times a day, oral oxycodone 2.5 mg four times a day, and placebo four times a day. Participants did not report a statistically significant decrease in breathlessness in any of the three interventions. The response to opioids was not associated with etiology, severity of CHF, or concurrent drug therapies. In addition, it was well tolerated without adverse effects. The study sample was small and the dose may not be enough to achieve relief from breathlessness.

BACK TO OUR CASE

The palliative care and intensive care teams discussed the prognosis of the patient and reviewed the current treatment for her dyspnea. The patient's fluid overload was managed by CVVHD and renal function was declining. The patient's hemoglobin was 9.5 mg/dL. Per the Seattle Heart Failure Model, the patient had an 86% chance of in-hospital mortality with an average life expectancy of six months. The palliative care team recommended a time-limited trial of morphine 2 mg IV every hour for two hours to see how that might affect her hemodynamic status as well as her dyspnea. Upon re-assessment, the patient reported a decrease in her breathlessness to a 5/10 using the NRS. The palliative care team then recommended transfusing one unit of packed red blood cells (PRBC) during the CVVHD and balancing the fluid of the PRBC with fluid to be taken off. The patient then reported a further decrease of dyspnea to 4/10, which was tolerable for her. She was subsequently discharged from the hospital with a home hospice referral.

| ! | TAKE AWAY POINTS |

- Heart failure is a complex and dynamic disease process that has many etiologies for alterations in cardiac structure and function that requires astute assessment to determine the underlying cause of dyspnea.
- Opioids may be beneficial but caution should be exercised so that they do not worsen the cardiac function, especially in acutely decompensating heart failure.
- Less is known about using opioids to treat HF associated dyspnea than is known about dyspnea associated with cancer or COPD.
- Oxygen may be helpful in patients with hypoxemia. In the setting of normoxemia, however, there may be a negative effect on hemodynamics.

| 📖 | REFERENCES |

[1] Hunt SA, Abraham WT, Chin MH, et al. Focused update incorporated into the ACC/AHA 2005 Guidelines for the Diagnosis and Management of Heart Failure in Adults. A Report of the American College of Cardiology Foundation/American Heart Association Task Force on Practice Guidelines Developed in Collaboration With the International Society for Heart and Lung Transplantation. *J Am Coll Cardiol*; Apr. 14, 2009; 53(15):e1–e90.

[2] Goodlin SJ. Palliative care in congestive heart failure. *J Am Coll Cardiol*; 2009; 54(5):386–396.

[3] Blum K. Heart failure. In: Morton PG, Fontaine DK, eds. *Critical Care Nursing. A Holistic Approach*, 9th edition. Philadelphia: Lippincott Williams & Wilkins; 2009; 437–466.

[4] The Criteria Committee of the New York Heart Association. *Nomenclature and criteria for diagnosis of diseases of the heart and great vessels*, 9th edition. Boston: Little, Brown; 1994.

[5] Levy WC, Mozaffarian D, Linker DT, et al. The Seattle Heart Failure Model: prediction of survival in heart failure. *Circulation*; Mar 21 2006; 113(11):1424–1433.

[6] Nakayama M, Osaki S, Shimokawa H. Validation of mortality risk stratification models for cardiovascular disease. *Am J Cardiol*; May 18, 2011.

[7] Dutka DP, Johnson MJ. Breathlessness in heart failure. In: Booth S, Dudgeon D, eds. *Dyspnoea in Advanced Disease. A Guide to Clinical Management*. Oxford, England: Oxford University Press; 2006; 39–54.

[8] Blinderman CD, Homel P, Billings JA, Portenoy RK, Tennstedt SL. Symptom distress and quality of life in patients with advanced congestive heart failure. *J Pain Symptom Manage*; June 2008; 35(6):594–603.

[9] Ospasich C, Gualco A, De Feo S. Physical and emotional symptom burden of patients with end-stage heart failure: What to measure, how and why. *Journal of Cardiovascular Medicine*; 2008; 9:1104–1108.

[10] Jessup M, Abraham WT, Casey DE, et al. 2009 focused update: ACCF/AHA Guidelines for the Diagnosis and Management of Heart Failure in Adults: a report of the American College of Cardiology Foundation/American Heart Association Task Force on Practice Guidelines. Developed in collaboration with the International Society for Heart and Lung Transplantation. *Circulation*; Apr 14 2009; 119(14):1977–2016.

[11] Johnson MJ, Oxberry SG, Cleland JG, Clark AL. Measurement of breathlessness in clinical trials in patients with chronic heart failure: the need for a standardized approach: a systematic review. *Eur J Heart Fail*; Feb 2010; 12(2):137–147.

[12] Guyatt GH, Nogradi S, Halcrow S, Singer J, Sullivan MJ, Fallen EL. Development and testing of a new measure of health status for clinical trials in heart failure. *J Gen Intern Med*; Mar-Apr 1989; 4(2):101–107.

[13] Davidson PM, Johnson MJ. Update on the role of palliative oxygen. *Curr Opin Support Palliat Care*; Jun 2011; 5(2):87–91.

[14] Cranston JM, Crockett A, Currow D. Oxygen therapy for dyspnoea in adults. *Cochrane Database Syst Rev*; 2008; (3):CD004769.

[15] Park JH, Balmain S, Berry C, Morton JJ, McMurray JJ. Potentially detrimental cardiovascular effects of oxygen in patients with chronic left ventricular systolic dysfunction. *Heart*; Apr 2010; 96(7):533–538.

[16] Lorenz KA, Lynn J, Dy SM, et al. Evidence for improving palliative care at the end of life: a systematic review. *Ann Intern Med*; Jan 15 2008; 148(2):147–159.

[17] Setoguchi S, Glynn RJ, Stedman M, Flavell CM, Levin R, Stevenson LW. Hospice, opiates, and acute care service use among the elderly before death from heart failure or cancer. *American Heart Journal*; Jul 2010; 160(1):139–144.

[18] Peacock WF, Hollander JE, Diercks DB, Lopatin M, Fonarow G, Emerman CL. Morphine and outcomes in acute decompensated heart failure: an ADHERE analysis. *Emerg Med J*; Apr 2008; 25(4):205–209.

[19] Johnson MJ, McDonagh TA, Harkness A, McKay SE, Dargie HJ. Morphine for the relief of breathlessness in patients with chronic heart failure—a pilot study. *Eur J Heart Fail*; Dec 2002; 4(6):753–756.

[20] Oxberry SG, Torgerson DJ, Bland JM, Clark AL, Cleland JG, Johnson MJ. Short-term opioids for breathlessness in stable chronic heart failure: a randomized controlled trial. *Eur J Heart Fail*; Jun 28 2011; volume 9, pages 1006–1012.

Case 2.6 Treating Dyspnea during Ventilator Withdrawal

Margaret L. Campbell

HISTORY

Estelle was an 83-year-old African-American woman who was admitted to the hospital via the emergency department (ED) with acute respiratory failure secondary to aspiration of gastric contents. Estelle resided in a nursing home and was in the terminal stage of Alzheimer's disease (AD). She was emergently intubated, placed on mechanical ventilation, and admitted to the medical intensive care unit (MICU).

Estelle's daughter was her health care surrogate and arrived at the hospital shortly after Estelle was admitted to the MICU. Discussions about treatment goals ensued and because of the advanced state of Estelle's AD a decision was made to cease intensive interventions, withdraw mechanical ventilation, and provide a focus on comfort. Regrettably, these goals had been previously established at the nursing home but no documentation was sent to the hospital with Estelle.

PHYSICAL EXAMINATION

Temperature: 38.2°C, blood pressure: 120/60, heart rate: 128, respiratory rate: 24

Central nervous system: Patient opens her eyes to verbal and tactile stimulation, withdraws from pain, does not follow commands

Case Studies in Palliative and End-of-Life Care, First Edition. Edited by Margaret L. Campbell.
© 2012 John Wiley & Sons, Inc. Published 2012 by John Wiley & Sons, Inc.

Head, eyes, ears, nose, throat: Right eye cataract, dry mucus membranes

Cardiac: S1 S2 and tachycardia, no S3 or S4, no murmurs

Lungs: Diminished sounds right lower lobe (RLL), coarse crackles throughout, copious thick secretions, oral endotracheal tube, SpO_2 94% on an FiO_2 of 0.50

Gastrointestinal: Scaphoid abdomen, normal bowel sounds, no tenderness

Genitourinary: Voiding, Foley catheter

Extremities: Cachectic, no pressure ulcers or deformities

DIAGNOSTICS

Chest X-ray: Bilateral infiltrates, consolidation RLL

CLINICAL QUESTION

What treatments may reduce dyspnea during ventilator withdrawal?

DISCUSSION

Ventilator Withdrawal

Withdrawal of life support precedes most intensive care unit (ICU) deaths. It is estimated that one in five (20%) of the 2.4 million people who die each year in the United States will do so in an ICU.[1] Most ICU deaths are preceded by decisions to withhold or withdraw life-sustaining therapies.[2,3] Yet little is known about optimal practices to prevent suffering in patients undergoing cessation of intensive care therapies or decreasing distress in surrogates who are involved in decisions about withdrawing therapy when poor prognosis can reliably predict death in ICU patients. Withdrawal of therapies, such as mechanical ventilation, often leads to patient suffering and distress and to high levels of psychological distress among family members if they are not performed correctly.

Invasive mechanical ventilation is provided through an artificial airway such as an endotracheal tube or a tracheostomy. Non-invasive mechanical ventilation entails a tight fitting mask over the nose or nose and mouth. Withdrawal of invasive mechanical ventilation is the focus of this case, consisting of reduction in mechanical ventilatory support until the patient is breathing spontaneously. This may be accomplished in one step by turning off the ventilator and removing the endotracheal tube, an approach commonly referred to as "terminal extubation." An alternative multi-step process, described as "terminal weaning," is completed using a step-wise incremental reduction of oxygen and ventilation over a period of several minutes to hours. It is concluded by turning off the ventilator; a subsequent decision to remove or maintain the endotracheal tube follows. Currently, there are no evidence-based guidelines for withdrawal of mechanical ventilation.

Care decisions are guided by clinician preferences rather than an evidence-based approach. Indeed, a survey of physician ventilator withdrawal practices indicated that surgeons and anesthesiologists preferred terminal weaning, compared to internists and pediatricians who preferred a single-step approach followed immediately by extubation.[2] It is interesting to note that physician rather than patient characteristics contributed to choice of method. There are no known investigations comparing one method to another. Ventilator withdrawal processes are not standardized. Small samples and largely retrospective chart reviews characterize the body of evidence about processes for ventilator withdrawal. Available evidence suggests there is (a) a lack of a common measure for detecting respiratory distress to guide the process, (b) high variability in initiation and escalation of opioids across studies of ventilator withdrawal, and (c) an inability to predict the method that best ensures patient comfort without hastening death.[4]

Characteristics of Patients Undergoing Ventilator Withdrawal

Cognitive impairment or unconsciousness typifies the period before death in the ICU. Thus, most patients are unable to reliably report any distress. Patients undergoing ventilator withdrawal are at risk for respiratory distress in response to respiratory failure. Patients who cannot self report symptom distress can be at risk for under treatment.[5] Conversely, mechanically ventilated patients may be vulnerable to over treatment of anticipated distress.

Patients undergoing ventilator withdrawal are heterogeneous. For example, patients choosing ventilator withdrawal for themselves are awake and aware and often completely dependent on the ventilator. However, a majority are critically ill and cognitively impaired or unconscious. Some patients have been intubated for only a short time and subsequent extubation of the endotracheal tube is not expected to produce airway complications. In other cases the patient has had an endotracheal tube for more than a few days or has other airway conditions, such as self-extubation laryngeal edema, that predict complications such as stridor or complete airway obstruction. Thus, the anticipated experience of the patient will vary greatly. A patient-centered algorithm that accounts for differences in patient characteristics, such as the one suggested in this case, is essential for improving the practice of withdrawal of mechanical ventilation. The ideal best practice process for conducting ventilator withdrawal across a heterogeneous population must account for the variance in patient experience and a patient-centered algorithm will provide the best guide.

Families are at risk for high levels of distress when mechanical ventilation is withdrawn because they are intimately involved in this process in a number of ways. Patients are usually unable to make the decision to withdraw ventilation and family members serve in a surrogate capacity. Patient death often occurs shortly after withdrawal and many families want to be with the patient at the time of death. Weigand reported that family members' experiences involved a variety of dimensions.[6] Lack of clear, timely, comprehensive communication from healthcare providers can contribute to the anxiety and distress reported by patients' families after a patient's death in the intensive care unit.[7] Uncertainty about the prognosis of the patient, concern about decisions that need to be made, what to expect during dying, and the extent of a patient's suffering pervade families' end-of-life experiences.[8] Family counseling, information, and support provided by the nurse are integral to the patient/family-centered algorithmic approach that we propose testing.

Interventions and Procedures

Assessment

The gold standard for measuring symptom distress is the patient's report. When the patient is severely cognitively impaired or unconscious self reporting becomes impossible. The Respiratory Distress Observation Scale (RDOS) is the only known tool for assessing respiratory distress when the adult patient cannot self report dyspnea. The RDOS has undergone rigorous clinical testing to establish scale reliability, inter-rater reliability, convergent validity, construct validity, and discriminant validity.[9-11] The RDOS is an eight-item ordinal tool to measure the presence and intensity of respiratory distress; each item is scored from zero to two points and the points are summed. Higher scores suggest higher intensity respiratory distress. The instrument is not valid for use in children or when the patient is undergoing neuro-muscular blockade or has amyotrophic lateral sclerosis.

Ventilator Withdrawal Algorithm

Complete the Following Pre-Withdrawal
- Cease neuromuscular blocking agents, if any; proceed with with-drawal after return of motor function.
- For hospitalized patients, notify Organ Procurement Organization (OPO) of plans to withdraw ventilation, postpone withdrawal until after OPO evaluation.
- Establish IV access if none previously.
- Prepare family.

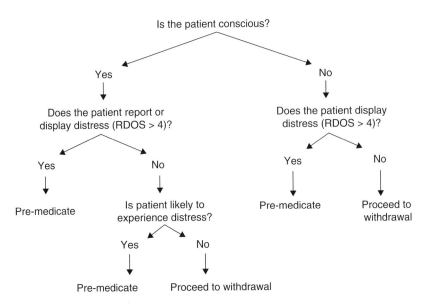

Figure 2.6.1. Pre-medication process.

- ○ Identify where family prefers to be during withdrawal, bedside or other.
- ○ Identify family preference for chaplain support.
- ○ Permit family private time with patient for last rituals, traditions if desired.
- ○ Secure chairs, water, tissues wherever family will be in the hospital.
- ○ Describe the process to family in lay terms.
- ○ Describe expected patient behaviors.
- ○ Describe permissible family behaviors.
- ○ Answer family questions.

Evaluate for Pre-Medication (Figure 2.6.1)
Pre-medication regimen: Administer morphine 5 mg intravenous bolus and lorazepam 1 mg intravenous bolus. Wait 15 minutes for peak effectiveness and proceed with ventilator withdrawal if RDOS less than or equal to 4. Re-administer morphine 5 mg if RDOS is greater than 4 and wait 15 minutes to re-assess for a therapeutic effect, that is RDOS less than 4.

Select a Withdrawal Method (Figure 2.6.2)
- T-piece
  Turn off ventilator, place room air T-piece, and assess RDOS.
- Rapid wean
  1. Decrease positive end-expiratory pressure to zero, wait two minutes if no distress (respiratory distress observation scale [RDOS] less than or equal to 4) proceed

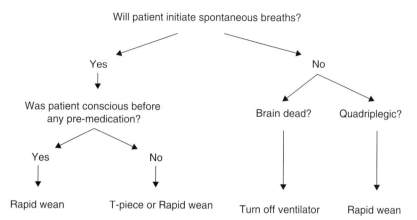

Figure 2.6.2. Withdrawal method.

2. Reduce FiO$_2$ by .20 every minute until .21, if no distress proceed
3. Change mode to synchronized intermittent mandatory ventilation/pressure support ventilation, wait two minutes, if no distress proceed
    a. Maintain tidal volume (Vt)
    b. Set frequency to 10 breaths/minute
    c. Set PSV to 5 cm
4. Reduce SIMV frequency by two breaths every two minutes until four breaths, if no distress proceed
5. Change mode to continuous positive airway pressure (CPAP) 0 cm, PSV 5 cm, wait two minutes, if no distress proceed
6. Turn off ventilator, place humidified room air T-piece

- Respond to distress
    1. Assess RDOS immediately after every ventilator change and after ventilator is turned off
    2. Cease wean progress whenever RDOS exceeds 4
    3. Bolus with morphine 5 mg, wait 15 minutes for peak effectiveness, if no distress proceed with rapid wean
    4. Re-bolus with morphine 5 mg and lorazepam 1 mg if distress persists and repeat every 15 minutes if needed until RDOS is less than or equal to 4.

- Continuous morphine infusion
    1. Begin infusion at conclusion of rapid wean, if pre-medication or medication administered during wean
    2. Initial dose = 50% of total bolus doses, e.g. bolus with 5 mg × 3 = 15 mg, begin infusion at 7.5 mg/hour
    3. Titrate infusion to maintain RDOS at or below 4 by administering morphine 5 mg bolus, increase infusion by 2.5 mg after each bolus

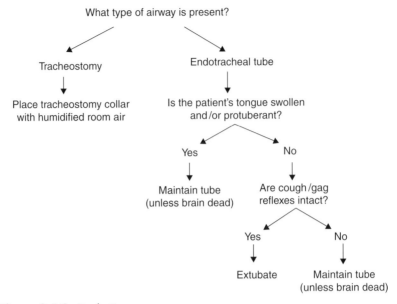

Figure 2.6.3. Extubation.

Make an Extubation Decision (Figure 2.6.3)
- Extubation
  1. Drape the distal end of the endotracheal tube.
  2. Cut tube ties and release air from the cuff.
  3. Suction until cough is elicited, if any.
  4. Withdraw the suction catheter and tube simultaneously while applying suction.
  5. Wrap catheter and tube in drape and discard out of sight of patient's family.
  6. Clean patient's mouth and face.
  7. Monitor patient for post-extubation stridor.
- Treat stridor
  Dilute racemic epinephrine 2.25% (22.5 mg/ml) 0.5 cc in 3 cc normal saline as an aerosol treatment, repeat once after first treatment if stridor persists

  Prewithdrawal process: Ceasing neuromuscular blocking agents, also known as paralytics, is a standard through expert consensus so that patient signs of distress are not masked.[12] Notification to the regional Organ Procurement Organization prior to ventilator withdrawal is a Center for Medicare and Medicaid Services requirement.[13] An intravenous access affords the rapid administration of medications that may be required to provide relief from distress. All other pre-withdrawal processes are directed at family preparation.[14]

Pre-medication: Pre-medication is recommended if respiratory distress can be anticipated.[12] The algorithm identifies medication decisions based on patient consciousness and ability to experience distress. Some patients undergoing ventilator withdrawal are comatose and not expected to be able to experience distress; thus, the algorithm provides guidance about which patients may benefit from pre-medication. Opioids and benzodiazepines are the most commonly used medications for this purpose, although reported doses in other investigations have been highly variable.[4] Opioids are the drug of choice for the treatment of dyspnea.[15] Benzodiazepines have utility in adjunct to opioids.[16] The doses in the algorithm are standard adult doses. Guidelines for titration to patient effect are included (see Figure 2.6.1.).

Withdrawal methods: Rapid weaning and turning the ventilator off without weaning (T-piece) are conventional withdrawal methods.[12] These methods have not been directly compared previously. Rapid weaning is suggested in cases in which the patient may experience distress because this process affords an opportunity to restore the patient to a previous ventilator setting while their her is relieved. The straight-to-T-piece method is reserved for unconscious patients who, in the clinical judgment of the practitioner, are unlikely to experience distress. The algorithmic guideline for treating distress takes into consideration the timing of the peak effect of morphine and/or lorazepam (see Figure 2.6.2.)

Extubation: Maintaining the endotracheal tube in the face of a swollen or protuberant tongue or absent cough/gag reflexes will minimize the occurrence of partial or complete airway obstruction which may be a source of patient and/or family distress. When a patient is withdrawn from the ventilator in the context of brain death there is no expectation of spontaneous breathing or coughing/gagging; hence, the endotracheal tube can be removed (see Figure 2.6.3).

BACK TO OUR CASE

Estelle was awake but severely cognitively impaired secondary to advanced state AD. Thus, she was unable to report about her respiratory comfort. The MICU staff relied on the RDOS to assess Estelle's respiratory comfort before, during, and after ventilator withdrawal.

After preparing Estelle's family the MICU nurse followed the algorithmic approach suggested previously. She gave Estelle morphine 5 mg as an intravenous bolus with lorazepam 1 mg. A rapid wean approach was used and Estelle maintained an RDOS below 4 throughout the process. She had only been intubated for one day and had no risk factors for post-extubation stridor; thus, she was extubated. A morphine infusion at 2 mg/hour was initiated to maintain respiratory comfort.

Estelle's family remained at her bedside and agreed with the nursing assessment that Estelle was in no respiratory distress. Respiratory rate gradually slowed and Estelle died peacefully four hours after the ventilator was turned off.

! TAKE AWAY POINTS

- Ventilator withdrawal is a commonly performed ICU procedure to afford a natural death.
- The process is not standardized and no studies to compare methods have been conducted.
- A patient-centered algorithmic approach is suggested.

REFERENCES

[1] Angus DC, Barnato AE, Linde-Zwirble WT, et al. Use of intensive care at the end of life in the United States: an epidemiologic study. *Critical Care Medicine*; 2004; 32:638–643.

[2] Faber-Langendoen K. The clinical management of dying patients receiving mechanical ventilation. A survey of physician practice. *Chest*; Sep 1994; 106(3):880–888.

[3] Prendergast TJ, Claessens MT, Luce J. A national survey of end-of-life care for critically ill patients. *American Journal of Respiratory Critical Care Medicine*; 1998; 158:1163–1167.

[4] Campbell ML. How to withdraw mechanical ventilation: A systematic review of the literature. *AACN Adv Crit Care*; October/December 2007; 18(4):397–403.

[5] Campbell ML, Templin T, Walch J. Patients who are near death are frequently unable to self-report dyspnea. *J Palliat Med*; Oct 2009; 12(10):881–884.

[6] Wiegand DL, Deatrick JA, Knafl K. Family management styles related to withdrawal of life-sustaining therapy from adults who are acutely ill or injured. *J Fam Nurs*; Feb 2008; 14(1):16–32.

[7] Nelson JE, Puntillo KA, Pronovost PJ, et al. In their own words: patients and families define high-quality palliative care in the intensive care unit. *Crit Care Med*; Mar. 2010; 38(3):808–818.

[8] Kirchhoff KT, Walker L, Hutton A, Spuhler V, Cole BV, Clemmer T. The vortex: families' experiences with death in the intensive care unit. *Am J Crit Care*; May 2002; 11(3):200–209.

[9] Campbell ML. Fear and pulmonary stress behaviors to an asphyxial threat across cognitive states. *Res Nurs Health*; Dec 2007; 30(6):572–583.

[10] Campbell ML. Psychometric testing of a respiratory distress observation scale. *J Palliat Med*; Jan-Feb 2008; 11(1):44–50.

[11] Campbell ML, Templin T, Walch J. A respiratory distress observation scale for patients unable to self-report dyspnea. *J Palliat Med*; Mar 2010; 13(3):285–290.

[12] Truog RD, Campbell ML, Curtis JR, et al. Recommendations for end-of-life care in the intensive care unit: a consensus statement by the American College [corrected] of Critical Care Medicine. *Crit Care Med*; Mar 2008; 36(3):953–963.

[13] Center for Medicare and Medicaid Services. Hospital conditions of participation about organ/tissue donation. http://www.cms.gov/manuals/downloads/som107ap_a_hospitals.pdf. Accessed November 6th, 2008.

[14] Wiegand DL. Withdrawal of life-sustaining therapy after sudden, unexpected life-threatening illness or injury: interactions between patients' families, healthcare providers, and the healthcare system. *Am J Crit Care*; Mar 2006; 15(2):178–187.

[15] Jennings AL, Davies AN, Higgins JP, Gibbs JS, Broadley KE. A systematic review of the use of opioids in the management of dyspnoea. *Thorax*; Nov 2002; 57(11):939–944.

[16] Navigante AH, Cerchietti LC, Castro MA, Lutteral MA, Cabalar ME. Midazolam as adjunct therapy to morphine in the alleviation of severe dyspnea perception in patients with advanced cancer. *J Pain Symptom Manage*; Jan 2006; 31(1):38–47.

Case 2.7 Cough Associated with COPD and Lung Cancer

Peg Nelson

HISTORY

Melanie was an 83-year-old woman admitted to the hospital with profound, intractable nonproductive cough, which interrupted her sleep and caused her chest to hurt. Her medical history included end-stage chronic obstructive pulmonary disease (COPD) complicated by a recent diagnosis of stage 4 non-small cell lung cancer. Melanie was living independently in a senior apartment and had been dependent on oxygen for two years. She was divorced and supported by her daughter, Peggy, who lived near and assisted when needed. She had been a three-pack/day smoker for 45 years, but quit smoking 20 years ago. One month prior to hospital admission, when she had learned about the lung cancer, which already had spread to her liver and bones, Melanie made the decision to not pursue palliative chemotherapy and was offered hospice care. Her Eastern Cooperative Oncology Group (ECOG) performance status was 2/5 at the time of diagnosis, but prior to hospital admission, her fatigue and cough had caused her status to increase to 3/5 and she was only able to do limited self care and was in bed or a chair more than half the day.

Melanie had tried over-the-counter cough syrup for her cough with no improvement. She reported that the cough was 10 out of 10 on a numeric rating system. She reported pain in the right side of her chest, which worsened with coughing. Her pain score was five out of 10 using the numeric pain scale (NPS). She had lost 15 pounds in the last month, reported fatigue, poor appetite, occasional vomiting with cough, and difficulty sleeping. She had no desire for heroics but she was open to

Case Studies in Palliative and End-of-Life Care, First Edition. Edited by Margaret L. Campbell.
© 2012 John Wiley & Sons, Inc. Published 2012 by John Wiley & Sons, Inc.

any treatment that might improve her cough and comfort. Melanie also reported chronic shortness of breath but said that she was used to that and had lived an OK life until this cough would not go away. The palliative care team was consulted to assist with control of her symptoms and the transition to hospice care. She used the following home medications: Spiriva® and albuterol inhalers and guaifenesin cough syrup.

PHYSICAL EXAMINATION

Temperature: 38.2°C, blood pressure: 144/54, heart rate: 108, respiratory rate: 24

General: Emaciated white woman, appearing older than stated age, finding it difficult to talk without coughing

Central nervous system: Alert, oriented, no focal deficits

Head, eyes, ears, nose, throat: Mouth dry, with no defects or abnormalities

Cardiac: Color pale, heart sounds: S1, S2 and mild tachycardia, no S3 or S4, no murmurs

Lungs: Large anterior-posterior diameter, coarse lung sounds, diminished right mid field to base, with percussed dullness, with expiratory wheeze on left, mild tachypnea, no accessory muscle use at rest, SpO$_2$ 90% on two liters humidified nasal cannula, cough is nonproductive

Gastrointestinal: Abdomen is flat, normal bowel sounds, no tenderness, palpable hard nontender liver edge

Genitourinary: Voiding without difficulty

Extremities: Cachectic, no pressure ulcers or deformities, skin warm and dry

DIAGNOSTICS

Chest X-ray: Increased pulmonary nodules with development of right-sided moderately large pleural effusion and suggestion of post obstructive atelectasis

Complete blood count (CBC): White blood cell: 18,000, hemoglobin: 12, hematocrit: 36, platelets: 200,000

Neutrophils: 80%

B–type natriuretic peptide (BNP): 120

CLINICAL QUESTION

What treatments may reduce cough associated with advanced COPD and or lung cancer?

✓ **DISCUSSION**

Physiology of Cough

Cough is a protective, normal mechanism that removes foreign material and/or mucus from the airway branches including the larynx, trachea, and bronchi. It is both a voluntary and an involuntary response mediated by the central and peripheral nervous system. The vagus nerve in the airways and the glossopharyngeal nerve in the pharynx elicit the cough reflex. These nerves are excited by various mechanisms including external stimuli such as smoke and internally by chemicals within mucus. The brainstem is critical to the cough reflex because it sends information to innervate the cough within the respiratory system.

Etiology

Many medical conditions are accompanied by cough. Possibilities to consider when looking for causes of persistent cough include:

- Heart failure
- Respiratory infections
- Tuberculosis
- Lung cancer
- Cystic fibrosis
- Bronchospasm
- COPD (asthma, chronic bronchitis)
- Pleural effusion
- Gastroesophageal reflux disease (GERD)
- Excessive respiratory secretions
- Common cold, postnasal drip
- Aspiration
- Allergies
- Medications including angiotensin-converting-enzyme (ACE) inhibitors, nonsteroidal anti-inflammatories (NSAIDS), beta-blockers, certain chemotherapy agents, and inhalant medications
- Smoking

Prevalence

At the end of life, 30% to 50% of all patients report cough; in lung cancer it is a common symptom in 47% to 86% of patients.[1] Patients with COPD report daily coughing on most days.[2] For patients with advanced COPD, cough is a chronic daily symptom that worsens during exacerbations of the disease and when it is complicated by other co-morbidities.

Assessment

The patient assessment and evaluation of cough begins with a very thorough medical history and understanding of the many conditions that are accompanied by and/or cause cough. Chest X-ray, CBC with differential, and BNP are initially helpful for diagnosis of underlying causes, as well as a review of medications that may be contributing to the cough and a comprehensive physical assessment. Depending on the goals of care and the likelihood of aggressive treatment, further evaluation with CT scan, magnetic resonance imaging (MRI), and arterial blood gases (ABG) may be helpful.

The impact of the coughing on the patient's quality of life is another important consideration during assessment. Cough can seriously disrupt the patient's comfort and cause further complications. Loss of appetite, nausea, vomiting, weight loss, headache, pathologic rib fracture, dyspnea, dizziness, sweating, insomnia, chest and throat pain, exhaustion, inability to communicate with loved ones, self-consciousness, social isolation, and family stress all have been noted with patients who suffer from chronic cough.[3]

Treatment

Underlying and reversible causes should be treated if possible. However, many patients, especially those who are at the end of life, will benefit from the symptomatic treatment of a cough while waiting for other therapy aimed at curing or reducing underlying etiology. Some causes of cough, specifically those from terminal disease, may not be manageable, and symptomatic treatment becomes the focus of care.

Symptomatic treatment of cough can be classified in two ways, the centrally acting antitussive medications and the peripherally acting agents. In a symptomatic patient with end-stage disease, opioids are the first-line treatment.[4] Opioids are the only clearly effective, central acting antitussive drugs that quiet cough by suppressing the brainstem cough center, likely through mu and kappa opioid receptor agonism.[4] All opioids have the potential ability to suppress cough and there is no strong evidence that one opioid is superior to another. Side effects of opioids include sedation, constipation, nausea, and confusion. The strongest evidence for centrally acting medications for cough are for codeine, hydrocodone, and dextromethorphan.

Codeine has been shown to be effective for acute and chronic cough in several placebo-controlled trials.[4] The usual adult dose is 10 to 20 mg every four to six hours, although the dose can be titrated to effect if side effects do not limit administration. Codeine elixir is available alone and in combination with the expectorant guaifenesin; codeine also is available as a tablet. Codeine induces constipation at a higher degree than other opioids, so a bowel regimen is essential.

Hydrocodone has been shown to be as effective as codeine in head-to-head studies but with fewer gastrointestinal side effects, such as constipation.[4] A typical starting dose is 5 to 10 mg every four hours. Hydrocodone is only available as a combination product in the United States. The tablet hydrocodone most commonly used is in combination with acetaminophen. The hydrocodone elixir is prepared as a short-acting medication with the anticholinergic drug homatropine or as an extended-release elixir with the antihistamine chlorpheniramine. The titration of hydrocodone is limited by the medications that are in combination.

Dextromethorphan is the most commonly used centrally acting antitussive. It has been confirmed to be as effective as codeine for cough in many studies.[4] It is typically dosed at 10 to 20 mg every four to six hours. Dextromethorphan is available alone or as an elixir with guaifenesin. It is important to note that dextromethorphan potentially interacts with many drugs. By inhibiting the cytochrome P450 system it can affect the metabolism of many drugs and it also may cause a serotonin syndrome if used with serotonergic drugs such as SSRI type antidepressants.

The American College of Chest Physicians (ACCP) evidence-based clinical guidelines for patients with chronic bronchitis (COPD) recommends central cough suppressants such as codeine and dextromethorphan for short-term symptomatic relief of coughing.[5] For patients with cough and lung cancer, the ACCP guidelines recommend the use of hydrocodone.[6]

It is unclear whether adding a second opioid for cough is beneficial when the patient is already taking an opioid for analgesia. One uncontrolled, open label study showed hydrocodone used as a second opioid to be helpful in this setting.[4]

Peripherally acting medications used for cough are found in many over-the-counter and prescribed medications. There is little evidence of their benefit. The most common are discussed below.

Benzonatate suppresses cough by anesthetizing the stretch receptors in the respiratory tract. It is dosed at 100 to 200 mg three times/day. There are no controlled studies to confirm its effectiveness, but multiple uncontrolled studies support its use. Side effects are rare but include sedation, bronchospasm, headache, and nausea. Expert opinion within palliative care recommends adding it to an opioid for distressing cough.[7]

Antihistamines and anticholinergics are often part of combination antitussive elixirs with or without an opioid or dextromethorphan. Especially within the elderly, these drugs when delivered by mouth can cause sedation and confusion. Evidence for these oral agents in the acute setting is limited and thus these agents are not recommended.

However, for patients near death with copious secretions that cause cough or respiratory discomfort, anticholinergics are helpful.[7] In addition, inhaled anticholinergic bronchodilators such as ipratropium bromide have been found to effectively decrease cough and are recommended in patients with acute or chronic bronchitis.[8]

Expectorants (also called mucolytics) are designed to thin bronchial secretions and ease expectoration. The most common, guaifenesin, is usually dosed 200 to 400 mg every four hours. The ACCP guidelines state that there is no evidence that the currently available expectorants are effective for patients with stable or acute exacerbation of chronic bronchitis and therefore should not be used.[9] For chronic coughs that are severe and productive, mucolytics are often empirically used, although there is little evidence to support this common practice. In addition, expectorants may increase fluid in the respiratory tract; therefore, they are not recommended in the dying patient whose cough reflex is reduced.[11]

Sweet syrups such as honey or sugar syrup have been studied in a few controlled trials and have been shown to reduce cough in patients who have upper respiratory infections.[12] Nebulized local anesthetics, such as 5 ml of 2% lidocaine every six hours or 5 ml of 0.25% bupivacaine every eight hours have been reported anecdotally to assist with cough. Bronchospasm is a potential side effect.[13] There have been no clinical trials.

Strategies under investigation

Strategies under investigation with animals for cough include capsaicin antagonists, new opioids that specifically target the cough reflex without other opioid actions, endogenous cannabinoids, 5-HT receptor agonists, and tachykinin receptor antagonists.[10]

BACK TO OUR CASE

Melanie's cough had many underlying causes. Initial actions included stopping her guaifenesin, which was ineffective, and tapping her pleural effusion for 1,500 ml of straw-colored fluid. She was also given steroids and ipratropium bromide for her COPD exacerbation. Because she had a fever, elevated WBC, and possible pneumonia, she was started on antibiotics. Although all these interventions helped with the cough, she still reported a cough score of five out of 10 and she was given codeine 15 mg every four hours PRN and started on benzonatate 100 mg every eight hours, which reduced her cough score to two out of 10, which she found acceptable. Melanie was able to be discharged home.

! TAKE AWAY POINTS

- Cough in the patient with end-stage COPD and/or lung cancer can be very distressing and cause a severe decline in quality of life.
- Initial treatment of cough should focus on correcting or improving the underlying cause of the cough if possible.
- Opioids, particularly codeine, are the most effective treatment in the terminally ill patient for suppressing a distressing cough.

REFERENCES

[1] Molassiotis A, Zheng Y, Denton-Cardew L, Swindell R, Brunton L, Wilson B. Symptoms experienced by cancer patients during the first year from diagnosis: patient and informal caregiver ratings and agreement. *Palliative Supportive Care*; 2010; 8:313–324.

[2] Braman SS. Chronic cough due to chronic bronchitis: ACCP evidenced-based clinical guidelines. *Chest*; 2006; 129(1):104s.

[3] Irwin RS. Complications of cough: ACCP evidenced-based clinical guidelines. *Chest*; 2006; 129(1):59s–62s.

[4] Homsi J, Walsh D, Nelson KA. Important drugs for cough in advanced cancer. *Supportive Care Cancer*; 2001; 9:565–574.

[5] Braman SS. Chronic cough due to chronic bronchitis: ACCP evidenced-based clinical guidelines. *Chest*; 2006; 129(1):113s.

[6] Kvale PA. Chronic cough due to lung tumors: ACCP Evidence-based clinical practice guidelines. *Chest*; 2006; 129(1):152s.

[7] Estfan B, LeGrand S. Management of cough in advanced cancer. *Journal of Supportive Oncology*; 2004; 2:523–527.

[8] Braman SS. Chronic cough due to chronic bronchitis: ACCP evidenced-based clinical guidelines. *Chest*; 2006; 129(1):110s.

[9] Braman SS. Chronic cough due to chronic bronchitis: ACCP evidenced-based clinical guidelines. *Chest*; 2006; 129(1):112s–113s.

[10] Boulet LP. Future directions in the clinical management of cough: ACCP evidenced-based clinical guidelines. *Chest*; 2006; 129(1):284s–285s.

[11] Schroeder K, Fahey T. Systematic review of randomized controlled trials of over the counter cough medicines for acute cough in adults. *BMJ*; 2002; 324:1–6.

[12] Paul IM, Beiler J, McMonagle A, Shaffer ML, Duda L, Berlin CM. Effect of honey, dextromethorphan, and no treatment on nocturnal cough and sleep quality for coughing children and their parents. *Archives Pediatric Adolescent Medicine*; 2007; 161:1140–1146.

[13] Lingerfelt BM, et al. Nebulized lidocaine for intractable cough near the end of life. *Journal of Supportive Oncology*; 2007; 7:301–302.

Case 2.8 Hiccups and Advanced Illness

Marian Grant

HISTORY

Charles was a tall, 71-year-old white man status post a large embolic stroke in the left side of his brain. This stroke occurred after emergency bypass surgery for an acute myocardial infarction. Charles had trouble waking up post operatively and, once he did, his neurological deficits were noted. He recovered well from the bypass surgery and was in stoke rehabilitation for several weeks. However, long term, he had paralysis on his right side, urinary incontinence, and moderate expressive aphasia and dysphagia. He was living at home with a percutaneous gastrostomy tube (PEG), tube feedings, an indwelling urinary catheter, a wheelchair, and hired nursing care during the day. Charles was able to transfer with great assistance and could answer simple questions by nodding or shaking his head. He seemed generally comfortable, although he was frustrated by not being able to speak or move independently. His wife of 32 years, Dorothea, was his primary caregiver, although she was much smaller than he and had osteoarthritis and scoliosis.

Several months after his first stroke, Charles' level of consciousness, aphasia, and dysphagia acutely worsened. He also developed severe hiccups that did not subside after several hours. Because of the hiccups, he was physically uncomfortable and unable to sleep. His tube feedings needed to be held due to vomiting from the hiccups. He looked miserable, was getting weaker, and neither he nor Dorothea were

Case Studies in Palliative and End-of-Life Care, First Edition. Edited by Margaret L. Campbell.
© 2012 John Wiley & Sons, Inc. Published 2012 by John Wiley & Sons, Inc.

getting any rest. She remembered Charles hiccupping in the hospital after his surgery and felt the hiccups were adding to the suffering he had already had to endure from his stroke.

PHYSICAL EXAMINATION

Temperature: 36.7°C, blood pressure: 142/76, heart rate: 72, respiratory rate: 14

Central nervous system: Awake, alert, follows commands, unable to speak clearly, unable to move right arm or leg

Head, eyes, ears, nose, throat: No significant deficits or abnormalities, reduced hearing bilaterally

Cardiac: Regular rate and rhythm, no abnormal heart sounds, trace edema bilateral ankles

Lungs: Clear to auscultation bilaterally, hiccups 10 times/minute, strong, and regular in rhythm

Gastrointestinal: Bowel sounds in all four quadrants, abdomen soft and non-tender

Genitourinary: Voiding via indwelling catheter

Extremities: Right hand contracted and in wrist splint, bilateral lower leg splints

DIAGNOSTICS

Blood tests for hiccups are typically not helpful.[1]

CLINICAL QUESTION

What treatment reduces persistent hiccups?

DISCUSSION

Natural Etiology of Hiccups

Hiccups are a type of respiratory complication. They are the result of sudden inspiration due to involuntary spasms and contractions of the diaphragm and intercostal muscles. The sound is caused by the sudden closure of the glottis. These rhythmic spasms involve the vagus and phrenic nerves, the sympathetic nervous system, and central nervous system areas within the brain, where there is a central hiccup area.[2] Hiccups are typically brief, lasting a minute or so, and self-limited.[2] However, when they last longer they can be problematic. Although there are no formal definitions for persistent hiccups, they are generally considered to be those that last for more than 48 hours.[2] Intractable hiccups are considered those that last for longer than one month.[2]

Persistent hiccups can obviously have significant quality of life implications for patients such as Charles and their caregivers. At a basic physiological level, they interfere with breathing, eating, speaking, and sleeping.[2] This can impair a person's daily life and communication, and affect caregivers who live with the patient. The spasms can cause nausea, vomiting, and dyspnea, all of which are distressing symptoms warranting palliative care. Hiccups that last for several days or longer can cause fatigue, pain, depression, weight loss, dehydration, and malnutrition.[2] Intractable hiccups can also cause serious medical complications. These can include wound dehiscence, if they happen post operatively, and potentially life-threatening complications such as arrhythmia, heart block, hypoxia, hypotension, aspiration, and pneumomediastinum.[2]

Persistent hiccups are rare, seen in only 2% of patients with advanced cancer.[3] Cymet reported patients with persistent hiccups were predominantly male, 50 years or older, and had underlying medical conditions thought to be the cause of the hiccups.[4] Hiccups have more than 100 causes, although the cause is sometimes not identifiable.[5] Major causes within the palliative care or end-of-life population include malignancies, particularly those of the gastrointestinal system, lymphadenopathy, metabolic and electrolyte imbalances, gastric distension, brain metastases, stroke, pneumonia, pericarditis, pleuritis, and myocardial infarction.[1] Any physical process that involves potential irritation to the diaphragm, such as esophageal or gastric lesions, mediastinal or thoracic lesions,[6] hepatic issues, and inflammation or infection can cause hiccups.[1] Gastric distension is considered the most likely cause in those with advanced cancer.[5] Neurogenic causes include multiple sclerosis, basilar artery aneurysm, and cerebellar hemagioblastoma.[1]

In addition to organic causes, hiccups can be caused by various medications. Many of the drugs commonly used in palliative care, such as benzodiazepines, anticholinergics, steroids, opioids, and antibiotics can contribute to hiccups.[1,2] Steroids are thought to lower the threshold for synaptic transmission in the brain and so may activate the hiccup center.[1] Ironically, some of these same medications are also used to treat hiccups.

Assessment

Patient Report

Transient hiccups may be just annoying to the patient, but any hiccups that last longer than 24 hours or recur frequently enough to impede eating, speaking, sleeping, etc. need to be thoroughly assessed to determine what other complications the patient may perceive with them.

Common Tools

Hiccups typically can be observed by their sound and rhythm. In patients who cannot self report, their accompanying distress can sometimes be assessed from respiratory difficulties or other physical distress.

Treatment

Treating persistent hiccups can be challenging. A 2010 Cochrane review found little evidence to support any particular treatment for them.[7] This is likely because the different causes of hiccups may each require a specific treatment. However, if a cause is identified, treating that cause is the first place to start. If the issue is gastric distension, for instance, then treatment should be focused on resolving that. If it is drug related, then the patient's medication list should be scrutinized and any new medications systematically held to see if the hiccups resolve.

Home Remedies

Behaviors such as drinking out of the opposite side of a glass or holding one's breath should be tried, but may not be effective or even possible for patients with physical or cognitive disabilities.[2] Other nonpharmacologic options include stimulating the pharynx or palate with a cotton swab, applying pressure on the tongue or raising the uvula with a tongue depressor, applying pressure over the eyebrow area, gargling ice water, swallowing crushed ice, eating granulated sugar, or biting a lemon.[2, 8] A Valsalva maneuver or breathing into a paper bag may stop the diaphragmatic spasms by increasing carbon dioxide partial pressure (pCO_2) and cerebral vasoconstriction, which may be the reason holding one's breath can also be effective.[2] Finally, vagal stimulation via digital rectal or carotid massage are an option.[2]

Pharmacological Treatment

There is only one medication approved by the Food and Drug Administration (FDA) for intractable hiccups, the antipsychotic phenothiazine chlorpromazine.[2] The recommended oral dose is 25 to 50 mg three to four times a day for up to three days or until the hiccups stop.[9] If chlorpromazine is not effective after three days, it should be discontinued and another medication tried.[9] Chlorpromazine can be contraindicated in patients receiving palliative care due to the potential side effects of hypotension, urinary retention, and delirium.[2] Common side effects are anticholinergic effects and sedation.[10]

 If chlorpromazine is not effective, other medications can be tried. Gabapentin may also provide a benefit, although evidence is limited to case reports.[6] An oral regimen of initially 400mg three times daily for three days and then 400mg daily for another three days was effective with 15 patients whose hiccups were related to brainstem lesions.[6] Baclofen has also been used as a treatment for intractable hiccups.[1] It is best started at low doses, such as 5mg orally three times a day, especially in those with renal insufficiency.[1] Baclofen is sometimes used as part of a multidrug hiccups regimen including omeprazole and cisapride.[1]

Table 2.8.1 lists a wide range of medications that have been used to treat hiccups. No suggested doses are provided because there is

TABLE 2.8.1. Possible medications to treat hiccups.

Medication
Amantidine
Amitriptyline
Baclofen
Carvedilol
Chlorpromazine
Cisapride (in combination with omeprazole and baclofen or gabapentin)
Clonazapam
Dexamthethasone
Domperidone
Dopamine agonists
Gabapentin
Haloperidol
Ketamine
Lidocaine infusions
Methylphenidate
Metoclorpramide
Midazolam
Nebulized saline or lidocaine
Nefopam
Nifedipine/nimodipine
Olanzapine
Phenytoin
Quinidine
Ranitidine
Sertaline
Simethicone
Valproic acid

Smith HS, Busracamwongs A. Management of hiccups in the palliative care population. *Am J Hosp Palliat Care*; Mar-Apr 2003; 20(2):149–154.

Marinella MA. Diagnosis and management of hiccups in the patient with advanced cancer. *J Support Oncol*; Jul-Aug 2009; 7(4):122–127, 130.

Perdue C, Lloyd Ash E. Managing persistent hiccups in advanced cancer 1: physiology. *Nurs Times*; Aug 26-Sep 1 2008; 104(34):24–25.

Wilcox SK, Garry A, Johnson MJ. Novel use of amantadine: To treat hiccups. *Journal of Pain and Symptom Management*; 2009; 38(3):460–465.

little evidence to support specific regimens. Many are also used for other symptoms in palliative care.

Nonpharmacological/Interventional Treatment

If hiccups are resistant to medication, interventional treatments might be an option if the patient's goals, prognosis, and health status make them appropriate. A nasal catheter inserted to the level of approximately the second cervical vertebra and rapidly moved may stop hiccups by blocking the hiccup impulse.[8] Phrenic nerve blocks via a local anesthetic were effective on a long-term basis in three of five patients with advanced cancers.[2] Phrenic and vagal nerve stimulation via a transcutaneous nerve stimulator have also been reported as successful.[11] Breathing pacemakers are another possible option.[1]

Complementary and Alternative Medicine Strategies

Acupuncture may be effective for persistent hiccups but may be difficult to implement given the patient's condition or the availability of experienced providers.[2] Acupressure using pressure points on the hand or ear may also be effective.[12]

Strategies Under Investigation

More data is needed to determine what the most effective approaches are, yet research in this area is challenging given the low prevalence of hiccups and the wide range of potential causes. Ideally, randomized controlled trials of some of the most commonly used medications should be conducted.

If hiccups are resistant to all treatment and causing great distress, palliative sedation may be considered once all other options have been exhausted. This involves careful discussions with the patients and families about goals and consequences of palliative sedation.

BACK TO OUR CASE

In Charles' case, the hiccups were likely due to brain injury or swelling from a subsequent stroke because he had not recently started any new medications. Several of the home remedies listed above were tried to no effect. The nurse practitioner then prescribed chlorpromazine and educated Dorothea about possible side effects. This medication made Charles very sedated and he was unable to be taken out of bed while he was on it. In his case, the hiccups went away after a day on the chlorpromazine and so he stopped taking the medication. The hiccups recurred periodically as he had what appeared to be subsequent small strokes. Sometimes they resolved on their own and in other cases he needed to take the chlorpromazine again for them.

| ! | **TAKE AWAY POINTS** |

- Hiccups are a rare but troublesome respiratory symptom seen in a wide range of illnesses and patients.
- Persistent or intractable hiccups can produce significant quality of life and medical complications.
- Treatment includes home remedies, medications, and interventional therapies.
- Chlorpromazine is the only FDA-approved medication for intractable hiccups, but it has potentially problematic side effects for patients. Other medications have only anecdotal or case study evidence to support their use.
- Treating persistent hiccups can be challenging, but is worth trying to improve the lives of both patients and families suffering from them.

| 📖 | **REFERENCES** |

[1] Smith HS, Busracamwongs A. Management of hiccups in the palliative care population. *Am J Hosp Palliat Care*; Mar-Apr 2003; 20(2):149–154.
[2] Marinella MA. Diagnosis and management of hiccups in the patient with advanced cancer. *J Support Oncol*; Jul-Aug 2009; 7(4):122–127, 130.
[3] Potter J, Hami F, Bryan T, Quigley C. Symptoms in 400 patients referred to palliative care services: prevalence and patterns. *Palliat Med*; Jun 2003; 17(4):310–314.
[4] Cymet T. Retrospective analysis of hiccups in patients at a community hospital from 1995–2000. *Journal of National Medical Association*; 2002; 94(6):480–483.
[5] Perdue C, Lloyd Ash E. Managing persistent hiccups in advanced cancer 1: physiology. *Nurs Times*; Aug 26-Sep 1 2008; 104(34):24–25.
[6] Tegeler ML, Baumrucker SJ. Gabapentin for intractable hiccups in palliative care. *Am J Hosp Palliat Care*; Feb-Mar 2008; 25(1):52–54.
[7] Moretto EN, Wee B, Wiffen PJ, Murchison AG. Interventions for treating persistent and intractable hiccups in adults. *Cochrane*; 2010(10).
[8] Perdue C, Lloyd E. Managing persistent hiccups in advanced cancer 2: treatment. *Nurs Times*; Sep 2–8 2008; 104(35):20–21.
[9] Chlorpromazine. NCBI; 2011. http://www.ncbi.nlm.nih.gov/pubmedhealth/PMH0000553/. Accessed April 10, 2011.
[10] Thorazine. Medscape Reference. http://reference.medscape.com/drug/chlorpromazine-342970#4. Accessed April 10, 2011.
[11] Schulz-Stubner S, Kehl F. Treatment of persistent hiccups with transcutaneous phrenic and vagal nerve stimulation. *Intensive Care Med*; Mar. 2, 2011; 2150–2153.
[12] Xianguo H, Xueci X. How to use external treatment measures to cure hiccup. *Journal of Traditional Chinese Medicine*; 2005; 25(2):160.

Case 2.9 Treating Nausea Associated with Advanced Cancer

Judy C. Wheeler

HISTORY

Gwen was a 58-year-old Caucasian woman first seen in the emergency department (ED) for complaints of headache, left side and back pain, and nausea and vomiting. Her history included liver cancer, hepatitis C, alcoholism, and diabetes mellitus type 2. Her last reported alcohol ingestion was two months prior to hospital admission. She lived at home with a relative who served as her caregiver, refused chemotherapy, and wished to be kept comfortable, although she was not enrolled in a hospice program. Medications included furosemide, hydrocodone/acetaminophen, hydromorphone, glipizide, omeprazole, and morphine sulfate long acting, all taken orally. Her general appearance was that of a chronically ill, emaciated female. She was alert and oriented times four, and aware of her diagnosis and prognosis.

PHYSICAL EXAMINATION

Blood pressure: 95/60, respirations: 18, pulse: 108, temperature: 35.6°C
Head, eyes, ears, nose, throat: No defects or abnormalities, dry mucosa
Cardiac: S1, S2 no adventitious sounds, tachycardia, symmetrical moderate pitting edema
Respiratory: Clear to auscultation, oxygen saturation at 94% on room air

Case Studies in Palliative and End-of-Life Care, First Edition. Edited by Margaret L. Campbell.
© 2012 John Wiley & Sons, Inc. Published 2012 by John Wiley & Sons, Inc.

Gastrointestinal: Shifting dullness, mild diffuse tenderness, firm, no palpable mass
Genitourinary: Voiding, normal appearing genitalia
Skin: Dry, without jaundice, intact

DIAGNOSTICS

Lipase: 315 units/liter
Ammonia: 61 micromole/L
Platelets: 114 K/CUMM
Hemoglobin: 8.8 gn/dL
Hematocrit: 25.5%

CLINICAL QUESTION

What are the best practice treatments for nausea and vomiting?

DISCUSSION

Nausea and vomiting serve a purpose in the healthy body. Emesis protects the viscera from noxious stimuli, including poisoning, vestibular stimulation, and overdistension. When nausea and vomiting occur in the healthy individual, they are generally time-limited, and resolve when the precipitating stimuli are controlled. In the patient with liver dysfunction, nausea and vomiting can be prolonged, resulting in ongoing discomfort and greatly diminished quality of life. When compared with other, more visible or more life-threatening symptoms, nausea and vomiting can appear to be a relatively minor nuisances, but can result in serious deficits in quality at the end of life.

Symptoms in the patient with liver cancer may occur as nausea or vomiting, or a combination of both. Serious complications, including malnutrition, dehydration, and electrolyte imbalance, may result fairly quickly, especially with protracted vomiting. Treatment of nausea and vomiting is multifocal and centers on the treatment of reversible causes, the use of nonpharmacologic interventions, the use of pharmacological interventions, and the treatment of relevant complications. Generally, in the patient in whom immediate comfort is the primary goal of treatment, management focuses on pharmacological interventions.[1]

Assessment

Nausea is a subjective symptom that is best measured by self-report, whereas vomiting can be observed and measured. Vomiting is the expulsion of gastric contents through the mouth caused by forceful and sustained contraction of the abdominal muscles and diaphragm, whereas nausea is the unpleasant feeling of needing to vomit, felt in the throat and epigastrum.[2] Nausea is often accompanied by uncomfortable symptoms such as sweating, salivation, tachycardia, and indigestion. There is no consensus in the field of palliative medicine as to how to measure emesis, and a review of available tools used to measure nausea, vomiting, and retching concluded that none of them was ideal, especially given the variability of cognitive impairment, fatigue, and debility in the palliative care patient population.[3] Nausea and vomiting occur to some extent in 21% to 68% of advanced cancer patients, either as a result of the disease process or treatment, or as a combination of both.[4] Patient reported outcomes are probably the most reliable source of data for symptom assessment.

A thorough history and physical examination is an essential component in determining potential causes of nausea and vomiting.[5] The history should focus on the characteristics of nausea, vomiting, and anorexia. Medication history is important as well, because many medications, including chemotherapies, can contribute to nausea and vomiting, as can palliative measures such as radiation therapy and surgery. Disease processes that are seemingly unrelated to gastric distress, such as diabetes, can be linked to autonomic dysfunction and delayed gastric emptying, and should be evaluated.

Bowel obstruction may contribute to nausea and vomiting in the patient with liver cancer. As hepatomegaly results in increased intra-abdominal pressure, partial or complete bowel obstruction may occur. Symptoms vary depending on the location of the obstruction, but most always include abdominal pain, nausea, vomiting, and anorexia. Mannix describes a "gastric stasis syndrome" whose symptoms include early satiety, epigastric fullness, heartburn, and hiccups.[6] A short period of nausea is generally followed by large-volume vomiting. Such large volume vomiting can quickly result in dehydration, further compounding the discomfort of vomiting. However, patients should be encouraged to continue to eat pleasure foods as tolerated as vomiting may occur with or without intake.

Treatment

Pharmacologic

The first step in management of intractable nausea and vomiting is to identify the neuro-mechanisms which are triggering the symptoms.[5] Four pathways provide input to the vomiting center in the brainstem:

(1) the chemoreceptor trigger zone (CTZ), which stimulates vomiting in reaction to toxins in the bloodstream and cerebrospinal fluid; (2) the cortex, which produces nausea in reaction to sensory input, anxiety, meningeal irritation and increased intracranial pressure; 3) peripheral pathways carrying stimuli from receptors in the gastrointestinal tract, serosa, and viscera and transmitted through the vagus and splanchnic nerves, sympathetic ganglia, and glossopharyngeal nerves, and (4) the vestibular system of the labyrinth, which is stimulated by motion to trigger the vomiting center via the vestibulocochlear nerve.

It is possible for just one, many, or all of these triggers to contribute to nausea. In the patient with liver cancer, nausea and vomiting is likely caused by a combination of all of these factors. Opiods commonly used to treat the pain associated with liver cancer can contribute to stimulation of the chemoreceptor zone, gastroparesis, and sensitization of the labyrinth. For the liver cancer patient receiving chemotherapy, stimulation of the chemoreceptor zone and irritation to the gastrointestinal (GI) mucosa with resultant stimulation of the vagus and splanchnic nerves can result in nausea and vomiting. Bowel obstructions stimulate peripheral pathways as a result of the irritation of bowel by accumulated fecal matter and fluids. The accompanying toxins and impaired motility of the gastrointestinal tract trigger the peripheral pathways by stretching and irritating the walls of the gastrointestinal tract.

Mannix identifies eight key steps in the palliation of nausea and vomiting. These include:[6]

1. Identify the likely cause.
2. Identify the pathways by which the vomiting reflex is triggered.
3. Identify the neurotransmitter receptor involved in that pathway.
4. Prescribe the most potent antagonist for each receptor identified.
5. Choose the route of administration that ensures the drug will reach its receptors.
6. Give the drug regularly and titrate the dose carefully.
7. If symptoms persist, review the steps.
8. Consider whether the trigger for nausea and vomiting can be removed.

General guidelines for the prescription of medications to treat nausea and vomiting follow (Table 2.9.1).[7]

All of these medications may be administered orally, and as the disease process progresses and oral medications become poorly tolerated, most can be given via the subcutaneous route.[8]

Studies specific to the palliation of nausea and vomiting at end of life are sparse, and studies specific to their management in the patient with liver cancer could not be found. A Cochrane review of literature related to the use of droperidol for treatment of nausea and vomiting in palliative care patients found only one study meeting the inclusion criteria

TABLE 2.9.1. General guidelines for the prescription of medications to treat nausea and vomiting.

Drug	Mechanism of action	Potential for use in nausea and vomiting
Haloperidol	Dopamine agonist	Chemically or metabolically induced nausea and vomiting (second line choice) Regurgitation Unclear or multiple causation
Metoclopramide	Dopamine agonist	Chemically or metabolically induced nausea and vomiting (front line choice) Gastric stasis, outlet obstruction Bowel obstruction (incomplete)
Levomepromazine	Antihistamine	Gastric stasis, outlet obstruction Regurgitation Bowel obstruction Unclear or multiple causation Cranial disease
Cyclizine	Antihistamine	Regurgitation Bowel obstruction Cranial disease Unclear or multiple causation
Lorazepam	GABA facilitator	Cortical nausea

for patients in the terminal stage of illness.[9] In this study of patients with lung cancer, droperidol along with dexamethasone and metoclopramide reduced the duration of nausea, although the reduction in duration of vomiting was found to be statistically insignificant. A review of the impact of haloperidol on nausea and vomiting in palliative care found no randomized controlled studies.[10]

Some benefit can be extracted from the examination of the few studies related to the palliative treatment of nausea and vomiting in general and then applying those findings to the specific etiologies of nausea and vomiting in the patient with liver cancer. A study regarding the efficacy of haloperidol on patients with cancer who experienced nausea and vomiting was terminated due to slow enrollment and high attrition, but descriptive analysis of the data concluded that haloperidol had some efficacy in these circumstances.[11] A "cocktail" of antiemetics, consisting of 10 mg of metoclopramide, 25 mg of diphenhydramine, and 4 mg of dexamethasone given via intravenous piggyback every six hours was found to result in symptom relief for 57 of the 63 palliative care patients to whom it was given,[12] but seemed to be less effective for patients with partial bowel obstruction, esophageal cancer, gastric cancer, pancreatic cancer, and liver cancer. Olanzapine has been demonstrated to provide relief of nausea and vomiting as well as contribute to increased appetite and weight gain in the palliative care population.[13]

Results from a prospective study on an in-patient population of 129 hospice patients with cancer indicated that etiology-based guidelines were helpful in the management of nausea and vomiting in patients with advanced cancer.[1] Severity of nausea and/or vomiting was assessed by a verbal rating scale, and reported by the patients. Management guidelines were based on the assessed etiology of nausea and/or vomiting, and medications were dosed according to prescribed protocols. Sixty-nine percent of the patients with vomiting reported their symptoms controlled within 48 hours of implementation of treatment, and 89% were controlled within one week. Patients with persistent vomiting actually fared better than patients with persistent nausea, in whom only 44% of nauseated patients reported control of symptoms at 48 hours and 56% at one week. A major hypothesis for lack of control in a significant number of patients with either nausea or vomiting was that physicians, who were asked to rate their degree of confidence regarding the causes for nausea and/or vomiting, were uncertain of the cause of the problem in 25% of the patients, resulting in uncertainty regarding the best plan for management. In addition, about 25% of the participants were thought to have more than one cause of nausea and vomiting, further complicating the management plan. The study concluded that etiology-based guidelines aided in, but did not assure, control of nausea and vomiting in cancer patients.

Nonpharmacological Treatment

Nonpharmacologic interventions are always appropriate in the initial phases of managing nausea and vomiting. Smaller, more frequent feeding of bland, non-odorous foods may help, although there are few studies to actually confirm the effectiveness of dietary modification on nausea and vomiting. High-carbohydrate foods are often more easily tolerated, and sour flavors may be preferred to sweet ones.[14] Studies related to physiological techniques, such as acupressure and acupuncture, and psychological interventions including hypnotherapy and guided imagery have also been conducted with some success.

Complementary and Alternative Treatments

Chinese medical herbs were the subject of a Cochrane review of chemotherapy side effects in colorectal cancer patients. For some patients, the Chinese herb Huangqi resulted in reduction in nausea and vomiting and improved white cell counts as compared with patients treated with chemotherapy alone. The authors recommended further trials to provide support for clinical use.[15] A review to determine whether the stimulation of acupuncture points could reduce chemotherapy-induced nausea and vomiting found mixed results. Acupressure reduced first day nausea but had no effects afterward, and had no impact on vomiting. Electroacupuncture also reduced first day vomiting but manual acupuncture did not.[16]

Two protocols published in the Cochrane Library may have future use in the palliation of nausea and vomiting. The first will investigate the impact of aromatherapy on nausea and vomiting in post operative patients[17] and perhaps may have some bearing on the use of aroma therapy in palliative care. Another Cochrane protocol regarding interventions for the treatment of nausea and vomiting during initiation of chronic opioid therapy[18] may also have some generalizability to the palliative care population. Investigators plan to review the impact of any investigated therapeutic intervention, pharmacologic or nonpharmacologic, of any duration, on concomitant opioid use.

In rare instances, palliative sedation has been used to manage intractable nausea and vomiting at the end of life.[19] A goal for palliative sedation is reaching a state of conscious sedation where symptoms are controlled but the patient is still able to communicate. The authors conducted a survey of reported use of propofol in palliative care patients to determine indications, doses, and effects with use. Intravenous propofol was used for 13 patients for intractable nausea and vomiting, with three of the patients reporting moderate relief and nine reporting good relief; one patient was withdrawn from the study due to lack of sedation from propofol. The authors concluded that propofol showed superior use in cancer patients with nausea and vomiting for whom traditional methods of control had failed, with the effects on nausea being better than for vomiting. They recommend that use of propofol be reserved for patients for whom nausea is the major distressor.

BACK TO OUR CASE

Gwen was initially treated with haloperidol 3 mg every 24 hours for relief of potential chemical causes for nausea and vomiting related to hepatotoxins. Haloperidol is also known to be effective for opioid-induced nausea as well as for relief of nausea caused by obstruction. Metoclopramide 10 mg every six hours was added to aid in reduction of any stimulation of vomiting caused by bowel obstruction and impaired gastric emptying. When those two medications relieved but did not eliminate her nausea, and her fear of eating or drinking resulted in uncomfortable dehydration, a surgical placement of an indwelling paracentesis "pigtail" catheter aided in decompression contributing to bowel obstruction. Because Gwen was often dehydrated and fearful of eating or drinking, she was encouraged to take small frequent feedings of pleasure foods and fluids as desired and tolerated. She died shortly after enrollment in hospice at home, without complete relief of nausea but also without prolonged and painful vomiting.

! TAKE AWAY POINTS

- Interventions for the patient experiencing nausea and vomiting must always begin with a comprehensive assessment to determine the cause or causes of vomiting. Failure to properly assess the cause of nausea and vomiting is a major contributor to ineffective treatment.
- Effective treatment of nausea and vomiting is often multi-faceted, and may include one or more medications in combination with diet and lifestyle changes, and possibly surgical intervention.
- These is little data on the effectiveness of various interventions in relief of nausea and vomiting, and further research on the effectiveness of specific interventions in specific clinical circumstances is indicated.

REFERENCES

[1] Stephenson J, Davies A. An assessment of aetiology-based guidelines for the management of nausea and vomiting in patients with advanced cancer. *Support Care Cancer*; 2006; 14:348–353.

[2] Glare P, Dunwoodie D, Clark K, Ward A, Yates P, Ryan S, Hardy J. Treatment of nausea and vomiting in terminally ill cancer patients. *Drugs*; 2008; 68(18):2576–2590.

[3] Saxby C, Ackroyd R, Callin S, Mayland C, Kite S. How should we measure emesis in palliative care? *Palliative Medicine*; 2007; 21:369–383.

[4] Abernethy A, Wheeler J, Zafar S. Detailing of gastrointestinal symptoms in cancer patients with advanced disease: new methodologies, new insights and a proposed approach. *Current Opinion in Supportive and Palliative Care*; 2009; 3(1):41–49.

[5] Wood G, Shega J, Lynch B, Von Roenn J. Management of intractable nausea and vomiting in patients at the end of life. *Journal of the American Medical Association*; 2007; 298(10):1196–1207.

[6] Mannix K. Palliation of nausea and vomiting in malignancy. *Clinical Medicine*; 2006; 6(2):144–147.

[7] Shoemaker L, Estfan B, Induru R, Walsh T. Symptom management: an important part of cancer care. *Cleveland Clinic Journal of Medicine*; 2011; 78(1):25–34.

[8] Dahlin C, Lynch M, Szmuilowicz E, Jackson V. Management of symptoms other than pain. *Anesthesiology Clinics of North America*; 2006; 24:39–60.

[9] Dorman S, Perkins P. Droperidol for the treatment of nausea and vomiting in palliative care patients. *Cochrane Database of Systematic Review*; 2010; Issue 10.

[10] Perkins P, Dorman S. Haloperidol for the treatment of nausea and vomiting in palliative care patients. *Cochrane Database of Systematic Reviews*; 2009 Issue 2.

[11] Hardy J, O'Shea A, White C, Gilshenan K, Welch L, Douglas C. The efficacy of haloperidol in the management of patients with cancer. *Journal of Pain and Symptom Management*; 2010; 40(1):111–116.

[12] Kumar G, Hayes K, Clark R. Efficacy of a scheduled IV cocktail of anti-emetics for the palliation of nausea and vomiting in a hospice population. *American Journal of Hospice & Palliative Medicine*; 2008; 25(3):184–189.

[13] Licup N, Baumrucker S. Olanzapine for nausea and vomiting. *American Journal of Hospice & Palliative Medicine*; 2010; 27:432–434.

[14] Walker J, Lane P. Challenges and choices: an audit of the management of nausea, vomiting and bowel obstruction in metastatic ovarian cancer. *Contemporary Nurse*; 2007; 27(1):39–46.

[15] Wu T, Munro A, Guanjian L, Liu G. Chinese medical herbs for chemotherapy side effects in colorectal cancer patients. *Cochrane Database of System Reviews*, 2008, Issue 1.

[16] Ezzo J, Richardson MA, Vickers A, Allen C, Dibble S, Issell BF, Lao L, Ramirez G, Roscoe JA, Shen J, Shivnan JC, Streitberger K, Treish I, Zhang G. Acupuncture-point stimulation for chemotherapy-induced nausea or vomiting. *Cochrane Database of Systematic Reviews*; 2011; Issue 3.

[17] Steels H, Chang A, Gibbons K. Aromatherapy for treatment of postoperative nausea and vomiting. *Cochrane Database of Systematic Reviews*; 2009; Issue 1.

[18] Koetter K, Kranke P. Prevention and treatment interventions for nausea and vomiting during initiation of chronic opiod therapy. *Cochrane Database of Systematic Reviews*; 2009; Issue 3.

[19] Lundstrom S, Zachirisson U, Furst J. When nothing helps: propofol as sedation and antiemetic in palliative cancer care. *Journal of Pain and Symptom Management*; 2005; 30(6):570–577.

Case 2.10 Nausea Associated with Bowel Obstruction

Terri L. Maxwell

HISTORY

Janice was a 48-year-old white woman admitted to the in-patient palliative care unit with symptoms of bowel obstruction. She reported a three-day history of intractable nausea and vomiting and intermittent crampy abdominal pain, rated as an eight on a scale of zero to 10. Her appetite was very poor and for the few days prior to admission she was only taking sips of fluids. Her last bowel movement was five days prior to admission; she normally moved her bowels every few days. She was extremely weak and tired. Janice was accompanied to the hospital by her husband and sister.

Janice was diagnosed with stage IV ovarian cancer two years ago. Despite undergoing surgery and multiple courses of chemotherapy, her disease was progressing. A CT scan of the abdomen and pelvis performed four weeks prior to admission revealed extensive peritoneal metastasis, new liver lesions, and ascites. Her oncologist recommended that she enroll in hospice, but she deferred, stating that she was looking forward to her son's high school graduation in four months.

Janice lived at home with her husband and two sons, ages 18 and 15. She formerly worked outside the home as a bank teller until she became too ill to work. Janice was spending much of her time in bed. Janice's husband John worked long hours running a landscaping business. He appeared tired and anxious. Janice's sister Kate lived nearby and was spending much of her time at Janice's house while John was at work. Janice's two sons were busy with school and sports and did not help much around the house. John remarked that it seems like the boys are "hardly ever home anymore."

Case Studies in Palliative and End-of-Life Care, First Edition. Edited by Margaret L. Campbell.
© 2012 John Wiley & Sons, Inc. Published 2012 by John Wiley & Sons, Inc.

PHYSICAL EXAMINATION

Temperature: 38.4°C, blood pressure: 92/60 supine and 78/50 when standing, heart rate: 114, respiratory rate: 24

Central nervous system: Alert, oriented, and in obvious distress

Head, eyes, ears, nose, throat: Mucosa intact but dry and tongue coated, neck veins flat in supine position

Cardiac: S1, S2 and tachycardia, no S3 or S4, no murmurs

Lungs: Breath sounds clear on the left but diminished at right base; no wheezes, crackles, or accessory muscle use

Gastrointestinal: Abdomen markedly distended and tender with guarding to light palpation but no rebound guarding. Palpable masses in all four quadrants. Abdominal skin taut with striae and prominent dilated veins; well-healed midline scar. Bowel sounds hypoactive and hyperresonant on percussion over the abdomen. Positive fluid wave and shifting dullness for ascites was appreciated. Rectal exam negative for impaction, stool negative for occult blood

Genitourinary: Voiding small amounts of dark yellow urine

Extremities: Cachectic with 4+ pitting ankle edema bilaterally

DIAGNOSTICS

CT of the abdomen and pelvis: Confirmed widespread metastases with new right lung nodule and right mesenteric mass and dilated small bowel suspicious for obstruction

White blood count: 3.2, hemoglobin: 9.1, hematocrit: 45%, sodium: 145, potassium: 3.4, creatinine: 5.2

CLINICAL QUESTION

What treatments may reduce severe nausea and vomiting associated with small bowel obstruction?

DISCUSSION

Malignant bowel obstruction, especially affecting the small bowel, is a relatively common complication of abdominal and pelvic carcinomas such as colon or ovarian cancer.[1] Bowel obstruction can be partial or complete and may occur at more than one site. Most obstructions involve the small bowel, although in some cases, both are involved.[1] Compression of the bowel usually develops slowly and often remains partial.

Bowel obstruction occurs when gastric and intestinal contents are blocked as a result of poor bowel motility or by a mechanical occlusion. Mechanical causes of bowel obstruction include adhesions from surgery or previous radiation therapy, tumors blocking the intestines, intussception, volvulous (twisting of the colon), and impacted stool. In patients with ovarian cancer, tumor cells spread by peritoneal seeding that results in multiple sites of obstruction.

Malignant bowel obstruction is not a predictor of imminent death and decisions regarding its treatment are rarely urgent. Therefore, it is important to take the time necessary to consider what management strategy is best for the patient based upon her prognosis and goals.

Assessment

Evaluation of bowel obstruction includes physical exam, history, and imaging tests. When obtaining a history, questions to ask include:

- When did the symptoms begin to occur?
- Are the symptoms new or have they occurred in the past?
- Is the pain continuous or intermittent? What triggers the pain?
- When was your last bowel movement?
- Are you having nausea, vomiting, diarrhea, constipation, or blood in your stool, or fever?
- What are you vomiting?
- Have you had abdominal surgery or radiation to your abdomen?

The signs and symptoms of bowel obstruction vary depending on the underlying cause and site and extent of obstruction. Common symptoms of bowel obstruction include colicky, crampy abdominal pain; abdominal distention and fullness; nausea; vomiting; constipation; diarrhea; and an inability to pass stool or gas. Pain and vomiting occurs early in obstructions involving the small bowel and later in those with large bowel obstruction. Physical exam may reveal a distended, tender abdomen with or without palpable masses, although in patients with extensive mesenteric and omental spread, abdominal distension may be less prevalent.[1] Bowel sounds may be high pitched, diminished, or absent.

Imaging tests used to confirm a diagnosis of bowel obstruction include plain abdominal radiographs, contrast radiography, and abdominal CT. These studies help to define the site and extent of obstruction, as well as the underlying cause. Typically, abdominal X-rays reveal loops of intestines distended with gas. Abdominal CT also helps to determine the extent of disease to assist in the decision regarding management.

Treatment

Although there is no consensus on the management of malignant bowel obstruction, there is a growing evidence base to guide clinical practice guidelines.[1]

Surgery

Surgery remains the treatment of choice in cases where it is not contra-indicated due to clinical situations or status.[2] However, surgery is not advised for patients with end-stage cancer due to high operative mortality and high rates of complications.[1] In particular, patients with known diffuse metastatic cancer, involvement of the proximal stomach, or diffuse palpable masses, or who have massive ascites that rapidly recurs after drainage, are not recommended for surgery.[1] Relative contraindications to surgery include those with nonsymptomatic extensive metastatic disease, poor nutritional and/or performance status, or advanced age, or patients who have undergone previous radiation therapy to the abdomen or pelvis.[1] These patients should instead be offered supportive and palliative treatments aimed at reducing their symptoms and improving their quality of life.

Nasogastric Decompression

Because nasogastric tubes (NGT) are so distressing to the patient, they should be used only as a temporary measure until other treatments take effect. Initial decompression can be performed by placing an NGT to reduce the amount of secretions before pharmacological therapy is initiated or during the first few days of therapy. However, NGTs fail to control symptoms in the majority of cases and they are not recommended for long-term use.

Pharmacological Management

Pharmacologic management of partial bowel obstruction is focused on relieving pain, nausea, and vomiting. Anti-emetics are usually given in combination with anti-secretory agents to control vomiting.[1] Recommended anti-emetics include the prokinetic agent metoclopramide 60 to 120 mg administered parenterally to increase peristalsis and gastric emptying. Metoclopramide may be helpful in patients with partial obstruction due to its positive effect on gastric emptying in addition to its anti-emetic properties. It should be avoided in patients with complete obstruction because it may worsen vomiting or exacerbate colic.

No clinical trials have compared different anti-emetics in the management of malignant bowel obstruction and drugs from a variety of classes are frequently used alone or in combination. Phenothiazines and other antipsychotics such as haloperidol are commonly used to control emesis in these patients. Haloperidol can be administered orally, intravenously, and subcutaneously.[4] Chlorpromazine is equally effective, but is generally reserved for those who benefit from its sedating properties.[4] Corticosteriods, such as dexamethasone, are frequently administered as adjunct therapy for nausea and vomiting in patients with obstruction. While data are not conclusive, the anti-inflammatory properties of corticosteroids are also believed to reduce peritumoral edema;[5] initial doses of dexamethasone range from 4 to 12 mg daily.[2] Anticholinergics such as hyoscyamine or glycopyrrolate are used to relieve vomiting by decreasing secretions. They also help to minimize colic by reducing gastrointestinal smooth muscle spasm.[3]

Octreotide is a somatostatin analogue that is prescribed to patients who continue to have large volume emesis.[6] Octreotide has multiple mechanisms of action that are beneficial for treating obstruction, including decreasing gastrointestinal secretions, inhibiting the release of gastric hormones that contribute to obstruction and its symptoms, and facilitating water and electrolyte absorption by the gut wall.[2] Octreotide 0.2 to 0.9 mg/day is administered via continuous subcutaneous or intravenous infusion or in divided doses three times a day.[2] Patients with severe inoperable obstruction may benefit from the addition of scopolamine butylbromide which acts to further decrease secretions through a different mechanism of action.[3]

Opioid analgesics should be administered to manage abdominal pain. A trial of intravenous hydration is sometimes administered to palliate symptoms of thirst or dehydration.[1]

Venting Procedures

Some patients may benefit from a percutaneous venting procedure if the above measures fail to provide adequate relief and the patient is expected to live weeks to months. In these cases, a gastrostomy tube is placed in the stomach and attached to a drainage bag to allow for decompression of air and fluid. Patients can close the valve and eat or drink by mouth, although this does not result in effective feeding because the food drains directly into the bag.[3]

BACK TO OUR CASE

Janice was diagnosed with a partial small bowel obstruction due to widespread intraabdominal metastasis. Due to the progressive nature of her cancer, despite multiple courses of chemotherapy coupled with a poor performance status, a palliative approach using medications to manage symptoms was recommended. Metoclopramide 20 mg IV QID and dexamethasone 8 mg IV q day were initiated in addition to IV hydration. Morphine 5 mg IV q three hours PRN pain was also prescribed. Over the next three days, Janice's nausea, vomiting, and abdominal pain improved and she was able to take sips of fluids and eat small amounts of food.

The hospital's palliative care team, along with Janice's oncologist, held a family meeting with Janice, her husband, and her sister. Janice's oncologist reviewed Janice's current clinical status, including evidence of further disease spread on the recent CT scan. Her oncologist again recommended against additional chemotherapy, stating that it would be poorly tolerated and ineffective. He explained that due to the extensiveness of her cancer, she was not a surgical candidate. The palliative care team discussed Janice's goal to be home with her family as long as possible and agreed to home hospice support. A referral was made to hospice and Janice was discharged to home after she was successfully converted from IV to PO medications. Medications on discharge included metoclopramide 20 mg PO QID, morphine sulfate 20 mg/ml, 20 mg PO every three hour PRN pain, and glycopyrrolate 1 to 2 mg PO every eight hours.

! TAKE AWAY POINTS

- Malignant bowel obstruction is a common complication in patients with advanced abdominal or pelvic cancers.
- Symptoms of bowel obstruction vary depending upon the site and extent of obstruction, but nausea, vomiting, inability to pass stool, and colicky abdominal pain are common.
- Surgical intervention, including gastric decompression, is dependent upon the extent of obstruction and the patient's functional status, prognosis, and goals of care.
- Palliative management includes a combination of anti-emetics, anti-secretory agents, octreotide, and opioids for pain control.
- Most patients with irreversible bowel obstruction can be comfortably managed at home with a comprehensive plan for controlling symptoms and providing emotional and spiritual support.

REFERENCES

[1] Ripamonti C, Twycross R, Baines M, Bozzetti F, Capri S, De Conno F, Gemlo B, et al. Clinical-practice recommendations for the management of bowel obstruction in patients with end-stage cancer. *Support Care Cancer*; 2001; 9:223–233.

[2] Ripamonti C, Mercande S. How to use octreotide for malignant bowel obstruction. *Supportive Oncology*; 2004; 2(4):357–364.

[3] Hardy JR. Medical management of bowel obstruction. *British Journal of Surgery*; 2000; 87,1281–1283.

[4] Gare PA, Dunwoodie D, Clark K, Ward A, Yates P, Ryan S, Hardy, JR. Treatment of nausea and vomiting in terminally ill cancer patients. *Drugs*; 2008; 68(18):2575–2590.

[5] Shih A, Jackson KC. Role of corticosteroids in palliative care. *Journal of Pain and Palliative Pharmacotherapy*; 2007; 21:4,69–76.

[6] Prommer EE. Established and potential therapeutic applications of octreotide in palliative care. *Supportive Cancer Care*; 2008; 16:1117–1123.

Case 2.11 Nausea Related to Uremia, Dialysis Cessation

Linda M. Gorman

HISTORY

Clarence was a 69-year-old African-American man with end-stage renal disease (ESRD). He had been receiving hemodialysis for the past five years. He had type II diabetes and was insulin dependent for the 20 past years. He also had peripheral vascular disease and had his left leg amputated in the year prior to hospitalization. His right foot was cool to the touch; he was admitted to the hospital to evaluate for another amputation. Clarence lived in an assisted living facility and was visited regularly by his devoted grandson. When admitted to the hospital, Clarence informed his doctors and grandson that he did not want another amputation and wished to discontinue dialysis. He reported his quality of life was extremely poor and he did not wish to prolong his life in this state.

Clarence spent the next two days in the hospital preparing to be discharged with hospice enrollment. He began eating a few favorite foods such as orange juice that were previously forbidden; thereafter, he began complaining of continuous nausea. He rated the nausea as 10 out of 10 on a numeric rating system. Clarence was hoping to return home and have a few good days before lapsing into unconsciousness. The nausea was very distressing and he feared he would not have a peaceful death.

Case Studies in Palliative and End-of-Life Care, First Edition. Edited by Margaret L. Campbell.
© 2012 John Wiley & Sons, Inc. Published 2012 by John Wiley & Sons, Inc.

PHYSICAL EXAMINATION

Temperature: 38°C, blood pressure: 180/110, heart rate: 120, respiratory
    rate, 20
Central nervous system: Alert, oriented
Head, eyes, ears, nose, throat: No deficits
Cardiac: S1, S2 present; muffled S3 and S4; diastolic murmur; jugular
    vein distention
Lungs: Distant lung sounds, diminished at bases, rhonchi, SpO_2 90%
Gastrointestinal: Normal bowel sounds, no tenderness
Genitourinary: No urine output
Extremities: Cachectic, 4+ pitting edema in right leg, toes on right foot
    are discolored and cool to touch

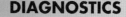

DIAGNOSTICS

None at this point, though can consider monitoring electrolytes

CLINICAL QUESTION

What treatments will prevent or reduce nausea in patients with uremia?

DISCUSSION

Nausea and Uremia

Nausea remains one of the most uncomfortable and distressing symptoms
that impacts all aspects of the patient's life.[1,2] It is a subjective symptom
involving an unpleasant sensation experienced in the back of the throat
and epigastrium and may or may not lead to vomiting, which is a separate
phenomonon.[3] It can be described as feeling "sick to my stomach" or
queasy. The pathways and mechanisms involved in nausea are less well
understood than vomiting.[4] The vomiting center in the brain receives
stimulation from the chemoreceptor trigger zone, vestibular system, and
vagal innervations in the gastrointestinal tract as well as input from the
midbrain. For nausea there is an association with cortical involvement that
would help to explain the highly aversive nature of nausea.[4] Nausea in the
absence of vomiting may arise from stimuli that excite the vomiting center
without sufficient amplification to trigger the vomiting cascade.

Nausea is frequently seen in the patient with ESRD[5] and it can be experienced by patients receiving hemodialysis.[6,7] It is also seen in uremic patients who are managed conservatively without dialysis[8] and those who discontinue dialysis.[9,10] In one investigation, 36% of patients who discontinued dialysis complained of nausea.[11] Though death from uremia is usually described as painless, nausea can occur as toxins accumulate, creating a high level of discomfort.[12] Saini et al. found that ESRD patients had similar a symptom burden and quality of life as patients with terminal malignancies.[13] These symptoms included nausea and pruritus. Uremia is believed to stimulate the chemoreceptor trigger zone. In addition, the multiple complications from uremia can contribute to nausea. Emotional factors, including anxiety and negative associations with certain stimuli such as odors, can also contribute to nausea.

Etiology of Nausea in This Population

- Metabolic impact of kidney failure, including electrolyte imbalance (particularly hypercalcemia, hyperkalemia, and hyponatremia)
- Hypercalcemia during dialysis
- Gastroparesis and distention of the stomach
- Side effect of multiple medications
- Stimulation of the chemoreceptor trigger zone by the accumulation of toxins in uremia
- Reaction to dialysate or too rapid removal of fluid during dialysis
- Complications from co-morbidities
- Constipation
- Association with negative stimuli from dialysis or other negative stimuli

Assessment

Regular assessments of this symptom as well as self-report tools that guide patients to track their symptoms are an important part of nausea assessment. The Edmonton Symptom Assessment System, Northern Alberta Renal Program, and the Dialysis Symptom Index have been used by nephrology professionals to rate nausea on scales of zero to 10 and zero to five, respectively.[14,15] Two assessment tools frequently used in oncology may also be useful. These include the Morrow Assessment of Nausea and Emesis (MANE) and Rhodes Index of Nausea and Vomiting Form 2 (INV-2).[16] Assessment should include the following:

- Pattern of nausea related to timing, association with food, position changes, dialysis, other stimuli
- Symptom triggers, including emotional factors
- Examination of the mouth
- Assessment of the abdomen for bowel sounds

- Bowel pattern assessment
- Review of labs for electrolyte abnormalities including hyponatremia, hypercalcemia, hyperkalemia
- Review of current medications and side effects

Treatment

Identifying and treating the underlying cause is the most effective treatment. However, because many ESRD patients have many co-morbidities and have multiple organs involved due to the effects of the renal failure, this can be difficult to determine.

Pharmacological Treatment

Choosing an anti-nausea medication is best achieved if the cause of nausea is known, so the drug with the appropriate pathway that triggered the symptom can be addressed. Limited research has been conducted on the effectiveness of various anti-nausea drugs in this population.[17] There are no studies of head-to-head comparison of different anti-nausea medications in uremia.[18] Knowledge of how the drug is metabolized is important in the presence of renal failure. Drugs that are metabolized via the kidneys accumulate toxic effects if the patient is not receiving dialysis. Drugs that are metabolized via the liver are generally used to avoid toxic side effects. In addition, because these patients are on a large number of medications and have multiple co-morbidities, they are prone to side effects or toxic effects when new medications are added. Doses may need to be reduced for these patients.

Because the nauseous patient may be unable to tolerate oral medications, alternate routes such as IV, rectal, or sublingual may be better tolerated; therefore, this is another factor that must be taken into account when selecting the appropriate medication. See Table 2.11.1 for a summary of commonly used anti-nausea medications.

Haloperidol is recommended for uremia-induced nausea at 50% of normal dose;[4,18] it works at the chemoreceptor trigger zone. Caution needs to be used in patients with heart disease because this drug can prolong the QT interval; this may not be relevant if the patient has hours to days to live. Metoclopramide may also be helpful. Patients with ESRD may be prone to extrapyramidal symptoms, so caution should be used.[18]

For patients who are discontinuing dialysis and who have nausea, effective treatment is usually haloperidol, metoclopramide, prochlorperzine, or ondansetron.[17] Benzodiazepines have no specific anti-nausea effect but may be useful and are usually well tolerated by patients with uremia. For the patient discontinuing dialysis, new medications should not be added until it is clear the patient is symptomatic to avoid adding any unnecessary medications which could produce side effects.

TABLE 2.11.1. Commonly used anti-nausea medications.

Drug	Dose	Rationale	Notes
Haloperidol	0.5 to 2 mg PO Q 8 hours	Inhibits nausea caused by stimulation of chemoreceptor trigger zone	Watch for extrapyramidal reactions
Metoclopramide	2.5 to 5 mg PO Q 4 hours prior to meals	Treats delayed gastric emptying	CKD patient prone to extrapyramidal reactions
Prochlorperazine	25 mg PR Q 8 hours 5 mg PO Q 6 to 8 hours	Antagonizes dopamine receptors at chemorector trigger zone	CKD patient prone to extrapyramidal reactions
Dexamethasone	2 to 4 mg PO 3 to 4 times/day	Block prostaglandins	Diabetic patients need to have blood sugars monitored closely
Ondansetron Granisetron	4 to 8 mg PO 1 mg PO Q 12 hours	5HT3 blocker (serotonin receptor antagonist)	High cost may be prohibitive in some settings
Dronabinol	2.5 to 5 mg PO	Synthetic cannabinoid	Side effects of drowsiness, euphoria may be unacceptable for some patients
Lorazepam	0.5 to 2 mg PO/ SL Q 4 hours PRN	Benzodiazepine that acts on the cerebral cortex. Reduces anxiety	Monitor for sedation, fall risk

5-HT3 blockers such as ondansetron, granisetron, and dolasetron mesylate may be useful in uremic patients or those on dialysis, especially because there may be multiple etiologies for the nausea. These serotonin receptor antagonists are relatively safe with limited side effects. These receptors are in the chemoreceptor trigger zone and the vomiting venter and in the gut. Corticosteroids may be effective in reducing hypercalcemia and uremia symptoms in acute renal failure.[19] They are often used in combination with other anti-emetics.

Very little research has been done on the use of cannabinoids in chronic kidney disease but it may present effective treatment in the presence of uremia.[20]

Nonpharmacological Treatment

Non-pharmacologic interventions can be useful by themselves or in combination with anti-emetics. Ginger has been the most studied herbal treatment for nausea.[21] It can be taken as a capsule, extract, tea, or fresh root. Other herbal remedies include anise, nutmeg, and tonka bean.

Acupuncture and acupressure have been shown to augment the effect of anti-nausea medications during chemotherapy and to reduce post-operative nausea and vomiting.[4] Therefore, these may be additional treatments to offer the patient with nausea. Acupressure prolongs the effect of acupuncture. The acupuncture point is located in the midline of the palmar aspect of each wrist, approximately 3 cm from the palmar crease.

Behavioral interventions can be effective due to their ability to induce relaxation, provide distraction, and enhance a sense of control. Using slow deep breathing, biofeedback, relaxing imagery, and progressive contraction and relaxation of various muscle groups can be helpful for some patients.[3]

Patients may try various comfort measures to reduce the discomfort of nausea. Some of these include:

- Apply cold cloth to forehead, neck, and wrists
- Avoid strong odors
- Eat bland, cold foods in small quantities
- Avoid fatty or spicy foods
- Drink carbonated beverages

BACK TO OUR CASE

Clarence was started on haloperidol 1 mg every eight hours. Within eight hours his nausea was reduced to six out of 10. The patient remained very anxious and focused on his wish to not die in the hospital. Lorazepam 0.5 mg every four hours PRN was added. Hospice was arranged and he was discharged from the hospital that day. On the initial hospice visit the nurse reviewed the current regimen with the medical director and it was decided to stay on the same medications; Clarence was satisfied with them. The social worker visited and suggested some relaxation breathing exercises in addition to helping with some life review. The staff of the assisted living brewed a ginger tea which he took every few hours. On the second day home his nausea was rated as a two. He continued on this regimen until he lapsed into unconsciousness five days later and died the following day with his caregivers from the assisted living facility and his grandson at his side.

| ! | **TAKE AWAY POINTS** |

- Nausea is a very frequent symptom in ESRD, both in the patient who is uremic and those who are receiving dialysis.
- Nausea often has multiple etiologies, and the presence of multiple medications and co-morbidities in these patients can make determining the cause very difficult.
- Haloperidol has been shown to be the most effective agent for nausea management in the patient who is discontinuing dialysis.

| 📖 | **REFERENCES** |

[1] Cohen L, de Moor CA, Eisenberg P, Ming EE, Hu H. Chemotherapy-induced nausea and vomiting: incidence and impact on patient quality of life at community oncology settings. *Support Care Cancer*; May 2007; 15(5):497–503.

[2] Ballatori E, Roila F, Ruggeri B, et al. The impact of chemotherapy-induced nausea and vomiting on health-related quality of life. *Support Care Cancer*; Feb. 2007; 15(2):179–185.

[3] King C, Tarcatu D. Nausea and vomiting. In: Ferrell B, Coyle N, eds. *Oxford Textbook of Palliative Nursing*, 3rd edition. New York: Oxford University Press; 2010; 221–238.

[4] Mannix K. Palliation of nausea and vomiting. In: Hanks G, Cherny N, Christakis N, Fallon M, Kaasa S, Portenoy R, eds. *Oxford Textbook of Palliative Medicine*, 4th edition New York: Oxford University Press; 2010; 801–811.

[5] Chonchol M, Chan L. Chronic kidney disease: Manifestations and pathogenesis. In: Schrier R, ed. *Renal and Electrolyte Disorders*, 7th edition. Philadelphia: Wolters Klumer/Lippincott Williams and Wilkins; 2010; 389–425.

[6] Davison SN, Jhangri GS. Impact of pain and symptom burden on the health-related quality of life of hemodialysis patients. *J Pain Symptom Manage*; Mar. 2010; 39(3):477–485.

[7] Jablonski A. Level of symptom relief and the need for palliative care in the hemodialysis population. *Journal of Hospice and Palliative Nursing*; 2007; 9(1):50–58.

[8] Murtagh F, Addington-Hall J, Donohoe P, Higginson I. Symptom management in patients with established renal failure managed without dialysis. *EDTNA/ERCA Journal of Renal Care*; 2006; 93–98.

[9] Murtagh FE, Addington-Hall J, Edmonds P, et al. Symptoms in the month before death for stage 5 chronic kidney disease patients managed without dialysis. *J Pain Symptom Manage*; Sep. 2010; 40(3):342–352.

[10] Germain MJ, Cohen LM, Davison SN. Withholding and withdrawal from dialysis: what we know about how our patients die. *Semin Dial*; May-June 2007; 20(3):195–199.

[11] Chater S, Davison SN, Germain MJ, Cohen LM. Withdrawal from dialysis: a palliative care perspective. *Clin Nephrol*; Nov. 2006; 66(5):364–372.

[12] Neely KJ, Roxe DM. Palliative care/hospice and the withdrawal of dialysis. *J Palliat Med*; 2000; 3(1):57–67.

[13] Saini T, Murtagh FE, Dupont PJ, McKinnon PM, Hatfield P, Saunders Y. Comparative pilot study of symptoms and quality of life in cancer patients and patients with end stage renal disease. *Palliat Med*; Sep. 2006; 20(6):631–636.

[14] Edmonton Symptom Assessment System-Northern Alberta Renal Program. kidneyeol.org/edmontonassment.pdf. Accessed March 29, 2011.

[15] Dialysis Symptom Index, University of Pittsburgh Medical Center. kidneyeol.org/DSI/pdf. Accessed March 29, 2011.

[16] Rhodes VA, McDaniel RW. Nausea, vomiting, and retching: complex problems in palliative care. *CA Cancer J Clin*; July-Aug. 2001; 51(4):232–248; quiz 249-252.

[17] Davison S, Cohen L, Germain M. Palliative and supportive care. In: Wilcox C, Berl T, Himmelfarb J, Mitch W, Murphy B, Salant D, Yu ASL (eds). *Therapy in Nephrology and Hypertension, 3rd edition*. Philadelphia: Saunders Elsevier; 2008.

[18] Douglas C, Murtagh FE, Chambers EJ, Howse M, Ellershaw J. Symptom management for the adult patient dying with advanced chronic kidney disease: a review of the literature and development of evidence-based guidelines by a United Kingdom Expert Consensus Group. *Palliat Med*; Mar. 2009; 23(2):103–110.

[19] Bayraktar UD, Warsch S, Pereira D. High-dose glucocorticoids improve renal failure reversibility in patients with newly diagnosed multiple myeloma. *Am J Hematol*; Feb. 2011; 86(2):224–227.

[20] Davison SN, Davison JS. Is there a legitimate role for the therapeutic use of cannabinoids for symptom management in chronic kidney disease? *J Pain Symptom Manage*; Jan. 2011; 41:768–778.

[21] Skidmore-Roth L. *Mosby's Handbook of Herbs and Natural Supplements*, 4th edition. St Louis: Mosby Elsevier; 2010.

Case 2.12 Opioid-Induced Pruritus

Richelle Nugent Hooper

HISTORY

Sarah was a 65-year-old white woman who presented to the emergency department (ED) with chest pain and associated difficulty breathing. She was found to have newly diagnosed pathological fractures from an undiagnosed primary malignant condition. She was admitted to the hospital for further evaluation and pain control.

On examination, Sarah reported that her pain level was 7/10 on a numerical rating system and 10/10 on inspiration. She had been given intravenous morphine initially in the emergency room and several times since her admission, and she reported that this had worked fairly well for her pain but that it did not last very long. Within 30 minutes of the injection she was experiencing more pain. Twenty-four hours after initiation of the analgesia regimen she reported that in addition to the pain, she was having itching on her face. This started around her nose and spread along the side of her face. There was no rash apparent on examination, but Sarah reported that the "itching is driving me crazy."

PHYSICAL EXAMINATION

Temperature: 38.4°C, blood pressure: 145/70, heart rate: 115, respiratory rate: 28
Central nervous system: Alert, oriented, no focal deficits

Case Studies in Palliative and End-of-Life Care, First Edition. Edited by Margaret L. Campbell.
© 2012 John Wiley & Sons, Inc. Published 2012 by John Wiley & Sons, Inc.

Head, eyes, ears, nose, throat: No defects or abnormalities

Cardiac: S1, S2, and tachycardia, no S3 or S4, no murmurs

Lungs: Diminished breath sounds generally, although clear in all lung fields, tachypneic, accessory muscle use, guarding noted with deep inspiration, SpO$_2$ 93% on 4 liters humidified nasal cannula

Gastrointestinal: Soft abdomen, normal bowel sounds, no tenderness or organomegaly

Extremities: Thin, no pressure ulcers or deformities, no apparent rash

DIAGNOSTICS

Chest X-ray: Mass noted in right lower lobe, approximately 3×4 cm with spiculations. Lytic lesions noted sporadically across right lower ribs. Fractures present in these areas in ribs five to nine.

? CLINICAL QUESTION

How can discomfort from the pruritus related to opioid administration be alleviated?

✓ DISCUSSION

Pruritus is classified as a subjective sensation that can be both unpleasant and irritating. It arises from the superficial layers of skin provoking an urge to scratch. There are no specific peripheral receptors for pruritus, with the stimulus apparently related to connections at the spinal level. Although there is no one area of the brain that is responsible for the processing of this stimulus, it is apparent that there is substantial activation of the motor cortex. This sensation is transmitted along unmyelinated C-fibers distinct from those that transmit pain,[1] along the lateral spinothalamic tract to the thalamus. From here it travels to the cerebral cortex where the sensation of itch is caused.[2]

The exact mechanism of pruritus related to opioid administration is unclear; it is known that many substances induce pruritus by causing a release of histamine from mast cells in the skin; however, this does not seem to be the underlying mechanism with opioid administration. Although some opioids release histamine, there are others that do not, yet still may cause pruritus.[3] For example, morphine is reported to cause histamine release from mast cells, and accounts for the majority of cases of opioid-related pruritus, particularly when administered via the epidural or intra-thecal route.[3] However, other opioids such as fentanyl or oxymorphone, which have also been known to cause pruritus, are less likely to produce histamine release.[4] Incidences of pruritus are most often associated with acute administration of opioids but have been observed in up to 10% of patients receiving chronic opioids.[4] This side effect is not considered an allergic reaction, and there is no evidence that it is dose related; however, it can be very uncomfortable for patients and may limit opioid administration and consequently reduce quality of life as abatement of symptoms is unlikely in most patients.

Treatment

There are three general approaches to the treatment and management of opioid-related pruritus, one option is to decrease the dose of the opioid, another is to change the opioid or route of administration, and the other option is treat the condition symptomatically. The latter option is the most challenging, and often most frustrating since there are often no specific treatments available. There is also some difficulty in evaluating the efficacy of antipruritic agents because the placebo effect has been found to be as high as 50%.[4]

Pharmacological Treatment

Several pharmacological agents have been used for treatment of pruritus and its prevention (Table 2.12.1).[5] Despite the controversial role of histamine in the cause of this condition, antihistamines (H1 antagonists) are often the first line treatment, with varying degrees of efficacy.[4] Within this class of medication, hydroxyzine has been found to be more effective than diphenhydramine or cyproheptadine, although all are sedating.[6]

Chlorpheniramine is also widely used, and some have argued that the sedating side effects of these medications at least allow a good night's sleep. Nonsedating antihistamines have been found to be as or more effective than the sedating forms, though evidence regarding this is limited.[6] There is increasing evidence that this condition involves the mediation of sensation through central mu receptors[4] and thus mu receptor antagonists such as naloxone or nalbuphine have been used successfully in reversing the effects of opioid-related pruritus. Naloxone has been used since the 1970s, particularly with epidural administration of opioids in a low-dose infusion.[7] Naloxone use has become widely accepted, partly due to its efficacy, reliability, and cost-effectiveness; unfortunately, it may also reverse the opioid analgesic effect which presents another challenge for the patient. Recently there has been increased use of methylnaltrexone in treating opioid-related pruritus, which is a peripheral opioid antagonist and related to naloxone. It has been

TABLE 2.12.1. Medications for reducing pruritus.

Drug	Dose	Rationale	Notes on use
Diphenydramine	25 to 50 mg PO/ IV/IM Q 4 to 6 hours PRN itching	H1 antagonist, antihistamine works by blocking histamine release from mast cells	Can be used orally, intravenously, or intramuscularly Is very sedating
Hydroxyzine	25 to 100 mg PO 6 to 8 hours PRN itching	H1 antagonist, antihistamine works by blocking histamine release from mast cells	Found to be more effective than diphenhydramine Is very sedating
Chlorphenirimine	4 mg PO Q 4 to 6 hours PRN itching	H1 antagonist, antihistamine works by blocking histamine release from mast cells	Maximum 24 mg/24-hour period Sedating
Ondansetron	4 mg PO/IV Q 4 hours PRN itching	Direct 5-HT antagonist Because opioid and serotinergic systems interact closely with one another within the central nervous system, this medication down-regulates 5-HT receptors following initial release of serotonin	May be given routinely prior to administration of epidural or intrathecal opioids
Naloxone	0.1 to 0.2 mg IV every 5 minutes PRN (titrate to effect) 0.17 to 0.2 mcg/ kg/minute via infusion	Mu-receptor antagonist Acts by blocking mediation of sensation through central mu receptors	May also be administered via infusion Can cause decreased efficacy of analgesia
Methylnaltrexone	0.1 to 0.15 mg/ kg SC	Peripheral opioid antagonist related to naloxone	Shown to reduce itching sensation without decreasing analgesic effect

shown to significantly reduce itch without reducing the analgesic effect; its reduced lipophilicity limits the passage across the blood/brain barrier.

Serotonin (5-HT) receptor antagonists have been demonstrated to be useful. It is thought that this is because the opioid and serotinergic systems interact closely in the central nervous system; therefore, medications in these classes have been more closely studied over the past few years.[5] Clinical evidence suggests that ondansetron, a direct 5-HT antagonist, is effective for the treatment of pruritus. This has been particularly helpful for prophylaxis, by reducing the incidence of perinasal scratching. Recently paroxetine has been identified as a possible treatment for opioid-related pruritus. It is thought that the rapid down-regulation of the 5-HT receptors follows the initial release of serotonin. One case study identified it as being particularly useful in patients with cancer who are taking opioids on a more chronic basis.[8] Because benefits may not be apparent for up to seven days, it is not beneficial in acute situations, but could certainly be employed in conjunction with other medications for chronic challenges.

Dopamine (D2) receptors may also be involved in the genesis of pruritus, although there is limited evidence to suggest that medications such as prochloperazine or haloperidol have any benefit clinically in treatment of this condition. Doxepin has more potent H1 antagonist properties than either hydroxyzine or diphenhydramine and has been used in some patients with varying success.[9] Again, this can be very sedating, so may only be beneficial for nocturnal use.

Other medications that have been used with some success include propofol, nonsteroidal ant-inflammatory medications,[5] and more recently gabapentin. The latter has only been reported in case studies as being beneficial but it seems reasonable to initiate a trial when other medications have failed to be effective,[10] particularly in chronic opioid use. There is certainly room for further study in this subject area; no recent prospective studies have been found as of this writing.[4]

Nonpharmacological Treatment

Given the limited pharmacological options available for reliable treatment, opioid rotation or non-drug interventions may be better options for patients.[8] Although scratching or rubbing the skin can inhibit the sensation of pruritus, it is not desirable to have patients scratching constantly, perpetuating the itch-scratch cycle, possibly causing trauma and secondary irritation. Thus, it is imperative to teach appropriate skin care. General measures include keeping nails short and using an emulsifying ointment or aqueous cream rather than soap, which can be drying to the skin. The use of cool compresses can also be helpful for some patients,[8] in addition to the wearing of loose cotton clothing. Topical antipruritics such as camphor-based lotions or oatmeal baths may also provide temporary relief. Sarna® lotion, which contains phenol and menthol, appears to be useful in minimizing symptoms but evidence is limited in all of these interventions. It is known that the use of topical corticosteroids should be avoided in patients with no evidence of inflammation. Capsaicin has been used effectively to treat pruritus; however, its use is limited due to secondary skin irritation.

Complementary and Alternative Medicine Strategies

No particular strategies have been studied, but there may always be a role for complementary interventions in a patient's treatment. The use of aromatherapy, meditation, or massage for relaxation may alleviate the distress caused by the itching, mostly by shifting the focus of attention; evidence is lacking, however.

Strategies Under Investigation

Further studies into the classes of medications discussed continue, particularly the use of oral interventions for patients using opioids on a chronic basis. An oral form of methylnaltrexone is currently under investigation for use in opioid-related constipation, but also could be considered for use in pruritus.

BACK TO OUR CASE

Treatment options for our patient were related to the plan for her overall treatment, particularly with regard to her pain management regimen. Initially it might be reasonable to try ondansetron intravenously or even low-dose naloxone. Sarah will need to transition to an oral form of opioid medication prior to discharge. This would provide an option to switch to a different opioid to evaluate any potential reaction. Alternatively, if the decision is made to continue with morphine in an oral form, it would be prudent to consider possible interventions. In this case, paroxetine or ondansetron may be prudent options.

TAKE AWAY POINTS

- The mechanism of pruritus related to opioid administration is not well understood.
- Treatment of pruritus related to opioid administration is very challenging; the best options may be nonpharmacological interventions.
- There are three main classes of medications: antihistamines, serotonin receptor antagonists, and mu receptor antagonists.
- Changing the opioid or route of administration to eradicate the itching completely is an alternative of last resort.

REFERENCES

[1] Schmelz M, Schmidt R, Bickel A, et al. Specific C-receptors for itch in human skin. *Journal of Neuroscience*; 1997; 17:8003.

[2] Yosipovitch G, Greaves MW, Schmelz M. Itch. *Lancet*; 2003; 361:690.

[3] Hermens JM, Ebertz JM, Hanifin JM, Hirshman CA. Comparison of histamine release in human skin mast cells induced by morphine, fentanyl, and oxymorphone. *Anesthesiology*; 1985; 62:124.

[4] Ganesh A, Maxwell LG. Pathophysiology and management of opioid-induced pruritus. *Drugs*; 2007; 67(16):2323–2333.

[5] Swegle JM, Logemann C. Management of common opioid-induced adverse effects. *American Family Physician*; 2006; Oct 15, 74(8):1347–1354.

[6] Rhoades RB, Leifer KN, Cohan R, Wittig HJ. Suppression of histamine-induced pruritus by thee antihistamine drugs. *Journal of Allergy Clinical Immunology*; 1975; 55:180.

[7] Friedman JD, Dello Buono FA. Opioid antagonists in the treatment of opioid-induced constipation and pruritus. *Annals of Pharmacotherapy*; 2001; 35:85.

[8] Tarcatu D, Tamasden C, Moryl N, Obbens E. Are we still scratching the surface? A case of intractable pruritus following opioid analgesia. *Journal of Opioid Management*; 2007; May/June, 167–170.

[9] Greene SL, Reed CE, Schroeter AL. Double-blind crossover study comparing doxepin with diphenhydramine for the treatment of chronic urticaria. *Journal of American Academy of Dermatology*; 1985; 12:669.

[10] Yesudian PD, Wilson, NJ. Efficacy of gabapentin in the management of pruritus of unknown origin. *Archives of Dermatology*; 2005; 141:1507.

Case 2.13 Pruritus in End-Stage Renal Disease

Linda M. Gorman

HISTORY

Rose was an 86-year-old woman with a history of advanced heart failure, diabetes, and stage 5 chronic kidney disease (CKD). She was admitted to the hospital due to her rising creatinine and symptoms of extreme fatigue, shortness of breath, reduction in urine output, nausea, discoloration of her skin, and most recently severe itching. Rose was a recent widow with one daughter involved in her care. The nephrologist had asked the patient to consider dialysis given that she was in stage 5 CKD. The nephrologist explained that dialysis should reduce some of her symptoms, including the itching. The patient lived alone, though it had become increasingly difficult to care for herself. She had been aware for some months that dialysis would be the next step, as her condition continued to deteriorate. She was aware that dialysis would reduce some of her symptoms but dialysis three times a week would be burdensome. She had not made up her mind on whether she wanted to try dialysis. Her daughter was very supportive and assured her mother that whatever she decided the daughter would support.

Rose reported the itching covered her whole body and rated it as a 10/10 on a numerical scale. It was particularly bothersome at night and she had not slept well since the itching started one week prior to hospital admission. Her quality of life had decreased significantly since the itching began.

Case Studies in Palliative and End-of-Life Care, First Edition. Edited by Margaret L. Campbell.
© 2012 John Wiley & Sons, Inc. Published 2012 by John Wiley & Sons, Inc.

PHYSICAL EXAMINATION

Temperature: 39°C, blood pressure: 170/110, heart rate: 90, respiratory rate: 18
Central nervous system: Alert, oriented,
Head, eyes, ears, nose, throat: No defects or abnormalities
Cardiac: S1 and S2 present, no murmurs
Lungs: Distant lung sounds, diminished at bases, SPO_2 90% on room air
Genitourinary: Voiding small amounts of light colored urine
Extremities: Skin has multiple areas of redness and scratch marks, several areas on her legs are bleeding from scratching, legs with 4+ pitting edema
Psychosocial: Anxious, depressed

CLINICAL QUESTION

What treatments are available to reduce the symptom of itching for uremic patients?

DISCUSSION

Pruritus comes from the Latin word for itch. Physiological itch is the short-lived cutaneous response to the usual events of living, whereas pruritus is more closely associated with pathological itch.[1] In health care these two terms can be used interchangeably when discussing pathophysiology and they will be used interchangeably in this case. Use of the term pruritus represents the symptomatic level or quality of itch that is defined as an intense cutaneous discomfort occurring with pathological change in the skin or body and eliciting vigorous scratching. Itching is one of the most common dermatological symptoms. The itch receptors are unmyelinated brushlike nerve endings found exclusively on skin, mucous membranes, and the cornea; itching can occur with or without a rash. Scratching the itch leads to inflammation, and new nerve endings release histamine, leading to a vicious cycle of itching and scratching. Scratching leads to altered skin integrity, excoriation, redness, and infection.[2] Both pain and itch are induced by noxious stimuli and therefore are designated nociceptive.

Itching is a very common symptom in end-stage renal disease (ESRD). ESRD may also be referred to as stage 5 of chronic kidney disease (CKD). Itching in ESRD, termed uremic pruritus, is prevalent in the dialysis population as well as those with uremia, including patients discontinuing dialysis or uremic patients managed conservatively without dialysis. It is poorly understood and there are limited treatment options. Few epidemiological studies have been done on this topic, yet it impacts a large percentage of patients. Studies have found a range of frequency of this symptom, from 22% to 90% of the dialysis population.[3-5] One of the largest scale studies found 42% incidence of moderate to severe itching independent of patient age, sex, ethnicity, type of dialysis, or cause of renal disease.[6] It is generally not observed in the acute renal failure population so some nephrologists propose that it may not be related to uremia.[7] Patel suggests a better term would be CKD associated pruritus or CKD itch.[7]

When dialysis is discontinued at the end of life, pruritus may be one of the uncomfortable symptoms.[8,9] Along with pain, dyspnea, nausea, and agitation, itching impacts comfort. Germain, Cohen, and Davison note that symptoms such as pruritus, nausea, dyspnea, agitation, and twitching due to accumulation of toxins may become more troublesome in the final days of life and need to be anticipated and treated.[8] Stage 5 CKD patients managed conservatively without dialysis are also prone to itching. Murtagh et al. found it to be the third most common symptom after fatigue and pain.[10,11] Saini et al. found that quality of life and symptom burden, including itching, were similar to those of patients with terminal cancer.[12]

The presence of itching in this population affects all aspects of quality of life, particularly sleep. Itching is usually worse at night due to fewer distractions. This contributes to daytime fatigue, agitation, and depression. Because poor sleep quality may be associated with poorer outcomes for dialysis patients, pruritus must be assessed throughout the patient's treatment.[6]

A number of theories on etiology for pruritus in this population have been developed.[11,13-15] They include:

- Immune system derangement leading to an inflammatory state
- High calcium and phosphate levels leading to formation of calcium/phosphate crystals
- Abnormal afferent pain fibers related to hyperactive parathyroid hormone
- Neuropathic injury caused by uremia
- Accumulation of endorphins, perhaps related to itching after opioid administration
- Hypersensitivity to dialysate
- Inadequate dialysis
- Hypersensitive nerve fibers related to dermal histamine and cytokine release

Assessment

Itching most commonly occurs on the torso, limbs, or the whole body.[13] Often the itching occurs in large, non-dermatomal areas with striking bilateral symmetry.[5] Pisoni's group found that use of the McGill pain questionnaire to assess pruritus was reliable.[6] In addition, the Edmonton Symptom Assessment tool has been adapted for symptoms common in renal failure to include rating itching from zero to 10.[16] The Dialysis Symptom Index from the University of Pittsburgh Medical Center asks the patient to rate renal symptoms including itching and dry skin from one to five.[17–19] Assessment of itching should include the following:[6, 20]

- Duration
- Frequency
- Character
- Location
- Factors that exacerbate or relieve the symptom
- Timing of symptom (especially important in patients being dialyzed) because the symptom may be related to the effectiveness of dialysis or hypersensitivity to dialysate
- Rate itching from zero to 10
- Track effect of itching on sleep and daily activities
- Examine for dry skin, scratch marks, reddening, nodules
- Identify other possible causes besides uremia

Treatment

There is no consensus on the most effective treatment regimen for pruritus for end-stage renal disease.[21]

Skin Creams

A number of skin creams and ointments have been studied and tried by patients. The most studied include capsaicin cream (0.25%), hydrourea cream, and tacrolimus ointments.[14,22] These have shown some success. Others include emollients with high water content; they may be effective in mild uremic pruritus. Skin treatments are often continued along with the following treatments.

Ultraviolet B phototherapy

Ultraviolet B phototherapy has been used for some years with some success.[11,14,15] An ultraviolet B light lamp is set up and the patient's affected areas are exposed to the light for a short period several times a week.[11] This may be somewhat impractical and not available in all settings.

Medications

Traditionally antihistamines have been given to many patients. These have limited success, though they may help the patient to sleep.[15] Small studies have looked at ondansetron, thalidomide, and gabapentin with mixed results.[11] Gabapentin has probably had the most success and reinforces the theory of a neuropathic mechanism in uremic pruritus.[6]

Interventions should be in place to address this symptom if the patient is stopping dialysis and had itching prior to dialysis withdrawal. If itching occurs after dialysis is stopped, use of creams along with sedation may be necessary so this distressing symptom can be controlled quickly. This is not the place for trials of interventions that may not be effective.

Complementary and Alternative Medicine/Alternative Approaches

Oatmeal baths have been reported by some patients to be particularly effective. Goldenseal, which can be used as a topical poultice, has also been reported to help with pruritus.[23]

BACK TO OUR CASE

Rose was very ambivalent about starting dialysis but agreed to applications of capsaicin cream to the affected areas and diphenhydramine for the itching. The antihistamine helped the patient sleep, which improved her mood. She reported the itching was reduced to six out of 10. A trial of gabapentin was added and within three days the symptom was rated as four. Once the itching was more tolerable and she was sleeping, Rose agreed to a trial of dialysis. After two dialysis treatments, the itching reduced to a two to three and she was taken off gabapentin. The patient agreed to continue hemodialysis as long as her quality of life remained in its current state. She was seen by a palliative care team and was able to clarify her future goals and minimal acceptable outcomes for her doctors and her daughter.

TAKE AWAY POINTS

- Pruritus related to uremia is a very frequent symptom of many patients with ESRD (with and without dialysis).
- This symptom has received limited examination in the literature, so research for effective treatments are limited.
- If first line treatment of skin creams and ointments are ineffective, then a trial of ultraviolet B phototherapy and gabapentin should be tried.
- For the patient withdrawing from dialysis who has a life expectancy of a few days or a week, aggressive symptom management with sedation may be required because the other interventions may not be effective immediately.

📖 **REFERENCES**

[1] Pittelkow R, Loprinzi C. Pruritus and sweating. In: Hanks G, Cherny N, Christakis N, Fallon M, Kaasa S, Portenoy R (eds). *Oxford Textbook of Palliative Medicine*, 4th edition. New York: Oxford University Press; 2010; 934–951.

[2] Smeltzer SC, Bare BG, Hinkle JL, Cheever KH. *Brunner & Suddarth's Textbook of Medical-Surgical Nursing*, 11th *edition*. Philadelphia: Lippincott Williams & Wilkins; 2008.

[3] Jablonski A. Level of symptom relief and the need for palliative care in the hemodialysis population. *Journal of Hospice and Palliative Nursing*; 2007; 9(1):50–58.

[4] Narita I, Alchi B, Omori K, et al. Etiology and prognostic significance of severe uremic pruritus in chronic hemodialysis patients. *Kidney Int*; May 2006; 69(9):1626–1632.

[5] Mathur VS, Lindberg J, Germain M, et al. A longitudinal study of uremic pruritus in hemodialysis patients. *Clin J Am Soc Nephrol*; Aug. 2010; 5(8):1410–1419.

[6] Pisoni RL, Wikström B, Elder SJ, et al. Pruritus in haemodialysis patients: International results from the Dialysis Outcomes and Practice Patterns Study (DOPPS). *Nephrol Dial Transplant*; Dec. 2006; 21(12):3495–3505.

[7] Patel TS, Freedman BI, Yosipovitch G. An update on pruritus associated with CKD. *Am J Kidney Dis*; July 2007; 50(1):11–20.

[8] Germain MJ, Cohen LM, Davison SN. Withholding and withdrawal from dialysis: what we know about how our patients die. *Semin Dial*; May-June 2007; 20(3):195–199.

[9] Chater S, Davison SN, Germain MJ, Cohen LM. Withdrawal from dialysis: a palliative care perspective. *Clin Nephrol*; Nov. 2006; 66(5):364–372.

[10] Murtagh F, Addington-Hall J, Edmonds P, et al. Symptoms in advanced renal disease: A cross-sectional survey of symptom prevalence in stage 5 chronic kidney disease managed without dialysis. *Journal of Palliaitve Medicine*; 2007; 10(6):1266–1276.

[11] Murtagh F, Addington-Hall J, Donohoe P, Higginson I. Symptom management in patients with established renal failure managed without dialysis. *EDTNA/ERCA Journal of Renal Care*; 2006; 93–98.

[12] Saini T, Murtagh FE, Dupont PJ, McKinnon PM, Hatfield P, Saunders Y. Comparative pilot study of symptoms and quality of life in cancer patients and patients with end stage renal disease. *Palliat Med*; Sep. 2006; 20(6):631–636.

[13] Weisshaar E, Matterne U, Mettang T. How do nephrologists in haemodialysis units consider the symptom of itch? Results of a survey in Germany. *Nephrol Dial Transplant*; Apr. 2009; 24(4):1328–1330.

[14] Chambers E. Palliative medicine in end stage renal failure. In: Hanks G, Cherny N, Christakis N, Fallon M, Kaasa S, Portenoy R (eds.) *Oxford Textbook of Palliativie Medicine*, 4th edition. New York: Oxford University Press; 2010; 1280–1290.

[15] Wang H, Yosipovitch G. New insights into the pathophysiology and treatment of chronic itch in patients with end-stage renal disease, chronic liver disease, and lymphoma. *Int J Dermatol*; Jan. 2010; 49(1):1–11.

[16] Edmonton Symptom Assessment System—Northern Alberta Renal Program. kidneyeol.org/edmontonassment.pdf. Accessed March 29, 2011.

[17] Dialysis Symptom Index, University of Pittsburgh Medical Center. kidneyeol.org/DSI/pdf. Accessed March 29, 2011.

[18] Novak MJ, Sheth H, Bender FH, Fried L, Piraino B. Improvement in Pittsburgh Symptom Score index after initiation of peritoneal dialysis. *Adv Perit Dial*; 2008; 24:46–50.

[19] Weisbord SD, Fried LF, Arnold RM, et al. Development of a symptom assessment instrument for chronic hemodialysis patients: the Dialysis Symptom Index. *J Pain Symptom Manage*; Mar. 2004; 27(3):226–240.

[20] Layegh P, Mojahedi MJ, Malekshah PE, et al. Effect of oral granisetron in uremic pruritus. *Indian J Dermatol Venereol Leprol*; Jul-Aug. 2007; 73(4):231–234.

[21] Claxton RN, Blackhall L, Weisbord SD, Holley JL. Undertreatment of symptoms in patients on maintenance hemodialysis. *J Pain Symptom Manage*; Feb 2010; 39(2):211–218.

[22] Davison S, Cohen L, Germain M. Palliative and supportive care. In: Wilcox C, Berl T, Himmelfarb J, Mitch W, Murphy B, Salant D, Yu ASL (eds). *Therapy in Nephrology and Hypertension*, 3rd *edition*. Philadelphia: Saunders Elsevier; 2008.

[23] Skidmore-Roth L. *Mosby's Handbook of Herbs and Natural Supplements*, 4th edition. St Louis: Mosby Elsevier; 2010.

Case 2.14 Opioid-Induced Constipation

Grace Cullen Oligario

	HISTORY

Thomas was a 74-year-old Caucasian male with hormone-refractory prostate cancer that had metastasized to his bone. His past medical history included sarcoidosis and chronic obstructive pulmonary disease. His medications included morphine sustained release 30 mg BID, morphine immediate release (IR) 15 mg Q three hours PRN for pain, Colace® 100 mg BID, bisacodyl 5 mg daily PRN for constipation, prednisone 5 mg daily, and Taxotere® Q three weeks. His course of chemotherapy was complicated by nausea and fatigue that resulted in a reduced dosage of his chemotherapy. He was referred to gastroenterology for persistent nausea and constipation and was placed on Zofran® PRN for his nausea and Miralax® 17 gm daily for his constipation. He suffered from bone pain and declined palliative radiation. He continued to have progression of his disease on modified doses of chemotherapy. The palliative care team's assistance was requested for symptom management and goals of care discussion.

During his initial visit with palliative care, Thomas reported using one to two of his breakthrough doses of his morphine IR daily for his scattered bone pain. He also complained of occasional abdominal pain that he attributed to his constipation. He reported using his Colace® and bisacodyl as prescribed without results. He said Miralax®

Case Studies in Palliative and End-of-Life Care, First Edition. Edited by Margaret L. Campbell.
© 2012 John Wiley & Sons, Inc. Published 2012 by John Wiley & Sons, Inc.

resulted in diarrhea and had been disruptive to his daily activities. He denied changes in his diet but reported cutting down on his fluid intake due to his problem with urinary incontinence and the inconvenience it caused when he was out of his house. His wife accompanied Thomas to his visit with palliative care and she reported that his appetite had been good. She also shared her observation that he had been spending more time sleeping at home and had stopped tending to their farm.

PHYSICAL EXAMINATION

Temperature: 98.3°C, pulse: 83, respiratory rate: 20, blood pressure: 110/70, pain: 0
General: Appears comfortable
Head, eyes, ears, nose, throat: Normocephalic, non-icteric, hearing adequate bilaterally, no rhinorrhea, oral mucosa appears moist, neck supple
Respiratory: Lungs clear to auscultation throughout
Cardiovascular: S1, S2, no murmur, no peripheral edema
Abdomen: Large but soft, non-tender on palpation, normoactive bowel sounds on all quadrants
Neurologic: No focal deficits
Digital rectal exam: No rectal masses or lesions, good rectal sphincter tone, small amount of stool noted in the rectal vault, no melena

DIAGNOSTICS

An abdominal X-ray was done on Thomas after he presented to the emergency room five days later with complaints of abdominal pain and distention. It showed severe constipation with no free intra-peritoneal air or obstructive bowel gas pattern.

An abdominal X-ray is also useful in performing a constipation scoring system (Figure 2.14.1). Using the film, transecting diagonal lines that meet at the umbilicus are drawn dividing the four abdominal quadrants where the ascending, transverse, descending, and rectosigmoid colons are. The amount of stool found in each quadrant is assigned a score: zero = no stool, one = stool occupies less than 50% of the lumen, two = stool occupies more than 50% of the lumen, and three = stool completely occupies the lumen. The scores are tallied and a total of seven or more indicates a severe case of constipation that requires immediate intervention.[1]

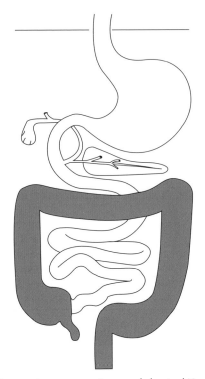

Figure 2.14.1. Constipation scoring system using an abdominal X-ray. Reprinted with permission from Alberta Health Services, Copyright 2012.

?	CLINICAL QUESTION

What interventions may prevent or eliminate constipation complicating malignancy?

✓	DISCUSSION

Etiologies of Constipation in Advanced Cancer

Conditions that have been linked to constipation in advanced cancer include:

- Metabolic disorders such as hypothyroidism, uremia, hypercalcemia, and hypokalemia
- Mechanical obstruction from the tumor
- Opioid use

- Medications such as anticholinergics, phenothiazines, antacids, and antidepressants
- Neurological lesions in cerebral tumors, cerebrovascular accident (CVA), spinal cord injury
- Immobility
- Autonomic neuropathy
- Cachexia
- Dehydration, poor oral intake
- Environmental factors such as inability to use the bathroom independently

The two most common causes found are side effects of opioid use and the sequelae of advanced disease.[2] Of patients on opioids for non-cancer pain, 15% to 90% have reported constipation. In patients with cancer, multiple causative and contributing factors have been linked to constipation such as dehydration, metabolic changes, and tumor burden, along with opioid use. It is estimated that about half of cancer patients on opioids have reported constipation along with other gastro-intestinal symptoms.[3] Opioids disrupt the normal forward propulsion of the gut wall, resulting in increased water reabsorption and longer stool transit time, which leads to harder and drier stool that is harder to pass. Opioid receptor activation also results in hormonal, molecular, and neuronal changes that inhibit intestinal secretions.[4]

Assessment

Patient Report

Common Tools

The Rome Criteria for constipation is used to diagnose functional constipation, which comprises about 30% of the total cases of constipation. It consists of the following diagnostic criteria that must have been present in the past three months and at least six months before diagnosis:

1. Must have two or more of the following conditions met:
    a. Straining during at least 25% of defecations
    b. Lumpy or hard stools in at least 25% of defecations
    c. Sensation of anorectal blockage or obstruction during at least 25% of defecations
    d. Sensation of incompletely evacuating following at least 25% of defecations
    e. Use of manual maneuvers to facilitate at least 25% of defecations
    f. Fewer than three defecations in a week
2. Rare presence of loose stools without laxative use
3. Criteria for irritable bowel syndrome is insufficiently met[3]

Constipation in patients with advanced disease tends to be accompanied by other symptoms. The use of opioids contributes to constipation by slowing down forward peristalsis and decreasing gastric secretions and intestinal fluid re-absorption.[5] There is an inverse relationship between the incidence of constipation and simultaneously prescribing a laxative with opioid therapy.[6]

Assessment for constipation is typically based on a patient's subjective report alone, whereas evaluation for effectiveness of therapies is derived from objective evaluation. Because constipation typically consists of a number of signs and symptoms, both a subjective and objective approach should be taken in diagnosing and post treatment re-evaluation.[7] The patient's abdomen may be distended on inspection. It typically has hypoactive bowel sounds on auscultation. On palpation, the abdomen may be firm and tenderness may or may not be present. Deep palpation may reveal a "sausage-like" mass. Rectal exam may show stool in the rectal vault.[8]

Treatment

Laxatives are commonly used to treat constipation (Table 2.14.1). Detergent laxatives, also known as stool softeners, work by promoting increased gastric secretions and intestinal fluid re-absorption; they usually become effective in one to three days. Stool softeners are typically not helpful in end-of-life care due to the patient's poor fluid intake and slowed gastric motility from inactivity and opioid use. Stimulant

TABLE 2.14.1. Drugs commonly used to manage constipation.

Drug	Dose	Rationale for use	Maximum recommended dose
Docusate	100 mg BID	Stool softener	500 mg in divided doses/day
Sennosides	8.6 mg, 2 tablets daily	Stimulant	12 tablets/day in divided doses
Bisacodyl	5-mg tablet every day	Stimulant	6 tablets/day in divided doses
Sorbitol	70 gm/100 ml, 15 ml BID	Osmotic	Can be titrated until results are obtained
Lactulose	10 gm/15 ml, 15 ml BID	Osmotic	Can be titrated until results are obtained
Polyethylene glycol	17 gm packet, 1 daily	Osmotic	Titrated to effect; fecal impaction, up to 8 packets/day
Methylnaltrexone	0.15 to 0.30 mg/kg subcutaneously	Reverses delayed cecal transit time	Titrated to effect

Thomas JR, Von Gunten CF. Management of constipation in patients with cancer. *Supportive Cancer Therapy.* 2004; 2(1):50. Reprinted from Pereira & Bruera, 2001, with permission from the Alberta Cancer Board.

laxatives promote peristalsis and fluid reabsorption, usually in six to 12 hours, but are associated with side effects that include abdominal cramping and pain. Sennosides and bisacodyl are among the most commonly used stimulant laxatives.[9] The combination of sennosides and docusate has not been shown to improve laxation or minimize the side effects associated with the use of sennosides alone.[10] Osmotic laxatives work by promoting fluid retention, resulting in improved peristalsis and softer stools with effectiveness usually apparent in one to two days. Potential side effects include electrolyte imbalance, abdominal cramping and distention, diarrhea, and flatulence. Sorbitol, lactulose, and polyethylene glycol are among the laxatives under this classification.[9]

Methylnaltrexone, a selective peripheral opioid receptor antagonist, has been found to reverse the delayed cecal-transit time caused by opioids. It does not affect the central nervous system and does not cause reversal of analgesia or opioid withdrawal. It is able to induce laxation within four hours when administered at doses ranging from 0.15 to 0.30 mg/kg subcutaneously.[11]

Regular exercise, including participation in physical therapy, helps prevent constipation and improves patients' quality of life but may not be an option when the patient is dying.[12] A diet high in fiber and fluids helps prevent constipation. Prune juice works as a natural stimulant laxative.[13]

Causative factors of constipation also can be modified. Electrolyte imbalances such as hypercalcemia, hyponatremia, and hypokalemia have been associated with constipation and can be corrected by supplementation or medications. The patient may be on medications besides opioids that can cause constipation. Consideration can be given to changing or discontinuing these medications if not contraindicated for the patient's condition. Among these medications are taxanes, anticholinergics, diuretics, and antidepressants. The use of transdermal opiates has been shown to result in less severe constipation than their oral counterparts but are associated with higher costs.

Allowing for privacy and providing supplies such as bedpans, bedside commodes, canes, walkers, or wheelchairs are helpful to a patient who has impaired mobility. It is helpful to involve the patient when creating a plan for their bowel care because they may have their own routines that are altered by a change in their environment such as hospitalization.[14]

Strategies under Investigation

Bifidobacterium and fructoligosaccharide, which are found in symbiotic yogurt, have been shown to improve constipation. Botulinum toxin, which has been used to treat chronic, refractory constipation in children, is being evaluated for effectiveness in treating adult constipation.[15] Prucalopride is currently only approved for use in Europe; it comes under the brand name Resolor®. It is used to treat chronic constipation for which laxatives have been ineffective. Prucalopride is a 5-HT4 receptor agonist and works by binding to the 5-HT4 receptors in the gastrointestinal tract to stimulate peristalsis. In three main European studies involving 1,999 patients, Resolor® was found to be 24% effective in treating constipation among patients compared to only 11% of patients who received a placebo.[16] Sacral nerve stimulation is also an emerging strategy.[15]

BACK TO OUR CASE

Thomas' Colace® and bisacodyl were discontinued. He was started on sennosides at two tablets BID and Miralax® 17 gm daily, as needed for constipation. His sennosides had to be increased to four tablets BID for better bowel regulation. He continued to consume inadequate amounts of fluid on days that he had to leave the house for appointments. He reported inconsistent use of his sennosides for fear of having diarrhea when he was running errands. He continued to have episodes of constipation every three to five days that was relieved by Miralax®.

TAKE AWAY POINTS

- Constipation can be a very distressing symptom and, unfortunately, very common.
- Prevention is key in handling constipation.
- Assessment plays a very important role in identifying constipation and its severity. This is also an opportunity to identify causative factors that can be eliminated or modified.
- Management of constipation should be tailored based on individual needs and may require a multi-modality approach.
- Involving patients in creating a plan for their care is very helpful because everyone's bowel habits are unique.

REFERENCES

[1] Dalal S, Del Fabbro E, Bruera E. Symptom control in palliative care—part I: Oncology as a paradigmatic example. *Journal of Palliative Medicine*; 2006; 9(2):395–396.
[2] Panchal SJ, Muller-Schwefe P, Wurzelmann, JI. Opioid-induced bowel dysfunction: Prevalence, pathophysiology and burden. *Int Journal of Clinical Practice*; 2007; 61:1181–1187.

[3] Stevens AM, Riley J. Managing and treating opioid-induced constipation in patients with cancer. *Gastrointestinal Nursing*; 2008; 6(9):16.

[4] Clark K, Urban K, Currow DC. Current approaches to diagnosing and managing constipation in advanced cancer and palliative care. *Journal of Palliative Medicine*; 2010; 13(4):473–474.

[5] Myotoku M, Nakanishi A, Kanematsu M, et al. Reduction of opioid side effects by prophylactic measures of palliative care team may result in improved quality of life. *Journal of Palliative Medicine*; 2010; 13(4):401.

[6] Lewicky-Gaupp C, Morgan DM, Chey WD, Meullerlie P, Fenner DE. Successful physical therapy for constipation related to puborectalis dyssnergia improves symptom severity and quality of life. *The ASCRS Textbook of Colon and Rectal Surgery.* 2008; 51:1686–1691.

[7] Noguera A, Centeno C, Librada S, Nabal M. Screening for constipation in palliative care patients. *Journal of Palliative Medicine*; 2009; 12(10):918–919.

[8] Ferrell BR, Coyle N. *Oxford Textbook of Palliative Nursing.* New York: Oxford University Press, Inc; 2010.

[9] Thomas JR, Cooney GA. Palliative care and pain: New strategies for managing opioid bowel dysfunction. *Journal of Palliative Medicine*; 2008; 11(1)(suppl):S7–S10.

[10] Hawley PH, Byeon JJ. A comparison of sennosides-based bowel protocols with and without docusate in hospitalized patients with cancer. *Journal of Palliative Medicine*; 2008; 11(4):575.

[11] Thomas J, Karver S, et al. Methylnaltrexone for opioid-induced constipation in advanced illness. *N Engl J Med*; 2008; 358:2332–2343.

[12] Thomas J. Optimizing opioid management in palliative care. *Journal of Palliative Medicine*; 2007; 10(suppl):S13.

[13] Benson AB, Stein R. *Cancer and Drug Discovery Development: Supportive Care in Cancer Therapy.* Totowa, NJ: Ettinger; 2009.

[14] Norlander L. *To Comfort Always. A Nurse's Guide to End-of-Life Care.* Indianapolis, IN: Sigma Theta Tau International; 2008.

[15] Kappor S. Management of constipation in the elderly: emerging therapeutics. *World Journal of Gastroenterology*; 2008; 14(33):5226–5227.

[16] http://www.ema.europa.eu/ema/index.jsp?curl=pages/medicines/human/medicines/001012. Accessed August 2, 2011.

Case 2.15 Depression in Advanced Disease

Todd Hultman

HISTORY

Henry was a 64-year-old African-American man with a history of Type 2 diabetes, dilated nonischemic cardiomyopathy (New York Heart Association [NYHA] class III/IV, ejection fraction [EF] 20%), and chronic renal insufficiency. He was status post placement of an implantable cardioverter defibrillator. He had refused hemodialysis on multiple occasions. Prior to this hospital admission for multiple falls he had been hospitalized for an exacerbation of heart failure.

Henry had lived at home prior to hospitalization for approximately four weeks, with cardiac home support that involved home telemetry for weight and blood pressure and regular calls from a heart failure nurse. He lived with his girlfriend and her two daughters. Prior to accessing disability money, he worked as an adult caregiver for handicapped adults. He reported no hobbies or sources of enjoyment. He denied any spiritual practice, claiming rebellion against his family for forcing him to go to church at a younger age.

Prior to hospital admission he was functionally independent, ambulating short distances outside and requiring no assistance for activities of daily living. At hospital admission he was limited to household distances with a rolling walker and assistance with washing and dressing; he had polyarthralgia from osteoarthritis. He reported feeling overwhelmed with managing his multiple disease processes and that he feared dying.

Case Studies in Palliative and End-of-Life Care, First Edition. Edited by Margaret L. Campbell.
© 2012 John Wiley & Sons, Inc. Published 2012 by John Wiley & Sons, Inc.

PHYSICAL EXAMINATION

Temperature: 96.7°F, blood pressure: 84/50, heart rate: 78, respiratory rate: 20

General: Frail male who appears older than stated age, lying in bed, alert and engaged, in no apparent distress

Head, eyes, ears, nose throat: Pupils equal, round, reactive to light, and accommodating, sclera clear; edentia, dry oropharynx

Cardiovascular: Regular rate and rhythm; S1, S2 with III/VI systolic murmur; extremities with 1+ edema and warm

Respiratory: Nonlabored, clear and diminished at bases, SpO_2 97% on room air

Gastrointestinal: Mildly distended, bowel sounds present, soft, nontender

Musculoskeletal: No deformities, tender right shoulder and bilateral knees

Skin: Without rash, poor turgor

Neurologic: Cranial nerves II to XII grossly intact, fine tremor in upper extremities

Neuropsychiatric: Oriented to person, place, and time, flat affect, adequate attention and concentration

DIAGNOSTICS

Drawn on admission: Blood urea nitrogen: 48, creatinine: 2.03, white blood count: 8.1, hematocrit: 33.4%, hemoglobin: 10.4

? CLINICAL QUESTION

What treatments may reduce depression associated with advanced heart failure?

✓ DISCUSSION

Depression in Cardiac Disease

Depression is one of the more common psychiatric diagnoses found in patients receiving palliative care.[1] While it is an ambiguous term, depression is a mood disorder that has an adverse effect on a person's ability to function at work, home, or school. For such patients, psychiatric illness almost always occurs in the context of other co-morbid advanced diseases. In the instance of heart failure, the prevalence of patients who meet diagnostic criteria for depression approaches 20%.[2] Much of the process for assessing and treating depression in patients with advanced disease is extrapolated from the general population. However, these co-morbid conditions are critical to consider because they shape both the assessment and intervention of the psychiatric illness, in this case, depression in the context of heart failure. Management of depression is critical given the implications for clinical outcomes related to disease management such as medication adherence, disease progression, and quality of life.[2,3]

Assessment

It is the standard of practice that all patients receiving palliative care be screened for psychiatric illness.[4] The simplest screening tool for depression is to ask the patient "are you feeling depressed?".[1] All positive responses warrant a follow-up. The conclusion that the patient has a good reason to be depressed does not justify failure to follow through with further investigation and treatment.[5]

When assessing a patient for depression beyond screening, the patient's co-morbid conditions shape the assessment process. Neuro-vegetative symptoms associated with depression such as anorexia, insomnia, psychomotor changes, and fatigue may be related to the disease process, in this case heart failure.[6] Therefore, when assessing for depression, the clinician should rely on the cognitive and affective components of depression. The components include feeling depressed, loss of interest in pleasurable activities, feelings of worthlessness, changes in ability to concentrate or think, and recurrent thoughts of death or suicidal ideation.[7]

The patient needs a full physical examination to rule out other sources of neuro-vegetative symptoms. Insomnia and poorly managed symptoms, especially pain, have been linked to a depressed mood.[8,9] The plan of care for depression must include aggressively intervening in these symptoms directly.[5]

A review of the patient's medication regimen is also warranted. Many medications necessary to manage advanced diseases have depressive-like side effects. For example, beta-blockers are linked to fatigue, insomnia, lethargy, decreased libido; alpha-blockers are linked to depressed mood; and thiazide diuretics have fatigue, weakness, and anorexia as known side effects.[10]

There are standardized self-report instruments for assessing depression. These instruments are not standardized for patients with advanced disease. Results must be extrapolated from the study populations. Recommended instruments include the Hospital Anxiety and

Depression Scale (HADS), Geriatric Depression Scale (GDS), and Beck Depression Inventory (BDI).[5] These instruments have adequate reliability and validity and do not require significant effort to complete.

Anhedonia means having no pleasurable activities in life; a report of anhedonia is as significant as a report of depressed mood when considering a diagnosis of depression.[7] Likewise, a patient report of insomnia and fatigue along with a sense of hopelessness are consistent with depression.

Treatment

Pharmacological interventions have emerged as first-line therapy for patients with major depression. When prescribing antidepressants it is important to consider the side effect profile and the context of advance disease states. Tricyclic antidepressants have served as the first line of treatment of depression for the general population for decades. In the context of cardiac disease, the side effect of orthostatic hypotension and the risk of QTc prolongation, with the chance of fatal cardiac arrhythmia such as torsades de pointe, preclude their use.[10]

Selective serotonin reuptake inhibitors, such as sertraline, have shown little to no cardiac side effects.[10] Newer drugs such as duloxetine, mirtazapine, venlafaxine, and bupropion have shown small increases in blood pressure, but not to the degree that they are considered contraindicated in heart disease. When considering selection of medication, it is useful to capitalize on known common side effects. For patients who also complain of insomnia in the context of depression, mirtazapine, with its sedation, may prove beneficial. Bupropion, well known for stimulation, may benefit patients who complain of feelings of fatigue. Duloxetine and venlafaxine have both shown varying degrees of success as adjuvant medication of pain involving neuropathy.[11,12] Any of this class of drugs are indicated for patients who have a prognosis of greater than two months. This indication is based on the time of onset of benefit.

Psychostimulants such as methylphenidate may be used with patients who have an estimated survival of less than two months. This medication has proven to be effective in supporting relief of mood disorders while also relieving fatigue and apathy.[13] Given stimulation as a common side effect, it should be used cautiously if at all in patients with risk of developing tachycardia or atrial fibrillation, often a concern for patients with advanced cardiac disease.

Sometimes prescribing an antidepressant medication is not indicated given the complex interplay of psychiatric illness, advanced disease, and medication regimen. There is longstanding evidence for the benefit of cognitive behavioral therapies for patients with depression. These therapies may also be used with cardiac patients.[14] Such interventions, which correct maladaptive beliefs and inaccurate information processing that are linked to depression, may be as effective as pharmacologic strategies.[15] No one cognitive behavioral therapy stands as superior to others.[5] However, such therapies are not indicated for use in patients who are in psychological crisis, such as when the patient is hospitalized in an acute care setting. Cognitive behavioral therapies may also be used in tandem with medications for a robust effect.

Although not specifically developed for the treatment of depression, dignity therapy has shown promise in ameliorating many of the affective and cognitive components of depression in patients with advanced diseases.[14] The purpose of dignity therapy is to allow patients to create meaning out of their experiences with their disease while promoting purpose, dignity, and quality of life.[16] Dignity therapy has the added benefit of contributing to family well being because the outcome of the patient's work can be shared with them during their time of bereavement.[17]

There are often psychological concerns that occur in tandem with depression in patients with advanced disease. As with psychiatric illness, it is the standard of practice to intervene in these issues. The distress from the loss of functional status or fears of distressing symptoms such as dyspnea in heart failure may be particularly frightening to patients.[3,5] Dignity therapy may also be used to address these concerns as they occur in the context of advanced disease.[16]

Beyond individual therapeutic interventions such as talk-based therapies, group therapies, in which the patient may establish a social network, have also increased the success of treatment plans for the management of the psychologic distress related to advanced disease.[18] Such support groups, when disease focused, may be better at ameliorating anxiety and psychologic distress rather than depression. To reduce depression, consider support groups that target the specific disease.[9]

Little work has been developed to provide support to family caregivers who care for patients with depression and advanced disease. The trajectory of diseases such as heart failure, with its radical and often unpredictable changes in the patient, including unexpected death, provide caregivers with significant challenges.[19] The addition of a co-morbid psychiatric illness can exacerbate any distress or fatigue the caregiver may experience. Given that the family is the unit of service in palliative care and that the standard of practice is to address all salient social concerns of the patient, any intervention in the management of depression must include an assessment of the family's experience of caregiving and the development of a plan of care that also meets their needs.[20,4]

BACK TO OUR CASE

In the case of Henry, the interview and exam showed ongoing arthralgia that required opioids for management. Henry reported having no pleasurable activities in his life, a condition known as anhedonia. Exacerbating his depression was a sense of existential distress related to his purported atheism. He feared dying secondary to fear of nothingness.

A medication review found diuretics were contributing to his sense of fatigue, but were necessary to manage his heart failure. As he endorsed anhedonia along with insomnia that was considered secondary to his cardiac disease, the decision was made to start mirtazapine. Given that mirtazapine also has an anxiolytic effect, it was also hoped that it would help Henry reduce some of his anxiety secondary to his existential distress. He was offered cognitive behavioral therapy on an outpatient basis when he came to see his cardiologist; he refused. Because he had no professed spiritual practice, he was also not open to spiritual support for his existential concerns. Supportive counseling was offered to Henry's girlfriend and her two daughters, which they accepted.

! TAKE AWAY POINTS

- All patients receiving palliative care must be screened for depression.
- Depression must be treated when identified.
- Assessment of depression in advanced disease should focus on cognitive and affective components.
- Rational selection of medication should capitalize on known side effects of the selected drug.
- Nonpharmacologic strategies should be incorporated in the plan of care when appropriate.

REFERENCES

[1] Block S. Psychological issues in end-of-life care. *Journal of Palliative Medicine*; 2006; 9(3):751–772.
[2] Rutledge T, Reis V, Linke SE, Greenberg, BH, Mills PJ. Depression in heart failure: A meta-analytic review of prevalence, intervention effects and associations with clinical outcomes. *Journal of the American College of Cardiology*; 2006; 48(8):1527–1537.
[3] Hallas CN, Wray J, Andreou P, Banner N. Depression and perceptions about heart failure predict quality of life in patients with advanced heart failure. *Heart & Lung*; 2011; 40:111–121.
[4] National Quality Forum. *A National Framework and Preferred Practices for Palliative and Hospice Care Quality*. Washington, DC: Author. 2006.
[5] Hultman TD, Reder EAK, Dahlin C. Improving psychological and psychiatric aspects of palliative care: The National Consensus Project for Palliative and Hospice Care. *Omega: Journal of Death and Dying*; 2008; 57(4):323–339.

[6] Miller M, Massie MJ. Depression and anxiety. *The Cancer Journal*; 2006; 12:388–397.

[7] American Psychiatric Association. *Diagnostic and Statistical Manual of Mental Disorders*, Revised 4th edition. Washington, DC: Author. 2000.

[8] Bolge SC, Joish VN, Balkrishnan R, Kanna H, Drake CL. Burden of chronic sleep maintenance insomnia characterized by nighttime awakenings among anxiety and depression sufferers: Results of a national survey. *Journal of Clinical Psychiatry*; 2010; 12(2);pii: PCC09m00824.

[9] Olaya-Contreras P, Persson T, Styf J. Comparison between Beck Depression Inventory and psychiatric evaluation of distress in patients on long-term sick leave due to chronic musculoskeletal pain. *Journal of Multidisciplinary Healthcare*; 2010; 3:161–167.

[10] Levenson JL. Psychiatric issues in heart disease. *Primary Psychiatry*; 2006; 13(7):29–32.

[11] Lunn MPT, Hughes RAC, Wiffen PJ. Duloxetine for treating painful neuropathy or chronic pain. *Cochrane Database of Systemic Reviews*. 2009; 4:Art. No.:CD007115. DOI: 0.1002/14651858.CD007115.pub2.

[12] Bradley RH, Barkin RL, Jerome J, DeYoung K, Dodge CW. Efficacy of venlafaxine for long term treatment of chronic pain with associated major depressive disorder. *American Journal of Therapeutics*; 2003; 10:318–323.

[13] Hardy SE. Methylphenidate for treatment of depressive symptoms, apathy, and fatigue in medically ill older adults and terminally ill adults. *American Journal of Geriatric Pharmacotherapy*; 2009; 7(1):34–59.

[14] Lorenz KA, Lynn J, Dy SM, et al. Evidence for improving palliative care at end of life: A systematic review. *Annals of Internal Medicine*; 2008; 148(2):147–159.

[15] Driessen E, Hollon SD. Cognitive behavioral therapy for mood disorders: Efficacy, moderators and mediators. *Psychiatric Clinics of North America*; 2010; 33:537–555.

[16] Chochinov HM, Kristjanson LJ, Hack TF, Hassard T, McClement S, Harlos M. Dignity therapy in the terminally ill: Revisited. *Journal of Palliative Medicine*; 2006; 9:666–672.

[17] McClement S, Chochinov HM, Hack T, Hassard T, Kristjanson LJ, Harlos M. Dignity therapy: Family member perspectives. *Journal of Palliative Medicine*; 2007; 10:1076–1082.

[18] Song Y, Lindquist R, Windenburg D, Cairns B, Thakur A. Review of outcomes of cardiac support groups after cardiac events. *Western Journal of Nursing Research*; 2011; 33:published online.

[19] Penrod J, Hupcey JE, Baney BL, Loeb SJ. End-of-life caregiving trajectories. *Clinical Nursing Research*; 2011; 20:published online.

[20] National Consensus Project for Quality Palliative Care. *Clinical Practice Guidelines for Quality Palliative Care, 2nd edition*. Pittsburgh, PA: Author; 2009.

Case 2.16 Treating Anxiety

Darrell Owens

HISTORY

Ann was a 56-year-old Caucasian woman with metastatic pancreatic cancer who was being seen in the palliative care clinic for follow-up on her cancer-associated pain. Ann had been followed in the palliative care clinic since her diagnosis two years prior. She was initially referred to the clinic for pain and symptom management while undergoing active treatment. Shortly after diagnosis she underwent a Whipple procedure, as well as concurrent chemotherapy and radiation therapy. She successfully completed all initial therapies, but approximately one year later, a routine post treatment CT showed evidence of recurrence with a new liver mass.

Unfortunately, Ann was misinformed by the radiation oncologist that her repeat CT did not show any further evidence of disease. Approximately two weeks later at a follow-up appointment with her medical oncologist, she was given the correct information which was that her disease was metastatic, news that she reported "blindsided" her. Immediately following her oncology appointment she began to experience insomnia, increased irritability with health care providers and her husband, and difficulty concentrating. These symptoms were in addition to worsening abdominal pain, nausea, and fatigue.

After three months of having hospice recommended by her nurse practitioner, Ann was admitted to a home hospice program. Her overall physical and psychological symptom burden fluctuated from day to

Case Studies in Palliative and End-of-Life Care, First Edition. Edited by Margaret L. Campbell.
© 2012 John Wiley & Sons, Inc. Published 2012 by John Wiley & Sons, Inc.

day, as did her overall symptom distress level. She reported that she was feeling more irritable, which she described as "everyone makes me angry." She also reported ongoing insomnia despite the use of medication, and that it was difficult for her to focus on reading books or the daily newspaper, two activities that she had always enjoyed. Ann reported that her physical pain was well controlled on methadone and that she had not experienced nausea or vomiting for several weeks. She endorsed significant fatigue and anorexia. When asked to describe how she thought she was doing, Ann responded that she believed she would die soon. She also expressed concern that her son, with whom she had no contact in five years because of a falling out over her drug usage, was planning on a visit. Additional issues included the fact that she had been reflecting back over her life, and had informed her nurse practitioner that "she did not like what she saw."

Review of Systems

Constitutional: Denied fever, chills, night sweats; reported insomnia—difficulty falling and remaining asleep

Edmonton Symptom Assessment Scale (modified): Pain at present: none, pain (over the past three days): mild, localized to abdomen, characterized as a dull, squeezing ache; unable to identify any aggravating or alleviating factors

Pain control: Acceptable

Activity level: Not active

Nausea: Not nauseated

Level of constipation: None

Last bowel movement: Today

Feelings of depression: Moderately depressed

Feelings of anxiety: Very anxious

Level of fatigue: Very fatigued

Appetite: Poor

Shortness of breath: Mild when walking stairs in apartment

PHYSICAL EXAMINATION

Temperature: 37.6°C, blood pressure: 104/58, heart rate: 88, respiratory rate: 14

General: Poorly groomed, cachectic woman in moderate emotional distress

Head, eyes, ears, nose, throat: Temporal wasting; poor dentition; pupils equal, round, reactive to light

Respiratory: Without increased work of breathing, lungs clear to auscultation bilaterally

Cardiac: Regular rate and rhythm, S1, S2, without murmurs, gallops, or rubs

Abdomen: Positive bowel sounds, soft, non-distended, painful to light palpation

Neurologic: Alert, oriented, speech clear and coherent, able to participate in discussion, recent and remote memory intact

Psychiatric: Affect ranges from tearful to anger

DIAGNOSTICS

No diagnostic studies were conducted during this visit

CLINICAL QUESTION

What treatments may reduce anxiety associated with cancer?

DISCUSSION

Natural History of Anxiety in Palliative Care

Anxiety, which is classified as a mood disorder, is defined as a normal human response to a threat that is real or perceived and is often a natural consequence of receiving a life-limiting diagnosis.[1,2] Mood disorders, which include both anxiety and depression, are the most commonly diagnosed psychiatric illnesses. In palliative care patients depression coexists with physical symptoms approximately 25% of the time. See Case 2.15 for a comprehensive discussion of depression. The exact prevalence of anxiety in this patient population is unknown, because it is commonly under diagnosed and subsequently under-treated.[3] It is believed that anxiety is either not diagnosed or not documented in the medical record in approximately 50% of patients receiving palliative care.[4]

Although anxiety has been studied less than depression, it is thought to be a common occurrence in patients receiving palliative care. In a study conducted by Delgado-Guay and colleagues, 44% of patients experienced anxiety. These findings were consistent with other studies that found anxiety was present in approximately 30% (range 11% to 62%) of patients in their last one to three weeks of life.[5] Anxiety in terminally ill patients can be associated with many factors including anorexia, depression, dyspnea, receiving inadequate information, and young adulthood. It occurs in children and adults, as well as in partners and relatives.[4]

It is common for anxiety to increase as one's illness progresses. Like inflammation, anxiety has a purpose, and is often considered the psychic equivalent of pain.[6] Anxiety has the ability to activate the sympathetic nervous system, specifically the fight or flight response. It can be constructive and beneficial, stimulating patients to adapt to a variety of circumstances and restore homeostasis.[6] In patients with a life-limiting illness, there are also times when anxiety, by activating the sympathetic nervous system and the subsequent fight or flight response, can prevent patients from participating in treatments or seeking care, which can place them at risk for significant harm.[6]

Etiologies of Anxiety in Palliative Care

Anxiety in patients receiving palliative care has many etiologies, and may arise from physical, psychological/emotional, social, or spiritual issues. In some patients anxiety may be a component of a preexisting primary psychiatric illness such as post traumatic stress disorder, affective disorder, or a generalized anxiety disorder.[5–7]

Potential physical causes of anxiety include pain and/or other distressing symptoms common in the patient, e.g., dyspnea, nausea, anorexia, and fatigue.[2,8] Organic diseases such as those involving the thyroid and parathyroid glands, as well as those of the central nervous system, have been identified as causes of both acute and chronic anxiety. Other common etiologies of acute anxiety include sepsis, hypoxia, and multi-system organ failure.[6,7] Medications, especially in the elder population, also have the potential to cause anxiety. Some common offenders include corticosteroids, benzodiazepines, opioids, and respiratory stimulants.[6–8]

There are also many potential psychological, emotional, and social etiologies of anxiety in patients receiving palliative care. People with life-limiting illness, and their families, experience multiple anxiety-producing issues as their disease progresses. Some of these may include experiencing a loss of control, self-esteem, and/or independence, as well as a loss of identity related to family and career roles. Other potential anxiety-provoking issues include a lack of information, or as noted in our case study, misinformation about one's condition, treatment options, and prognosis.[7]

Spiritual or existential issues also have the potential to cause anxiety. The inability to find meaning in one's life, illness, and death can cause tremendous anxiety, as can unresolved issues or unanswered questions regarding the afterlife. Guilt and blame associated with one's illness, such as might be seen in a smoker who developed lung cancer, are also potential causes of anxiety.

Assessment

Patients experiencing anxiety may report a number of symptoms. While some may be able to directly articulate that they are feeling anxious or worried, and subsequently rate their level of anxiety, others need a skilled provider who is familiar with common assessment findings, both subjective and objective. Common subjective findings of anxiety include reports of insomnia, irritability, inability to concentrate, and decreased ability to deal with or solve problems.[7,9] Patients may express that they are afraid, with or without a particular source, that they are unable to stop ruminating about a particular topic, or that they perceive a nonthreatening situation as a threat, e.g., discussion of advance care planning.[4]

The physical or objective findings associated with anxiety represent the body's response to psychological stressors. As the physical findings increase, the patient's functional abilities decrease. While functional ability in progressive disease is expected, a thorough assessment is indicated to assure that the decline is not related to undiagnosed anxiety.[7] The most common objective findings are trembling, tension, restlessness, diaphoresis, cold hands, nausea, diarrhea, palpitations, and tachycardia.[4,7]

There are a plethora of validated tools available for the assessment of anxiety. The Edmonton Symptom Assessment System (also referred to as the Edmonton Symptom Assessment Scale) is widely used in palliative care. While reliability for this tool has been well-established, emotional symptoms such as depression and anxiety are poorly captured.[10] For hospitalized patients the Hospital Anxiety and Depression Scale is frequently cited as a reliable tool.[5,11,12] Other assessment tools include the Memorial Symptom Assessment Scale, the Beck Anxiety Inventory, and the Generalized Anxiety Disorder Anxiety Tool (GAD-7). Regardless of the tool selected, it is important that the provider be competent with the administration and interpretation of the results.

Anxiety Treatment

It is important to note that most patients experience some degree of anxiety during the course of their illness. The majority of them do not require medical or pharmacological intervention, because they respond well to support and reassurance from family, friends, and health care providers.[8] Several different studies have identified the usefulness and non-usefulness of a formal palliative care consultation in the alleviation of anxiety, an intervention that is in need of more study.[13] As with any symptom, the first step to selecting an appropriate therapy is a good assessment. This is especially important with anxiety, because an accurate assessment may enable providers to identify contributing factors, such as misinformation that can then be immediately treated with education.

When treating anxiety, nonpharmcological interventions should always be considered first. Supportive measures such as encouraging patients to share their thoughts, feelings, hopes, and fears, as well as providing education and information through an open dialogue, is often all the therapy needed. A specific goal of supportive measures is to help patients identify anxiety triggers and then assist them with reframing those triggers to ones that do not provoke anxiety.[4] This reframing process is commonly referred to as cognitive behavioral therapy. Similar interventions include guided imagery, distraction, and relaxation.

For patients in whom supportive measures are ineffective, the addition of medication may be indicated.[13] Pharmacotherapy may provide the patient with the ability to tolerate supportive measures. Medication should always be considered complementary to supportive measures when treating anxiety.[6,13] Prior to the initiation of pharmacotherapy, it is important to assess for depression, which can be exacerbated by the use of anti-anxiety medications. For patients with symptoms of both anxiety and depression who have a prognosis that will allow them to experience the benefits of therapy, it is recommended that antidepressant medications be started first.[7] In patients who are without symptoms of depression, or for whom antidepressant therapy is ineffective, benzodiazepines are considered first-line therapy.[6-7,13-14]

Benzodiazepines are reported to be more effective in the treatment of anxiety than antidepressants, beta-blockers, or buspirone. They are considered the most effective medications in the treatment of both generalized and anticipatory anxiety.[6] Benzodiazepines are not without side effects and patients, especially the elderly, should be carefully monitored for confusion, memory and concentration impairment, somnolence, and delirium. Because many palliative care patients may have compromised renal and hepatic function, the most appropriate prescribing pattern is to start low and titrate slowly.

Short-acting benzodiazepines such as lorazepam for generalized anxiety and temazepam for sleep are more appropriate for patients with hepatic impairment because they are metabolized via conjugation and contain no active metabolites.[13] Lorazepam is considered first-line therapy in most settings due to its shorter half-life and lower side effect profile.[7] The usual starting dose is 0.5 mg to 1 mg PO TID to QID. The usual insomnia dose of temazepam is 30 mg PO at HS.[7] Clonazepam, which has a longer half-life and more mood-stabilizing effects, can be dosed less frequently while providing consistent relief.[13] Benzodiazepines can be administered via a variety of routes including oral, intranasal, intravenous, intramuscular, subcutaneous, rectal, and sublingual. Patients who have been receiving benzodiazepines for a prolonged period of time require a taper, because abrupt discontinuation can precipitate withdrawal symptoms.

There are several complementary and alternative medical (CAM) therapies available for the treatment of anxiety. Unfortunately, studies supporting their use in anxiety management are lacking. Several studies regarding the use of music therapy have been conducted, including a

2008 randomized controlled trial that demonstrated it was effective at reducing anxiety levels as measured by the Edmonton Symptom Assessment Scale.[9] CAM therapies that have been used in the treatment of anxiety include acupuncture, massage, hypnosis, and aroma therapy.[4] Their use in the treatment of anxiety, as well as other common symptoms in palliative care, is in need of further research.

BACK TO OUR CASE

Ann's nurse practitioner diagnosed her with anxiety and initiated therapy with lorazepam 1 mg PO every six hours PRN. After approximately one week she reported that she was taking four to six mg per day, that her sleep had improved, and that she was feeling less anxious and irritable. Her nurse practitioner added clonazepam 2 mg PO BID to her regimen, at which time her PRN usage of lorazepam decreased to 1 to 2 mg several times per week.

Despite improvement in her anxiety, Ann continued to report feelings of sadness, hopelessness, helplessness, and anhedonia. Her nurse practitioner diagnosed her with depression. The hospice team initiated weekly counseling visits from the social worker and chaplain, and based on her prognosis of greater than six weeks, a selective serotonin reuptake inhibitor was added to her medication regimen. Approximately four weeks later Ann reported that her overall mood was significantly better, that she had "reconnected" with her son, and that she was back to reading almost daily.

TAKE AWAY POINTS

- Anxiety is one of the most common mood disorders diagnosed in patients receiving palliative care.
- Anxiety is not diagnosed by health care providers in approximately 50% of patients who experience it.
- Anxiety and depression often coexist.
- Anxiety management includes both supportive and pharmacological therapies.

REFERENCES

[1] Emanuel L, Librach S. *Palliative Care Core Skills and Clinical Competencies.* Philadelphia: Saunders Elsevier; 2007.
[2] Rosenblatt L, Block S. UpToDate. In: Basow D (ed). *UpToDate.* Waltham, MA: UptoDate; 2011.

[3] Delgado-Guay M, Parsons HA, Li Z, Palmer JL, Bruera E. Symptom distress in advanced cancer patients with anxiety and depression in the palliative care setting. *Support Care Cancer*; 2009; 17:573–579.

[4] Dean M, Harris J-D, Regnard C. *Symptom Relief in Palliative Care*, 2nd edition. New York: Radcliffe Publishing; 2011.

[5] Teunissen SCCM, de Graeff A, Voest EE, de Haes JCJM. Are anxiety and depressed mood related to physical symptom burden? A study in hospitalized advanced cancer patients. *Palliative Medicine*; 2007; 21:341–346.

[6] MacLeod A. *The Psychiatry of Palliative Medicine: The Dying Mind*. New York: Radcliffe Publishing; 2007.

[7] Kinzbrunner B, Policzer J, eds. *End-of-Life Care: A Practical Guide*, 2nd edition. New York: McGraw-Hill; 2011.

[8] Bruera E, Higginson IJ, Ripamonti C, Gunten CV, eds. *Textbook of Palliative Medicine*. London: Hodder Arnold; 2006.

[9] Horne-Thompson A, Grocke D. The effect of music therapy on anxiety in patients who are terminally ill. *Journal of Palliative Medicine*; 2008; 11:582–590.

[10] Richardson LA, Jones GW. A review of the reliability and validity of the Edmonton Symptom Assessment System. *Curr Oncol*; 2009; 16:55.

[11] Mitchell AJ, Meader N, Symonds P. Diagnostic validity of the Hospital Anxiety and Depression Scale (HADS) in cancer and palliative settings: A meta-analysis. *Journal of Affective Disorders*; 2010; 126:335–348.

[12] Wilson KG, Chochinov HM, Skirko MG, et al. Depression and anxiety disorders in palliative cancer care. *J Pain Symptom Manage*; 2007; 33:118–129.

[13] Roth AJ, Massie MJ. Anxiety and its management in advanced cancer. *Curr Opin Support Palliat Care*; 2007; 1:50–56.

[14] Mystakidou K, Rosenfeld B, Parpa E, et al. Desire for death near the end of life: the role of depression, anxiety and pain. *General Hospital Psychiatry*; 2005; 27:258–262.

Case 2.17 Terminal Secretions

Terri L. Maxwell

HISTORY

Charles was a 64-year-old African-American male who was diagnosed with a glioblastoma two years prior to his death. After undergoing surgery, radiation, and chemotherapy, Charles' cancer was in remission until his tumor recurred. Despite a trial of experimental chemotherapy his disease continued to progress. A week prior to death, despite titrating doses of steroids, his symptoms worsened and he fell when trying to get out of bed. He became progressively more lethargic and confused, spending most of his time in a hospital bed set up in his living room. Respecting Charles' wishes to die at home, his family enrolled him in hospice.

Charles's condition rapidly deteriorated. He was not eating or drinking and he was difficult to arouse. Although he appeared comfortable, his breathing had slowed and he was making a gurgling sound with each breath. His wife and five adult children and extended family gathered around his bedside. They were upset about the noisy breathing and they asked the hospice nurse to please do something to prevent Charles from choking.

PHYSICAL EXAMINATION

Temperature: 37.5°C, blood pressure: 90/60, heart rate: 102, respiratory rate: 8 and irregular

---

Case Studies in Palliative and End-of-Life Care, First Edition. Edited by Margaret L. Campbell.
© 2012 John Wiley & Sons, Inc. Published 2012 by John Wiley & Sons, Inc.

Central nervous system: Obtunded

Head, eyes, ears, nose, throat: Tongue dry and coated, lips dry and slightly cracked, no other abnormalities

Cardiac: S1, S2 and tachycardia

Lungs: Coarse rhonchi throughout all quadrants, no wheezing or accessory muscle use, SpO_2 93% on room air

Gastrointestinal: Soft, nontender abdomen, normal bowel sounds

Genitourninary: Voiding concentrated amounts of urine into catheter bag attached to a condom

Extremities: 1+ lower extremity edema, heels slightly reddened, no pressure ulcers

DIAGNOSTICS

N/A

CLINICAL QUESTION

What causes noisy breathing and how can it be effectively managed?

DISCUSSION

Terminal secretions commonly occur during the final days or hours of a patient's life. The prevalence of terminal secretions varies widely, but it is estimated that it occurs in approximately 75% of patients in the final two days of life.[1-7] Patients with lung or brain malignancies, or those who have a prolonged dying phase, are at increased risk to develop terminal secretions.[1,6,7] Patients with conditions known to inhibit swallowing reflexes, such as head and neck or esophageal cancers, or those with neurodegenerative processes are also more likely to develop terminal secretions.[9]

Secretions accumulate in the lungs or oropharynx when the patient loses consciousness or is too weak to clear his own saliva or mucous. Excessive secretions in dying patients may also be a result of infection, pulmonary edema, and/or fluid overload. Air passing through or over these secretions during inspiration and expiration results in a noisy, rattling sound, which led to the term "death rattle."[1]

Terminal secretions are categorized as either type 1 or type 2, based upon their primary source.[1] Type 1 secretions (oropharyngeal) are due

TABLE 2.17.1. Death rattle intensity scale.[3]

0 = Not audible
1 = Only audible near patient
2 = Clearly audible at the end of the patient's bed in a quiet room
3 = Clearly audible at the door of a quiet room

Back IN, Jenkins K, Blower A, Beckhelling J. A study comparing hyoscine hydrobromide and glycopyrrolate in the treatment of death rattle. *Palliat Med;* July 2001; 15(4):329–336.

to the accumulation of and inability to clear saliva, whereas type 2 secretions (pseudo death rattle) primarily result from the accumulation of bronchial secretions caused by an underlying respiratory problem such as pulmonary edema, heart failure, or infection.[1] These subtypes were proposed to identify whether a patient's secretions were likely to respond to anticholinergic therapy. However, these subtypes have never been validated in a clinical study, and many patients may experience a combination of the two.

Terminal secretions may contribute to symptoms such as dyspnea, restlessness, and insomnia;[1,8] however, the majority of patients experiencing terminal secretions have a low level of awareness, so they usually are not distressed. However, the presence of secretions and associated sounds may upset caregivers.[9] Whereas some family members view the development of secretions as a helpful sign of impending death,[9] others believe that secretions are causing their loved one to choke or drown.[10] Because family members vary in their interpretations of and responses to terminal secretions, it is important to explain the cause and provide reassurance that their loved one is not suffering.[9,10]

Assessment

Standard assessment tools are rarely used in clinical practice to quantify or describe terminal secretions, and patients are usually not responsive enough to self report. Table 2.17.1 illustrates an example of a tool that can be used to score/quantify death rattle intensity.[3] The clinician should also assess the patient's ventilatory rate and breathing pattern and evaluate for signs of agitation, restlessness, or discomfort. The clinician can try to differentiate "real" death rattle from "pseudo" death rattle by auscultating the throat and chest to identify the regions most affected. The family can be asked when the secretions began and if they are continuous or intermittent. Because initiating therapy may be at the request of the family, the clinician may inquire how the symptom is affecting them and what they think is causing the problem. Lastly, the family's comfort goal should be identified.

Treatment

Nonpharmacological

Nonpharmacological interventions such as repositioning and decreasing fluids should be considered first line in the management of terminal secretions. Repositioning the patient to lateral recumbency with the head slightly raised may encourage drainage and decrease pooling of secretions. Hydration (parenteral or tube feedings) may contribute to pulmonary edema in frail, dying patients, which may worsen noisy breathing.[11] The family should be counseled to reduce fluid intake and discontinue or decrease parenteral fluids. Suctioning is not recommended except in instances where fulminate pulmonary edema is present.[11] Terminal secretions are usually inaccessible to suction and the procedure may result in additional discomfort to the patient and/or the volume is so small that suctioning is disproportionately burdensome.

Pharmacological

Anticholinergic agents are commonly used to reduce saliva and mucous production. They are less likely to be effective when secretions are of a pulmonary origin. Although anticholinergic agents inhibit secretion production, they do not have an effect on secretions that are already present.[3,6,11] For that reason, if anticholinergic therapy is indicated, an agent such as atropine that has a fast onset of action should be initiated at the first sign of congestion.

Well-controlled studies demonstrating the superiority of one anticholinergic over another are lacking,[12] and the response rate to anticholinergics varies greatly.[1-7,11] Therefore, selection of an agent should be based on its onset of action, duration of action, route of administration, adverse effect profile, and cost. Salivary (type 1) secretions are thought to be more likely to respond to anticholinergic therapy compared to bronchial (type 2) secretions.[11,13] A possible explanation for this difference is that bronchial secretions take longer to accumulate to a clinically noticeable volume.[3,11,14] Prophylactic treatment with anticholinergic therapy in high-risk patients may improve outcomes, but more research is needed to support this theory.[6] Because the use of anticholinergics may produce significant side effects, such as dry mouth, blurred vision, and constipation, among others, their benefits and burdens should be carefully considered, and for some patients, nonpharmacological options may be more appropriate.

Atropine, scopolamine, glycopyrrolate, and hyoscyamine are the most commonly used anticholinergics to treat terminal secretions. Atropine may be administered by oral (PO), intramuscular (IM), intravenous (IV), or subcutaneous (SC) routes at a starting dose of 0.4 mg every four to six hours as needed.[14-16] Atropine 1% eye drops may be given orally to the back of the throat or sublingually to reduce secretions.[16] The initial recommended dose for the oral administration of eye drops is one to two drops every four to six hours as needed.[16] Compared to other anticholinergics, atropine is the most cost effective agent for treating terminal secretions; however, similar to other medications in its class, it may produce unpleasant side effects.

Scopolamine may be administered by PO, IM, IV, and SC routes. Oral therapy is initiated at a starting dose of 0.4 mg every eight hours as needed, whereas parenteral dosage forms are initiated at a starting dose of 0.4 mg every four hours as needed. Scopolamine is also available as a transdermal patch, which is changed every 72 hours. There is limited evidence to support the application of more than one patch. The patch may take up to 12 hours for effect, making it a poor choice for actively dying patients.[8,12]

Glycopyrrolate may be administered by PO, IM, IV, and SC routes. The recommended parenteral starting dose is 0.2 to 0.4 mg three to four times daily as needed.[3] Oral glycopyrrolate, in the form of tablets or liquid, has slow, erratic absorption and usually requires higher starting doses, around 1 to 2 mg two to three times daily as needed for effect.[16]

Hyoscyamine is most commonly administered PO or SL. It is available as an immediate-release disintegrating tablet and oral liquid and as a sustained-release tablet/capsule. An injectable form also may be given IV, IM, or SC. The recommended starting dose for immediate-release oral and parenteral formulations is 0.125 to 0.25 mg every four hours as needed.[13] Use of hyoscyamine for terminal secretions is purely anecdotal and based on its anticholinergic mechanism of action.[14,15]

While anticholinergic medications may help to effectively manage some secretions, it is important to weigh the risks of potential side effects against the potential benefits. Elderly patients are particularly sensitive to side effects from anticholinergics. However, during the terminal phase of a patient's life when the patient is less responsive, the potential benefit of the drugs in reducing secretions and easing respirations may outweigh the burden of side effects.

BACK TO OUR CASE

Upon hearing Charles' family's concerns about the noisy breathing, the nurse explained why this was happening and reassured them that although the sound was disturbing, it was not causing direct distress to Charles. The family agreed that Charles looked peaceful, but they hated the sound. The nurse elevated the head of the bed to promote drainage and explained that suctioning would not likely be beneficial and may cause discomfort. Instead, the nurse obtained an order for atropine 1% ophthalmic drops 0.4 mg and administered them every four hours. The nurse explained that the medication will not work immediately, but would help to prevent additional accumulation of secretions. In addition, the nurse and nurse's aide provided frequent mouth care. Over time, the noisy breathing lessened and Charles passed peacefully with his family at his bedside.

! TAKE AWAY POINTS

- Terminal secretions occur in a large number of dying patients and are a strong predictor of impending death, generally present in the last 48 hours.
- Terminal respiratory secretions can be, but are not always, a source of distress to relatives. Providing education and reassurance about the cause and management of secretions may help relieve caregiver distress.
- Salivary secretions are more likely to respond to anticholinergic therapy than bronchial secretions (pseudo death rattle).
- When indicated, anticholinergic agents should be initiated as soon as congestion appears.
- There is no conclusive evidence that one anticholinergic agent is more effective than the others; selection should be guided by desired route of administration and cost.
- Consider the risk vs. benefit before starting anticholinergic therapy, especially in the elderly.
- Further comparative clinical trials and evidence-based guidelines are needed.

📖 REFERENCES

[1] Bennett MI. Death rattle: An audit of hyoscine (scopolamine) use and review of management. *J Pain Symptom Manage*; Oct. 1996; 12(4):229–233.
[2] Wildiers H, Menten J. Death rattle: Prevalence, prevention and treatment. *J Pain Symptom Manage*; 2002; 23(4):310–317.
[3] Back IN, Jenkins K, Blower A, Beckhelling J. A study comparing hyoscine hydrobromide and glycopyrrolate in the treatment of death rattle. *Palliat Med*; July 2001; 15(4):329–336.
[4] Hugel H, Ellershaw J, Gambles M. Respiratory tract secretions in the dying patient: A comparison between glycopyrronium and hyoscine hydrobromide. *J Palliat Med*; Apr. 2006; 9(2):279–284.
[5] Hughes A, Wilcock A, Corcoran R, Lucas V, King A. Audit of three anti-muscarinic drugs for managing retained secretions. *Palliat Med*; May 2000; 14(3):221–222.

[6] Kass RM, Ellershaw J. Respiratory tract secretions in the dying patient: A retrospective study. *J Pain Symptom Manage*; Oct. 2003; 26(4):897–902.

[7] Morita T, Tsunoda J, Inoue S, Chihara S. Risk factors for death rattle in terminally ill cancer patients: a prospective exploratory study. *Palliat Med*; Jan. 2000; 14(1):19–23.

[8] Spiller JA, Fallon M. The use of Scopoderm in palliative care. *Hosp Med*; 2000; 61(11):782–784.

[9] Wee BL, Coleman PG, Hillier R, Holgate SH. The sound of death rattle I: Are relatives distressed by hearing this sound? *Palliat Med*; 2006; 20(3):171–175.

[10] Wee BL, Coleman PG, Hillier R, Holgate SH. The sound of death rattle II: How do relatives interpret the sound? *Palliat Med*; 2006; 20(3):177–181.

[11] Clark K, Butler M. Noisy respiratory secretions at the end of life. *Current Opinion in Supportive & Palliative Care*; 2009; 3(2):120–124.

[12] Wee B, Hillier R. Interventions for noisy breathing in patients near to death. *Cochrane Database of Systematic Reviews*. 2008; 16.

[13] Bennett M, Lucas V, Brennan M, Hughes A, O'Donnell V, Wee B. Using anti-muscarinic drugs in the management of death rattle: Evidence-based guidelines for palliative care. *Palliat Med*; 2002; 16(5):369–374.

[14] Owens DA. Management of upper airway secretions at the end of life. *J Hosp Palliat Nurs*; 2006; 8(1):12–14.

[15] De Simone GG, Eisenchlas JH, Junin M, Pereyra F, Brizuela R. Atropine drops for drooling: A randomized controlled trial. *Palliat Med*; Oct. 2006; 20(7):665–671.

[16] Olsen AK, Sjogren P. Oral glycopyrrolate alleviates drooling in a patient with tongue cancer. *J Pain Symptom Manage*; Oct. 1999; 18(4):300–303.

Case 2.18 Fungating Wounds and the Palliative Care Patient

Laura C. Harmon

HISTORY

June was a 55-year-old woman with a significant medical history for uncontrolled hypertension, chronic kidney disease stage 3, and squamous cell carcinoma of the neck of unknown primary etiology status post tracheosotomy and percutaneous endoscopic gastrostomy (PEG) tube. June presented to the emergency department complaining of intermittent bleeding from the tracheostomy during suctioning. June stated that the bleeding had been present for one day prior to admission accompanied by fever, chills, fatigue, weight loss, and greenish sputum that was malodorous. June verbalized that she first noticed the neck mass that was initially the size of a golf ball, and within a few months the mass had increased to the size of a grapefruit, subsequently occluding her airway.

Excisional biopsy and tumor debulking was planned under general anesthesia with oral intubation; however, complications with intubation necessitated an emergent tracheostomy status post excisional biopsy of a 9- × 10-cm necrotic mass that revealed poorly differentiated invasive squamous cell carcinoma (Figure 2.18.1). A computed tomography (CT) scan of the chest with contrast revealed a 0.8 × 1.5-cm soft tissue density in the right apical lung, two or more nodules in the left lung, lytic lesions on the right 10th rib and first through fifth rib along with a 4.8-cm mass on the left ovary.

Case Studies in Palliative and End-of-Life Care, First Edition. Edited by Margaret L. Campbell.
© 2012 John Wiley & Sons, Inc. Published 2012 by John Wiley & Sons, Inc.

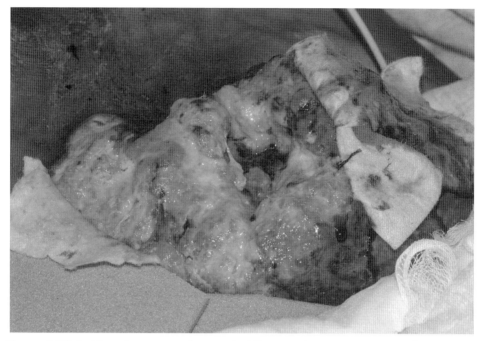

Figure 2.18.1. Necrotic mass revealing poorly differentiated invasive squamous cell carcinoma.

 PHYSICAL EXAMINATION

Temperature: 39.1°C, blood pressure: 146/70, heart rate: 120, respiratory rate: 24

Central nervous system: Alert and oriented, no focal deficits noted

Head, eyes, ears, nose, throat: Pupils equal, round, reactive to light and accommodation; extraocular movements intact, tracheostomy; neck with left sided fungating wound 5 × 6 × 4 cm; tissue bed 100% tan/brown, thick, moist, malodorous necrotic tissue, draining copious amounts of serous exudate; peri-skin macerated; pain 8/10 to touch and upon dressing changes

Cardiac: S1, S2/tachycardia, no S3, S4/murmurs noted

Respiratory: Breath sounds clear to auscultation anterior and posterior diminished bilateral bases, SpO₂ 98% on 28% humidified supplemental oxygen

Gastrointestinal: Positive bowel sounds, abdomen soft, nontender, nondistended with PEG tube left quadrant

Genitourinary: Independent voiding

Musculoskeletal: Ambulatory, moves all extremities, strength 5/5 upper and lower, no deformities

Integument: Skin warm and dry, no lesions or rashes

DIAGNOSTICS

White blood count: 15.2, red blood count: 2.61, hemoglobin: 8.0, hematocrit: 25.4%, platelets: 112,000, sodium: 141, potassium: 4.5, chloride: 109, CO_2: 26, anion gap: 13, glucose: 102, blood urea nitrogen: 35, creatinine: 1.3, calcium: 11.2

Chest X-ray: Left basilar consolidation and pleural effusion, right lung is clear, no pneumothorax on either side, no cardiomegaly; hila are normal, no evidence of heart failure; clinical correlation with CT scan recommended

CT thorax: Demonstrated tumor invasion into the pectoralis major muscle and periosteum of the ribs with multiple bilateral necrotic and cavitating pulmonary nodules, suspicious for metastases; differential includes septic emboli, but given the other findings metastases seems more likely; moderate to large left-sided pleural effusion with pleural metastasis; mediastinal lymphadenopathy.

? CLINICAL QUESTION

What are the treatment options for terminally ill patients with a malignant fungating wound?

✓ DISCUSSION

Fungating wounds are also known as malignant wounds, cutaneous malignancies, malignant cutaneous ulcers, or tumor necrosis. Fungating malignant wounds are one of the most devastating wound entities that patients must deal with. The wounds present a great challenge to the patient, their families, and caregivers for a multitude of reasons such as malodor, exudate, pain, and bleeding.[1] Malignant wounds are said to be a rare complication of cancer that usually signifies terminal disease and affects all dimensions of a patient's existence: physical, psychological, social, and spiritual.[1]

Fungating malignant wounds are caused by malignant cells that invade skin tissue and, if left untreated, will progressively invade and destroy adjacent areas.[2] Of patients with metastatic disease, 5% to 10% experience skin involvement that occurs during the last six to 12 months of life.[3] Sixty-two percent of malignant fungating wounds (MFW) originate from breast cancer, followed by head and neck 24%, genital and back 3%, and cancers of other areas 8%.[4]

The first phase of development occurs from a primary skin cancer that has been left untreated over a period of time such as skin tumors that are identified as squamous or basal cell carcinomas or malignant melanomas. The primary tumor has the ability to invade up into and through the skin.[4] A tumor that invades blood or lymph vessels has the potential for metastatic spread to the skin due to the presence of small capillaries which can trap circulating malignant cells. Tumor spread might also occur along tissue planes or via implantation or seeding of malignant cells during surgery.[4] The first sign of skin involvement is usually the development of discreet nontender skin nodules. The nodules may be skin-tone, pink, violet/blue, or black/brown in color and are a result of tumor cell proliferation within the structures of the skin.[4]

As malignant cells grow and divide, the nodules enlarge and start to interfere with local skin capillaries and lymph vessels. The growing tumor commonly has a disorganized micro-circulation and impaired blood clotting. This combination of features leads to poor skin perfusion, tissue hypoxia, and subsequently tissue death. The development of necrotic tissue in a fungating wound can be a significant problem due to aerobic and anaerobic organisms that thrive in non-viable tissue leading to progressive tissue destruction.[5]

Edema and malodor, which are additional characteristics of fungating wounds, occur when fatty acids that are released as a metabolic end product accumulate, creating stagnant exudate and thus odor.[5] Fungating wounds may appear as craters or nodules and contain multiple nodules with macerated, inflamed, and/or blistered peri-wound skin; hence, the name fungating because they often have a cauliflower-like appearance.[6]

Assessment

Every malignant wound is unique, not only in appearance but also in the presenting symptoms, with some patients having multiple symptoms and others having few.[4] Patients may present at an early stage or only when metastatic disease is evident, with diagnosis based on histological assessment.[7] Therefore, a comprehensive assessment is important, because malignant wounds are unique in presentation, multifactorial, difficult to treat, and capable of impacting dramatically on the patient's quality of life as well as the lives of those caring for them.[7]

All domains of the patient's illness experience, not just the wound, are explored and entail a detailed review of the patient's past medical history, social support systems, coping ability, and disease impact on her life and that of her family. Additionally, evaluation of nutritional status, ability to self-care, and psychosocial issues such as depression, body image, and sexuality are all discussed.[7] Facilitation of open communication with the patient is essential and sets the stage for the creation of an effective plan of care.[2] It is useful to begin the assessment by asking the patient about what aspect of the wound is most disturbing.[2] Care is then targeted toward the areas of most concern to the patient and family while maximizing the effects of the intervention.

In a qualitative study patients with malignant fungating wounds were interviewed to obtain an understanding of what an MFW means to cancer patients and how it influences their lives.[3] Five patient-centered themes were identified: declining physical well-being, wound-related stigma, need for expert help, strategies in wound management, and living positively with the wound.

Treatment

Management of fungating wounds is based upon achieving the objectives of symptom control and patient comfort rather than wound healing. Due to the terminal prognosis and poor healing potential for patients with malignant fungating wounds, wound healing may be an unrealistic goal in the setting of palliative care, whereas quality of life should be emphasized.[6]

Treatment options for patients with fungating wounds are aimed at treating the underlying pathology when appropriate, while simultaneously maintaining congruence with the goals and objectives identified during the physical and psychosocial assessment.[5] The choice of treatment depends on the type of cancer, the site and size of the tumor, how advanced the tumor is, the severity of symptoms, and patient choice.[5]

Commonly used therapies that may appear curative in nature are actually used to control symptoms; they include tracheostomy as a primary treatment modality or when therapy-resistant dyspnea occurs for the patient with a head or neck cancer.[8] These therapies may include PEG placement when dysphagia and/or aspiration ensue, radiotherapy to reduce tumor size, chemotherapy for tumor reduction, hormonal therapy to slow tumor growth in certain cancers such as breast and prostate, and finally surgery to remove the tumor, which is not always possible or desirable due to location or the risk of hemorrhage.[9]

When traditional cancer fighting treatments to control symptoms are not possible or are ineffective, then symptom control becomes paramount. Four main symptom management principles have been identified for patients with fungating wounds: management of excessive exudate production, control of wound odor, prevention and control of wound infection, and control of bleeding.[5]

Malodor associated with a malignant wound is often described by patients as the one symptom that causes the greatest amount of distress. Odor can be effectively controlled once the bacterial bioburden within the wound is reduced by eliminating necrotic devitalized tissue that is the source of the foul odor, either surgically or chemically.[6] However, it must be emphasized that use of debridement must be tailored to each patient's specific needs. For example, mechanical debridement may be contraindicated if the tissue within the wound is friable and bleeds easily because mechanical debridement is a non-selective therapy. Patients who are neutropenic or immunosuppressed do not benefit from debridement using autolysis, which is disintegration or liquefaction of tissue or cells by the body's own mechanisms, due to insufficient leukocytes and the increased production of exudate. Finally, in some situations removal of necrotic eschar could reveal or damage underlying structures; in this case, the eschar is maintained because it functions as a protective covering.[6]

Antimicrobial therapy with metronidazole 500 mg crushed to a powder consistency or metronidazole gel 0.75% applied to the wound bed can be effective in neutralizing wound odor, which may be due to the presence of necrotic or infected wound tissue. Additional odor-fighting therapies include activated charcoal as a primary or secondary dressing or silver-impregnated dressings that exist as a hydrofiber, giving the added benefit of odor and exudate control.[10]

Malignant fungating wounds can produce large amounts of exudate, sometimes in excess of a liter/day, making control of drainage exceedingly important. Reducing the amount of exudate produced by the wound decreases malodor; it is important to prevent soiling of bedding and clothing, thereby improving patient confidence and comfort.[3] Malignant wounds are often dressed with two or more layers. Ideally, the primary layer should be non-adherent, conformable, and capable of venting excess moisture to the secondary layer while allowing for atraumatic removal. The secondary layer should be highly absorbent and aesthetically acceptable; however, despite advances in wound management and the complex anatomic locations of fungating wounds, there is still no ideal dressing product available in the sizes or configurations required for these wounds.[2] Additionally, most dressing products are designed in accordance with the theory of moist wound healing for acute wounds and are not appropriate for fungating wounds, which are chronic in nature and excessively moist. As a result of the lack of appropriate dressing products and the complexity of malignant wounds, the nurse's creativity often becomes the major factor influencing the success of a dressing regimen in conjunction with a wound, ostomy and continence consultation.[2]

Dressing options consist of hydrocolloids for low exudate producing wounds, hydrofibers and foam for moderate to copiously draining wounds (i.e., Aquacel®), a high-absorbency dressing or calcium alginates (i.e., Kaltostat®, which provides haemostatic properties for control of bleeding), or foam non-border (a non-adhering dressing that can be used as a primary layer).[11]

Wound drainage pouches are another creative idea to consider for heavily exudative wounds that are characterized by dressing changes that are required more than two to three times per day, peri-skin deterioration secondary to maceration or skin stripping from tape removal, hampered mobility, or uncontrolled odor.[6] Pouching systems have many desirable features that make them a worthwhile option to consider due to their ability to provide collection of exudate and containment of malodor. Pouches come in various sizes and configurations ranging from systems with attached skin barriers, flexible adhesive surfaces, access windows for application of topical therapies, as well as drain spouts that allow the patient to attach the pouch to a nighttime drainage system so that fluid does not pool over the wound and potentially cause leakage.[4]

Control of pain is another key component that must be addressed when caring for patients with complex wounds. Caregivers must understand that pain is experienced differently by each patient. The physical sensation of pain in malignant wounds may be caused by a number of factors, such as pressure from the invading tumor, damage to surrounding nerves, exposure of dermal nerve endings, recurrent infections, swelling resulting from impaired lymphatic drainage, malodor causing nausea and vomiting, as well as the wound care procedure itself.[4]

It is important to remember that pain is not just physical; it is a combination of the lived experience of physical, psychological, social, and spiritual. Psychological factors such as anger, fear, anxiety, and depression can affect the experience of pain. To effectively intervene, a comprehensive pain assessment that identifies the type, severity, frequency, and duration of pain is completed. The goal is analgesia and topical non-adhering dressings that will do no harm. Administering analgesia on a scheduled basis with sustained-released oral morphine as well as short-acting analgesia before dressing changes is appropriate and effective. [6]

When malignant fungating wounds fail to respond to traditional standards of combination therapy such as radical surgery, radiotherapy, chemotherapy, and/or topical considerations and patient quality of life is at stake, additional investigational strategies should be considered. Very few level 1 randomized controlled trials have been conducted; thus, the majority of supporting evidence comes from case studies and theoretical papers. Support from this level of evidence can be found for the use of topical opioid drugs, such as diamorphine, combined with hydrogel for pain that does not respond to conventional analgesia or in combination with topical therapy. Diamorphine is mixed with hydrogel, which is a cross-linked polymer gel that is non-adherent, can be removed without trauma from the wound bed, and has the ability to provide moisture and debride necrotic tissue while simultaneously providing a soothing effect to the inflamed friable wound. The mixture of diamorphine and hydrogel is applied directly to the wound surface and covered with a non-adhering, absorbent secondary-layer dressing. The morphine concentration is a 1 to 1 mixture; 1 mg morphine to 1 gram of hydrogel. Metronidazole is another carrier option that can be used in conjunction with morphine to attain pain and odor control.[11]

Care of the terminally ill patient with a malignant fungating wound presents a myriad of challenges for the patient who not only must face the fact that life will be coming to an end, but must face it on a daily basis due to the complexity of the wound that is a never-ending reminder of her mortality. To create an effective patient-centered plan of care, staff must understand that the emphasis is on relieving suffering, maintaining function, and enabling patients to engage in activities that are important to them.[5]

BACK TO OUR CASE

June elected to change her goals of therapy to a comfort care focus with palliative wound care. The goals of June's wound care were to manage excessive exudate production, control wound odor, and prevent and control wound infection and bleeding. Metronidazole 500 mg tablets crushed to a powder consistency were applied to the wound bed with each dressing change to neutralize odor. The wound was then dressed with a non-adhering dressing made of fine mesh gauze lightly impregnated with Vaseline®. The fine mesh allowed drainage of wound exudate to the secondary dressing while the Vaseline® provided atraumatic removal. The additional dressings applied to the wound bed for exudate control consisted of calcium alginate, a heavy fiber dressing made from seaweed. Calcium alginates have the dual function of providing hemostasis in the event the friable wound bed began to bleed vs. absorption of moderate to heavy exudate. The calcium alginate was then covered with semi-permeable foam such as soft polyurethane dressing sheets to maximize absorption and prevent strikethrough, which was an important concern for June. The entire dressing was secured with a net tube dressing such as Surgilast®, which makes dressing changes less traumatic for the patient due to the absence of tape, which can cause skin striping and is very painful. With this regimen June achieved satisfactory wound management and pain and odor control prior to her discharge home with hospice. The hospice anticipated having a wound specialist as part of June's interdisciplinary hospice team.

TAKE AWAY POINTS

- Treat the underlying pathology when appropriate.
- Maintain congruence with the goals and objectives identified during the physical and psychosocial assessment.
- Treatment depends upon type of cancer, site, size, severity of tumor, and symptoms.

REFERENCES

[1] Alexander S. Malignant fungating wounds: epidemiology, aetiology, presentation and assessment. *Journal of Wound Care*; 2009; 18(7):273–280.

[2] Goldberg MT, McGinn-Byer P. Oncology-related skin damage. In: Bryant RA (ed). *Acute and Chronic Wounds*, third edition. St. Louis: Mosby. 2007; 374–379.

[3] Lo S, Hu W, Chang S, Hsu M, Wu L. Experiences of living with a malignant fungating wound: a qualitative study. *Journal of Clinical Nursing*; 2008; 17:2699–2708.

[4] Naylor W. Malignant wounds: aetiology and principles of management. *Nursing Standard*; 2002; 16(52):45–56.

[5] Alexander S. Malignant fungating wounds: managing malodor and exudate. *Journal of Wound Care*; 2009; 18(9):374–382.

[6] Naylor W. A guide to wound management in palliative care. *International Journal of Palliative Nursing*; 2005; 11(11):572–579.

[7] Collier M. The assessment of patients with malignant fungating wounds— a holistic approach: part 1. *Nursing Times*; 1997; 93(44):1–4.

[8] Sesterhenn A, Folz B, Bieker M, Teymoortash T, Werner J. End of life care for terminal head and neck cancer patients. *Cancer Nursing*; 2008; 31(2):40–46.

[9] Alexander S. Malignant fungating wounds: Key symptoms and psychosocial. *Journal of Wound Care*; 2009; 18(8):325–329.

[10] Benbow M. Fungating malignant wounds and their management. *Journal of Community Nursing*; 2009; 23(11):12–18.

[11] Grocott P. Care of patients with fungating malignant wounds. *Nursing Standard*; 2007; 21(24):57–66.

Case 2.19 Pressure Ulcer Care in Palliative Care

Laura C. Harmon

HISTORY

Theresa was an 82-year-old woman who presented to the hospital from her long-term care facility for work-up and treatment of altered mental status, fever, and failure to thrive. Her past medical history was significant for dementia, Alzheimer's type, type II diabetes mellitus, hypertension, and chronic kidney disease stage 4. On admission to the hospital she was awake and lethargic and unable to verbalize or follow simple commands. Per the nursing home, at baseline the patient was bed-bound and able to verbalize and respond to simple commands. However, for the weeks prior to hospital admission, the staff noticed a steady decline in Theresa's appetite with a decrease in mental status and a fever spike the day before admission to 39°C.

On evaluation in the emergency department, lab analysis identified a leukocytosis with an abnormal urinalysis. A CT of the head for altered mental status identified a right hemorrhagic lesion, calcified mass, and cerebral edema with midline shift and hydrocephalus. An MRI of the brain demonstrated four peripheral ring enhancing masses with intra-tumoral hemorrhage. The largest tumor was in the right frontal lobe causing a subfalcine herniation with a 0.9-cm midline shift to the left causing compression of the ventricles. The findings represented brain metastasis, primary site unknown.

Case Studies in Palliative and End-of-Life Care, First Edition. Edited by Margaret L. Campbell.
© 2012 John Wiley & Sons, Inc. Published 2012 by John Wiley & Sons, Inc.

PHYSICAL EXAMINATION

Temperature: 38.7°C, blood pressure: 170/86, heart rate: 60, respiratory rate: 20

Central nervous system: Patient awake and lethargic, unable to verbalize or respond to simple commands; moans and groans with movement

Head, eyes, ears, nose, throat: Head normocephalic, pupils equal, round, reactive to light, extraocular movements intact, neck supple, no jugular vein distention

Cardiac: S1, S2, regular, no S3, S4 or murmurs noted

Respiratory: Breath sounds clear to auscultation, nonlabored on room air, SpO$_2$ 95% on room air

Gastrointestinal/genitourinary: Hypoactive bowel sounds, abdomen soft, with pain on palpation right upper quadrant, voiding incontinent with diaper use

Musculoskeletal: Moves all extremities weakly and intermittently; strength 3/3 upper and lower

Integumentary: Skin warm and dry with positive pedal pulses, bilateral lower extremities with multiple areas of skin alteration:

- Left inner knee ulcer, stage 3, 10×9.5×2.5 cm. Wound is 60% pink tissue with 40% tan, moist slough; peri-skin intact, draining a large amount of purulent exudate with malodor.
- Left heel ulcer unstageable, 8×6 cm with 90% black, hard, stable eschar and 10% visible pink tissue
- Right heel ulcer unstageable 10×7 cm with 80% black hard, stable eschar and 20% pink tissue
- Left lateral foot 9×2 cm healed with intact re-surfaced skin, pigmented
- Left posterior leg ulcer unstageable, 15×3 cm total; wound comprised of 100% black, hard, stable eschar with intact peri-skin
- Sacral ulcer stage 3, with 80% pink non-granulating tissue and 20% moist, tan slough with intact peri-skin, moderate serosanguinous exudate with malodor.

DIAGNOSTICS

CT head: Right hemorrhagic lesion, calcified mass, and cerebral edema with midline shift and hydrocephalus

MRI: Four peripheral ring enhancing masses with intratumoral hemorrhage

?	**CLINICAL QUESTION**

What is the appropriate management for terminally ill patients with chronic pressure ulcers when comfort is the focus of care?

✓	**DISCUSSION**

The Wound Ostomy and Continence Society defines pressure ulcer development as a localized area of injury to the skin and/or underlying tissue usually over a bony prominence, as a result of pressure, or pressure in combination with shear and/or friction.[1] In today's health care arena, clinicians are caring for an increasing number of patients that are living longer with a number of co-morbid conditions that place them at risk for the development of pressure-related skin injuries. The prevalence of pressure ulcers in health care facilities has been on the rise for a number of years with pressure ulcer incidence rates varying considerably by clinical setting.[2]

Pressure ulcer prevalence (the percentage of patients with pressure ulcers at any one point in time) in acute care is estimated to be about 15%, while incidence (the rate at which new cases occur in a population over a given time period) is estimated to be about 7%.[2] Prevalence rates range from 2.2% to 23.9% in long-term care, and 0% to 17% in home care with an astronomical 2.5 million patients/year requiring pressure ulcer treatment at a cost as high as $70,000 for the management of a single full-thickness pressure ulcer; the total cost for treatment of pressure ulcers in the U.S. is estimated at $11 billion/year.[3]

Etiology

The development of a pressure ulcer is a devastating and complex physical outcome secondary to serious illness that can cause considerable harm to patients, hindering their functional recovery due to pain, lack of mobility, serious infections, sepsis, extended length of stay, and mortality. An estimated 60,000 hospitalized patients per year die from the complications of facility-acquired pressure ulcers.[2]

Development of pressure ulcers is a complex process that entails a number of contributing and confounding factors, the first of which begins with the cellular alteration that occurs as a result of impaired blood flow. While the initial insult to the skin is pressure related, the underlying pathophysiologic changes are due to impaired blood flow.[4] The deep tissue damage that pressure can create is more significant than the skin impairment that is initially often not visible and not indicative of the degree of injury that lies beneath. Clinicians must remember that although the damage to the skin's surface is a concern, the real problem is the degree of muscle damage that occurs when inadequate blood flow is not restored.[4]

The pathophysiologic effect of excessive pressure on soft tissue can be attributed to intensity of pressure, which is the minimal amount of pressure required to collapse the capillaries, thus decreasing blood flow with subsequent tissue anoxia if the pressure is not relieved.[5] Pressure applied to the skin in excess of the arteriolar pressure (32 mmHg) prevents the delivery of oxygen and nutrients to the tissue, resulting in tissue hypoxia, which is the accumulation of metabolic waste products and free radical generation.[6] In healthy individuals, this is not an issue, because patients that have intact sensory perception are able to shift their weight in response to the discomfort associated with capillary closure and tissue hypoxia.[5]

Duration of pressure, which is evaluated together with intensity, is said to exist as an inverse relationship where tissue hypoxia is created. For example, low-intensity pressure over a prolonged period of time can create tissue damage, just as high-intensity pressure over a short period of time will also lead to the same degree of tissue destruction. Pressures are greatest over bony prominences where weight-bearing points come in contact with the external surface.[5] A patient lying on a standard hospital mattress may generate pressures of 150 mmHg; chair sitting produces even higher pressures up to 300 mmHg, specifically over the ischial tuberosities. Animal studies conducted on rats as far back as 1959 found that continued pressure in excess of 70 mmHg for two hours resulted in irreversible tissue damage.[6]

Tissue tolerance is the ability of the skin and its supporting structures to endure pressure without adverse outcome; tissue tolerance is patient specific. A standard of every two-hour turning for one patient may not work for another who requires more frequent turning.[5] Nurses must stop the "blame game";[4] skin damage is not always evident when we first encounter a patient. The initial insult could have been underway well before the patient's admission, e.g., the patient was found down at home, time down unknown. The cellular insult could already be in process when the patient enters the setting; however, the insult is not known because the damage is not immediately visible.[4]

Once cellular injury is underway with subsequent tissue hypoxia, contributing factors that aid in the development of pressure-related ulcers are friction and shear. Friction is the force of rubbing two surfaces against one another. Friction without pressure is known as a "sheet burn," which is damage to the epidermis and upper dermal layers of the skin. Shear, on the other hand, typically goes hand in hand with friction; it is the result of gravity pushing down on the patient's body plus resistance between the body and the surface, i.e., the bed or a chair.[4]

Moisture, incontinence, and inadequate nutrition are additional contributing factors that enhance friction and shear leading to the development of pressure ulcers. Patients who are either severely ill, such as those who are intubated and sedated or those with cognitive deficits such as dementia or delirium, are at increased risk for incontinence. Urinary or fecal incontinence or third space edema results in over-hydration or maceration of the perineal skin. Macerated skin compromises the skin's ability to function as an effective barrier and thus over-hydrated skin is at greater risk for erosion and impairment of skin integrity.[6]

The final component, impaired nutritional intake, which many studies have identified, is an independent predictor for pressure ulcer development secondary to protein deficiency and malnutrition. Protein deficiency alone affects edema formation, causing the soft tissues to be more prone to the effects of pressure; it affects the diffusion of oxygen and nutrients as well as alters the response of the immune system, rendering a patient more susceptible to infection.[7]

The confounding factors that make up the other side of this complex picture are the associated age of the patient; co-morbid diseases such as hypertension, heart failure, renal failure, diabetes, and neurologic disease; and immobility that heavily impacts the skin's ability to survive. The clinician must care for this complex patient by providing a systematic, holistic assessment of the patient that addresses the multiple concomitant factors that may precipitate the development of pressure ulcers.[7]

Prevention

Pressure ulcer prevention in at-risk adults is a health care priority. The Agency for Health Care Policy and Research (AHCPR) recommends four goals for the care of patients at risk for the development of pressure ulcers:[8]

- Identifying at-risk individuals who require preventive intervention, i.e., scheduled turning, pressure redistribution surfaces, heel suspension, and protection of bony prominences
- Maintaining and improving tissue tolerance to pressure to prevent injury
- Protecting against the adverse effects of external mechanical forces, i.e., pressure, friction, and shear
- Reducing the incidence of pressure ulcer development through education

Assessment

Once a pressure ulcer has developed, the standard of care for wound healing begins with identification and staging of the wound, which provides the provider with a description of the degree of tissue destruction.[9] The National Pressure Ulcer Advisory Panel revised the

TABLE 2.19.1. Wound staging.

(Suspected) deep tissue injury	Purple or maroon localized area of discolored, intact skin, or blood-filled blister due to damage of underlying soft tissue from pressure or shear. The area may be preceded by tissue that is painful, firm, mushy, boggy, warm, or cooler than adjacent tissue.
Stage I	Intact skin with nonblanchable redness of a localized area, usually over a bony prominence. Darkly pigmented skin may not have visible blanching, but its color may differ from the surrounding area.
Stage II	Partial thickness loss of dermis, presenting as a shallow open ulcer with a red/pink wound bed, without slough. It may also present as an intact or open/ruptured serum-filled blister. Further descriptions: This stage should not be used to describe skin tears, tape burns, perineal dermatitis, maceration, or excoriation. Bruising indicates suspected deep tissue injury. Furthermore, the depth of a stage III pressure ulcer varies by anatomical location. For example the bridge of the nose, ear, occiput, and malleolus do not have subcutaneous tissue; thus, a stage III ulcer here can be shallow.
Stage III	Full thickness tissue loss. Subcutaneous fat may be visible, but bone, tendon, or muscle is not exposed.
Stage IV	Full thickness tissue loss with exposed bone, tendon, or muscle. Slough or eschar may be present, along with undermining and tunneling.
Unstageable	Full thickness tissue loss in which the base of the ulcer is covered by slough (yellow, tan, brown, gray, or green nonviable tissue) and/or eschar (tan, brown, or black) within the wound bed. Further description: Until enough slough and/or eschar are removed to expose the base of the wound, the true depth, and therefore the stage cannot be determined. Stable (dry, adherent, intact, without erythema or fluctuance) eschar on the heels serves as the body's natural (biological) cover and should not be removed.

Pieper B. Mechanical forces: Pressure, shear, and friction. In: Bryant RA (ed). *Acute and Chronic Wounds*, 3rd edition. St. Louis: Mosby; 2007.

universal pressure ulcer staging system. Each stage reflects the type and depth of observed damage.[10] Staging is intended to demonstrate the amount of tissue damage, not healing, and is just one facet of the assessment. Documentation should focus on the anatomic location of the wound; stage of tissue destruction (Table 2.19.1); assessment of the wound bed (color, presence of granulation tissue, slough, eschar, or tunnels); wound edges for undermining; peri-wound skin for the presence of skin tears, maceration, or excoriation; and dimension of the wound in centimeters. Once a wound has been identified and assessed, principles of therapeutic wound healing are incorporated into the patient's plan of care.[7,10]

An in depth assessment of the wound must be completed and takes into account healthy viable tissue that is pink, red, or beefy red. The amount and type of wound exudate determines the type of primary dressing used. Topical dressings that need to absorb are selected for a highly exudative wound (gauze, hydrofibers, or foam). Alternatively, select a topical dressing that donates moisture to the wound when the wound is dry, such as saline moist gauze, hydrogel, or moisture retentive dressings. Additionally, the wound must be assessed for the presence of non-viable tissue and the possible need for chemical vs. sharp surgical debridement, based on the patient's condition and goals of therapy.[9]

Treatment

As stated previously, the principles of effective wound management must incorporate a holistic approach that identifies and addresses all of the patient's physiologic needs. In the case of a terminally ill patient, the overall treatment goals give direction to the aggressiveness of wound management.[11]

Creation of a physiologic local wound environment entails prevention and/or management of infection, wound cleansing with normal saline, removing non-viable tissue (debridement), maintenance of a moist wound bed, elimination of dead space by lightly filling areas of depth with appropriate filler material, odor control, elimination or minimization of pain and protection of the peri-wound skin.[11] Therefore, a wound care dressing is created to achieve a physiologic wound environment that promotes healing in the absence of the epidermis and dermis mimicking the body's normal skin.[7] The dressing must promote adequate moisture (not too wet and not too dry), temperature control, pH regulation, blood supply, and control of the bacterial bioburden.[4]

The desired outcome when caring for the patient with a pressure ulcer is for the wound to heal and progress toward closure. Wound healing is defined as restoration of the integrity of the skin, or more specifically the resurfacing of the wound.[7] However, for some patients this is neither possible nor realistic, because wound healing depends on numerous factors, most importantly the patient's condition. When issues such as insufficient arterial perfusion, sepsis, and poor nutritional status are present, as may be the case in terminal illness, then complete wound healing is not always possible and requires a treatment plan that is goal directed. Goals for wound healing should be used to guide decisions concerning wound management so that the interventions selected are realistic and appropriate for the patient's situation.[11]

When the primary goal of care is palliation, the aim is to promote quality of life for the terminally ill patient and her family. For patients who are already suffering from a terminal illness, the presence of pressure ulcers intensifies their suffering, reduces their quality of life, and increases health care costs.[12] The main aim of palliative wound care for the patient who has selected a comfort care approach entails strategies that prioritize symptomatic relief and wound improvement ahead of wound healing. Thus, palliative wound care is an evolving body of knowledge and skills that take a holistic approach to relieving suffering and improving quality of life for patients with chronic non-healing wounds.[12] Many of the treatment options discussed previously were geared toward wound healing; in the setting of comfort, these same strategies can hinder patient comfort, causing greater pain. For example, maintaining an every-two-hour turn schedule for a patient with pressure ulcers on almost every turn surface would cause increased pain and suffering with each movement. Treatments should avoid focusing on the deterioration of the pressure ulcers, i.e., wounds with non-viable necrotic tissue, which would normally be treated with a chemical debriding agent. Instead, in palliative care, the focus is on pain control and management of infection, malodor, exudate, and bleeding. This is achieved with dressings that are conformable, comfortable, and capable of extensive wear-time to minimize painful daily dressing changes.[12] Assessment of the patient's condition should always drive the decision making for palliative wound care, where the primary focus is on patient comfort.[11]

↻ BACK TO OUR CASE

Theresa is terminally ill with a poor prognosis and her family has elected to change her goals of therapy to a comfort care focus with palliative wound care. The plan is as follows:

- Atraumatic dressing changes weekly to no more than every three days using extended wear materials that are non-adhering, absorbent, conformable, and atraumatic, specifically if the wound is highly exudative and requires a daily dressing. For example, non-adhering dressings made of fine mesh gauze lightly impregnated with Vaseline® may be used. The fine mesh allows drainage of wound exudate to the secondary dressing such as gauze or foam, as well as atraumatic removal during dressing changes. Semipermeable foam, such as soft polyurethane dressing sheets, maintain a moist environment and absorb moderate exudate. They are not recommended for non-draining wounds, sinuses, or tunneling. Dressing may be changed up to three times per week except for fillers, which may be changed daily. Hydrogel, which is a clear, viscous wound gel that is water based and contains glycerin, is available in a tube or impregnated in a gauze dressing; it maintains a moist environment, absorbs minimal exudate, may donate moisture to the wound, and assists in promoting autolysis of devitalized tissue. It requires a secondary dressing to fill wound depth. It usually requires fewer dressing changes than saline-moistened gauze.

- Control of bleeding, which may occur if there is erosion of capillaries within the wound bed, is a consideration. Consider hydrofibers such as calcium alginates, heavy fiber dressing made from seaweed. These agents maintain a moist environment, absorb moderate to heavy exudate, and may be used to fill wound cavities. They may be used in bleeding wounds/sites for hemostasis. They assist in promoting autolysis of devitalized tissue. Usually one sheet or six inches of rope is needed and is changed daily. Do not moisten dressing before application; irrigate with normal saline before removal.

- Odor control can be achieved with the use of silver impregnated hydrofiber, which is useful for colonized wounds or those at risk of infection. Wound drainage activates antimicrobial activity to decrease the bioburden. The highly absorbent material interacts with wound exudate to form a soft gel to maintain a moist environment. This may be used in dry wounds covered with saline-moistened gauze as a secondary dressing to maintain moisture. It is difficult to remove due to the gelatinous consistency. To do so, cleanse the wound with normal saline and replace. Antimicrobial therapy with metronidazole 200 mg tablets crushed to a powder consistency or metronidazole gel 0.75% applied to the wound bed with each dressing change can be effective in neutralizing wound odor, which may be due to the presence of necrotic or infected wound tissue. Metronidazole can be applied in combination with calcium alginate, hydrofiber, or foam dressings.

! TAKE AWAY POINTS

- Palliative wound care management entails strategies that prioritize symptomatic relief and wound improvement ahead of wound healing.
- Maintenance of a physiologic wound environment with dressings that are comfortable and conformable and possess the ability to control odor, exudate, bleeding, infection, and pain is the ideal.

- Pressure redistribution surfaces, i.e., static or low air-loss equipment which provides pressure relief, comfort, and aid in the prevention of newly acquired pressure ulcer development should be employed.
- Turning must be unscheduled and based on patient desire and comfort.
- Nutrition should be as desired for pleasure and appetite.

REFERENCES

[1] Wound Ostomy and Continence Nurses Society. Position statement: Pressure ulcer staging. Mount Laurel, NJ: WOCN; 2007.

[2] Redelings MD, Lee NE, Sorvillo F. Pressure ulcers: More lethal than we thought? Advances in Skin and Wound Care; 2005; 18(7):367–372.

[3] Keelaghan E, Margolis D, Zhan M, Baumgarten M. Prevalence of pressure ulcers on hospital admission among nursing home residents transferred to the hospital. NIH Public Access. Author Manuscript. 2008; 16(3):331–336.

[4] Clay K. *Evidence-Based Pressure Ulcer Prevention: A Study Guide For Nurses*, 2nd edition. Marblehead, MA: HCPRO; 2008.

[5] Pieper B. Mechanical forces: Pressure, shear, and friction. In: Bryant RA (ed). *Acute and Chronic Wounds*, 3rd edition. St. Louis: Mosby; 2007.

[6] Benton N, Harvath T, Flaherty-Robb M, Medcraft M, McWhorter K, McClelland F, Joseph C, Mambourg F. Managing chronic, nonhealing wounds. *Journal of Gerontological Nursing*; 2007; 33:38–45.

[7] Rolstad B, Ovington L. Principles of wound management. In: Bryant RA (ed). *Acute and Chronic Wounds*, 3rd edition. St. Louis Mosby; 2007.

[8] Agency for Health Care Policy and Research, U.S. Department of Health and Human Services. *Pressure ulcers in adults: Prediction and prevention.* AHCPR Publication No. 92-0047. Rockville, MD; 1992.

[9] Berlowitz D. Pressure ulcers: Epidemiology; pathogenesis; clinical manifestations; and staging. Uptodate. 2011; 1–10.

[10] National Pressure Ulcer Advisory Panel. *Pressure ulcer definition and stages.* Washington, DC: NPUAP; 2007.

[11] Bryant RA, Goldberg MT. Managing wounds in palliative care. In: Bryant RA. *Acute and Chronic Wounds*, 4th edition. St. Louis: Mosby; 2011.

[12] Hendrichova I, Castelli M, Mastroianni C. Pressure ulcers in cancer palliative care patients. *Palliative Medicine.* 2010; 24(7):669–673.

Case 2.20 Treating Ascites

Darrell Owens

HISTORY

Lydia was a 55-year-old African-American woman with a 16-month history of hepatocellular carcinoma (HCC). She was followed by a nurse practitioner in the primary palliative care clinic of the local public hospital. The etiology of her HCC was believed to be hepatitis B and C secondary to a long history of substance abuse which remained an active issue throughout the duration of her life. Lydia was eventually transferred to a skilled nursing facility after she was no longer able to live safely in her public housing apartment where she had been followed by home hospice. Lydia's nurse practitioner managed her primary and palliative care needs and saw her monthly via a home visit program. Upon transfer to the nursing facility her overall health and functional status declined significantly. She was found to have worsening ascites and was started on low dose diuretic therapy, and her transdermal fentanyl patch dose was increased.

Despite these changes Lydia's condition continued to decline, resulting in increased abdominal pain and ascites. Upon interview she reported that her abdominal pain had increased from a 4/10 to a 10/10. It was localized to the entire abdomen, characterized as cramping and squeezing. She was unable to identify any aggravating factors, and reported that PRN oxycodone 60 mg only reduced it to a 7 to 8/10. She

Case Studies in Palliative and End-of-Life Care, First Edition. Edited by Margaret L. Campbell.
© 2012 John Wiley & Sons, Inc. Published 2012 by John Wiley & Sons, Inc.

denied constipation, but reported feeling full all of the time, and that her stomach was much larger and tighter.

At that time she was receiving spironolactone 100 mg PO QD and furosemide 40 mg PO QD which had been started one month prior. Her opioid regimen was fentanyl transdermal 300 mcg/hour, and oxycodone 30 mg to 60 mg PO every two hours PRN. She had been placed on a fentanyl patch when living alone, because she had been unable to remember to take scheduled opioids, and had a history of crushing or trading other long-acting opioids. In addition to the above medications, she was also on a bowel regimen, and had several other comfort oriented PRN medications.

PHYSICAL EXAMINATION

Temperature: 37°C, blood pressure: 144/84, heart rate: 90, respiratory rate: 16

General: Lying in bed, poorly groomed, in moderate distress

Head, eyes, ears, nose, throat: Temporal wasting; pupils round, reactive to light; poor dentition

Respiratory: Mild increased work of breathing, lungs clear to auscultation bilaterally

Cardiac: Regular rate and rhythm, S1 S2, without murmurs, gallops, or rubs

Abdomen: Hypoactive bowel sounds; distended, tense, and tender to palpation

Gastrointestinal: Scaphoid abdomen, normal bowel sounds, no tenderness

Neurologic: Alert, oriented ×4, speech clear and coherent, able to participate in discussion without difficulty

DIAGNOSTICS

Given Lydia's desire for no invasive interventions, no diagnostic studies were ordered on the day of exam; however, blood urea nitrogen and creatinine had been obtained four weeks earlier when the diuretic therapy had been initiated. The results where 12 mg/DL and .6 mg/DL, respectively. Liver studies from approximately one year prior were aspartate aminotransferase (AST): 90, alanine aminotransferase (ALT): 47, alkaline phosphatase: 127, bilirubin (total): 0.7, protein (total): 10.6, albumin: 2.7. Prior CT, ultrasound, and needle biopsy of the liver results were all consistent with HCC.

? **CLINICAL QUESTION**

What treatments may reduce recurrent ascites and improve overall abdominal pain?

✓ **DISCUSSION**

Malignant ascites is associated with cancer and accounts for approximately 10% of all ascites.[1] The onset, progression, and/or recurrence of malignant ascites is associated with an overall decline in quality of life.[1] The diagnosis is often suspected based on history and physical alone. Confirmation requires accuracy of the physical exam, which can vary depending on the volume of fluid present, the specific technique used to examine the patient, and the actual clinical setting.[2]

Ascites can be a common problem in palliative care, with one study finding that 3% to 6% of patients admitted to a palliative care unit experienced problems associated with the diagnosis.[3] Malignant ascites is most commonly associated with primary tumors of the breast, ovary, colon, stomach, and pancreas, as well as with primary or metastatic tumors of the liver.[4] The presence of ascites is detectable at initial diagnosis in greater than 50% of patients.[3] The median survival time after the diagnosis of malignant ascites is one to four months; however, it may be longer in women with breast and ovarian cancer if chemotherapy options are available.[5] Currently there are no clinical predictors to identify which patients will develop malignant ascites, and therefore no preventative measures are available.[1] Despite the fact that this is a common problem in both palliative care and oncology, no widely accepted management guidelines have been developed based on randomized controlled trials.[6]

Cirrhosis and chronic liver disease account for greater than 80% of all ascites.[1,2,4] Cirrhosis represents the late stages of hepatic disease and is generally considered irreversible. Ascites is the most common complication, and as with malignant ascites it increases the risk of infection and renal failure.[7] Along with chronic liver disease, cirrhosis accounts for more than 25,000 deaths and 373,000 hospitalizations in the United States annually.[8]

Etiologies of Ascites

Ascites is the accumulation of fluid in the peritoneal cavity.[3,4,8,9] In approximately 5% of cases, there is more than one etiology. Common coexisting causes of ascites include cirrhosis/chronic liver disease plus either cancer, heart failure, diabetic nephropathy, or some combination of one or all.[2] Complications secondary to obesity such as diabetes and right heart failure are also common causes, and obesity itself can make it more difficult to make an accurate diagnosis due to excess abdominal adipose tissue. Patients with multiple etiologies are more difficult to diagnose, because they may have a diagnosis that alone is not sufficient enough to cause the retention of fluid, but when combined with other diagnoses may cause ascites.[2]

There are two primary causes of malignant ascites. The first is an increase in hepatic venous pressure secondary to multiple hepatic lesions, or a single large tumor that impairs hepatic blood flow. The increase in venous pressure results in fluid leakage into the peritoneum from the sinusoids, and from an increase in plasma renin, causing an increase in the retention of sodium and water by the kidneys.[3] The fluid that accumulates from this mechanism is similar to that which is found in ascites secondary to cirrhosis, because both causes are obstructive in nature. The second etiology is believed to be the result of high concentrations of plasma proteins secondary to increased permeability of tumor vascular systems.[3] The vascular systems of tumors are known to leak fluid, which in peritoneal tumors contributes to the formation of ascites. This etiology is less well understood by researchers.

Ascites secondary to cirrhosis has multiple etiologies, with splanchnic vasodilatation being the primary cause. Portal hypertension, formation of collateral veins, and the shunting of blood to the systemic circulation are all well documented etiologies.[7] Hypertension of the portal vein causes an increased production of vasodilators that subsequently leads to dilatation of the splanchnic artery. For patients with advanced disease, this vasodilatation is so severe that it causes significant decreases in arterial blood volume and mean arterial pressure (MAP). The body's compensatory mechanism attempts to restore the MAP via the retention of sodium and fluid. When these two factors combine, intestinal capillary pressure and permeability are altered, resulting in ascites.[7] Four types of ascites have been identified.[4]

The first is raised hydrostatic pressure, described above. The etiologies of this type include cirrhosis, right heart failure, inferior vena cava obstruction, hepatic vein occlusion, compression from tumors, and metastatic disease in the liver or abdomen.

The second is decreased osmotic pressure, which is caused by protein depletion such as can occur in nephrotic syndrome, reduced protein intake such as can occur in malnutrition, or reduction of protein production such as that commonly seen in cirrhosis.

The third type is when fluid production exceeds resorptive capacity such as occurs in infection or tumors of the abdomen.

The fourth type is chylous, which is ascites due to the obstruction and subsequent leakage of the abdominal lymphatic system.

Assessment

The first step in the assessment of ascites is to determine if it is causing the patient distress. When ascites does cause distress, the subjective symptoms are most commonly related to increased intra-abdominal pressure such as abdominal wall pain, early satiety, esophageal reflux, nausea with or without vomiting, insomnia related to the discomfort of lying flat, groin pain, and lower extremity edema.[3] Dyspnea is the primary reason for which patients with ascites seek medical care. Patients often report symptoms similar to those with right heart failure including dyspnea with exertion and sleeping in a semi-Fowler position.

Patients with ascites are usually dehydrated and have decreased urine output that is highly pigmented, high in osmolarity, and low in sodium.[7] There is often muscle wasting with thin extremities, increased abdominal girth with visible dilated abdominal veins, a positive fluid wave, and jugular venous distention. One of the earliest signs, dullness to percussion, is not present until at least two liters of fluid has accumulated. Additional objective findings can include pleural effusions and peritonitis.[7-9]

The International Ascites Club has proposed a grading system for ascites.[2] The system, which is included here, has yet to be validated with research: Grade 1: mild ascites detectable only by ultrasound, grade 2: moderate ascites manifested by moderate symmetrical distention of the abdomen, grade 3: large or gross ascites with marked abdominal distention.

Common Diagnostic Studies

Upon initial presentation of suspected ascites in the absence of a known diagnosis, imaging should be performed to confirm the presence of ascites, cirrhosis, or malignancy.[2,8] The most common diagnostic imaging test is ultrasound, which is the most cost-effective and does not require exposure to radiation or contrast. If more specific imaging is needed based on ultrasound results, a CT or MRI scan should be obtained. Performing an abdominal paracentesis with subsequent fluid analysis is the most proficient way to diagnose ascites and the etiology, as well as determine the presence of infection.[8] Despite popular belief that performing a paracentesis is dangerous, there is a very low incidence of serious complication, even in the setting of coagulopathy.[8]

Treatment

Once a patient develops clinically significant ascites, it is unlikely to resolve without treatment, and even then in some situations it remains resistant to therapies. The three mainstays of treatment, despite weak evidence, are diuretics, paracentesis, and peritoneovenous shunting.[4]

Diuretics have long been used in the treatment of ascites secondary to cirrhosis. Prior to initiating diuretic therapy it is important to understand the potential risks of overly rapid fluid removal and electrolyte imbalances. The rate of removal of ascitic fluid in cirrhosis depends on the presence or absence of peripheral edema.[10] When initiating dieresis, the initial volume of fluid lost originates in the vascular space and is subsequently replenished from edema fluid which is mobilized secondary to the decrease in intravascular volume. In patients with peripheral edema, patients are better able to tolerate rapid diuresis.[10] In patients without peripheral edema, the only option for fluid remobilization comes from the peritoneum, which limits the amount of ascitic fluid that can be removed to 300 to 500 ml/day to avoid plasma volume depletion and azotemia.[10] The primary electrolyte imbalance of concern is hypokalemia. In patients with ascites secondary to cirrhosis, hypokalemia can increase ammonia production, increasing the risk of encephalopathy and hepatic coma.

Malignant ascites does not respond as well to diuretic therapy as ascites from other causes. Patients with malignant ascites secondary to portal hypertension due to liver tumor involvement are more likely to respond to diuretics.[5] A serum-ascites albumin gradient of greater than 11 g/L is a good indicator that diuretics may be effective.[4] Spironolactone is the diuretic of choice for patients with high-gradient ascites due to the fact that they have activation of the renin/angiotensin system secondary to circulating blood volume depletion.[4]

The combination of spironolactone and furosemide in the treatment of ascites has well established evidence.[4,7,8,10] The starting dose is spironolactone 100 mg and furosemide 40 mg PO daily. This ratio usually maintains a normal serum potassium level. In at least one study these diuretics were more effective in combination than alone.[11] The doses can be doubled daily to achieve a clinical response up to a maximum of spironolactone 400 mg and furosemide 160 mg. The goal of therapy is fluid loss of 0.5 to 1 kg/day, higher if peripheral edema is present.

For up to 90% of patients, paracentesis can provide immediate relief of symptoms. A large volume of fluid (4 to 6 liters) can be removed safely and quickly in the outpatient setting. The use of ultrasound is only indicated for loculated fluid pockets.[5] Unfortunately, the symptom relief experienced from paracentesis is often only temporary, lasting days to weeks depending on disease severity. The safety of paracentesis has been proven in randomized clinical controlled trials.[10] Radiologically placed tunneled peritoneal catheters are another safe and effective treatment option for the chronic management of ascites.[12] The catheters allow for continuous gravity drainage or intermittent drainage via the use of a stopcock valve.

Peritoneovenous shunts are most effective in patients with breast and ovarian cancer, and least effective in those with gastrointestinal cancers.[4] These shunts, which are inserted percutaneously and drain into the internal jugular vein, return the ascites into the vascular system.[4,10] The history of complication rates for them has essentially eliminated their use except in cases of resistant ascites and hepatorenal syndrome.[10]

BACK TO OUR CASE

The etiology of Lydia's ascites is most likely her HCC. However, given her history of hepatitis B and C, cirrhosis could also be a contributing factor. At the time of Lydia's diagnosis she elected not to pursue any further invasive studies beyond the initial imaging and biopsy, and wanted no further oncology follow-up. She was referred to the primary palliative care clinic, where, based on the current clinical evidence (imaging, functional status, and biopsy results) as well as her stated goals of care to remain out of the hospital, she was referred to hospice. Other than treatment for a leg ulceration which required an overnight hospital stay for antibiotics, Lydia's wishes were honored and her goal of remaining out of the hospital was met. Her overall decline in condition was expected and was consistent with the progression of her HCC. Based on the clinical findings, including Lydia's cancer diagnosis and clinical presentation, her worsening ascites was most likely the primary contributing factor of her increased discomfort. Evaluation and management of her ascites required treatments that coincided with Lydia's previously stated goals to avoid invasive testing and remain out of the hospital.

Her diuretic therapy was increased over time to spironolactone 400 mg PO daily and furosemide 160 mg PO daily. Just after two weeks on the maximum diuretic dosage Lydia developed acute renal failure which resolved after the diuretics were discontinued. She declined a paracentesis and placement of a tunneled peritoneal catheter. Her fluid accumulation progressed slowly, and after a detailed discussion of the risks and benefits of intermittent diuretic therapy, Lydia elected for periodic short courses of diuretic therapy (three-day duration) of spironolactone 200 mg PO daily and furosemide 80 mg PO daily. Her transdermal fentanyl was titrated up to 325 mcg every 72 hours over a period of six weeks. Scheduled oxycodone 30 mg PO QID was also added due to the difficulties of receiving PRN medication in the nursing facility. Lydia died peacefully in her nursing facility having never returned to the hospital and reporting good pain control.

! **TAKE AWAY POINTS**

- Malignant ascites accounts for approximately 10% of all ascites and is less responsive to diuretic therapy.
- Ascites secondary to cirrhosis and chronic liver disease accounts for approximately 90% of all ascites, and is more responsive to diuretic therapy.
- Spironolactone and furosemide combined are more effective in treating ascites than either agent alone.
- Paracentesis provides rapid but temporary relief of symptoms.

📖 **REFERENCES**

[1] Ayantunde A, Parsons S. Pattern and prognostic factors in patients with malignant ascites: a retrospective study. *Annals of Oncology*; 2007; 18:945–949.

[2] Diagnosis and evaluation of patients with ascites. Up to Date, 2010. http://www.uptodate.com.offcampus.lib.washington.edu/contents/diagnosis-and-evaluation-of-patients-with-ascites?source=search_result&selectedTitle=3%7E150#H39. Accessed March 22, 2011.

[3] Bruera E, Higginson IJ, Ripamonti C, Gunten CV, eds. *Textbook of Palliative Medicine*. London: Hodder Arnold; 2006.

[4] Dean M, Harris J-D, Regnard C. *Symptom Relief in Palliative Care*, 2nd edition. New York: Radcliffe Publishing; 2011.

[5] Evaluation and management of malignant ascites. Medical College of Wisconsin, 2009. http://www.eperc.mcw.edu/fastfact/ff_176.htm. Accessed April 2, 2011.

[6] Mullard AP, Bishop JM, Jibani M. Intractable malignant ascites: An alternative management option. *Journal of Palliative Medicine*; 2011; 14:251–253.

[7] Owens D. Compendium of Treatment of End Stage Non-Cancer Diagnoses—Hepatic. Dubuque: Kendall Hunt; 2005.

[8] Overview of the complications, prognosis, and management of cirrhosis. Up to Date, 2010. http://www.uptodate.com.offcampus.lib.washington.edu/contents/overview-of-the-complications-prognosis-and-management-of-cirrhosis?source=search_result&selectedTitle=2%7E150. Accessed March 25, 2011.

[9] Saud B, Baltodano JD. Ascites. In: Stuart M, Green H, eds. Decision Making in Medicine, 3rd edition. Philadelphia: Mosby; 2010; 192–193.

[10] Initial therapy of ascites in patients with cirrhosis. Up to Date, 2010. http://www.uptodate.com.offcampus.lib.washington.edu/contents/initial-therapy-of-ascites-in-patients-with-cirrhosis?source=search_result&selectedTitle=2%7E150#H5. Accessed March 25, 2011.

[11] Angeli P, Fasolato S, Mazza E, et al. Combined versus sequential diuretic treatment of ascites in non-azotaemic patients with cirrhosis: results of an open randomised clinical trial. *Gut*; 2010; 59:98–104.

[12] Akinci D, Erol B, Ciftci TT, Akhan O. Radiologically placed tunneled peritoneal catheter in palliation of malignant ascites. *European Journal of Radiology*; in press, corrected proof.

Case 2.21 Delirium Management in Palliative Care

Kerstin McSteen

Eleanor was a 68-year-old woman who was diagnosed with non-Hodgkin lymphoma with bowel metastases nine months prior to hospital admission. She had completed a course of chemotherapy that included cisplatin a week prior to admission. Subsequently, Eleanor developed symptoms of nausea, weakness, lethargy, anorexia, and low-grade fever. Her granddaughter, Jane, who lived with her, became especially concerned after Eleanor did not wake up at her usual time and then did not recognize Jane when she checked on her. Jane brought her to the emergency department and Eleanor was admitted to the oncology ward of the hospital. Within hours of admission, Eleanor was transferred to the intensive care unit (ICU) when she became hypotensive and was diagnosed with urinary tract infection and septic syndrome. She was not intubated but did require vasopressors. She responded well to antibiotic therapy; her condition stabilized and three days later she was able to transfer back to the oncology unit.

The ICU nurse transfer report noted that Eleanor had been fairly somnolent while in the unit, which had been attributed to a few doses of morphine and lorazepam she had received, but she seemed to be waking up and was, in the words of the nurse, "becoming kind of a spitfire." The oncology nurse went in to Eleanor's room to complete her assessment and found her laying naked in the bed, with one leg hanging over the side rail. She had pulled her oxygen cannula off and her IV out

Case Studies in Palliative and End-of-Life Care, First Edition. Edited by Margaret L. Campbell.
© 2012 John Wiley & Sons, Inc. Published 2012 by John Wiley & Sons, Inc.

and blood was oozing from the site. Eleanor startled when she saw the nurse and screamed, "Get out of my house! I'll call the police! Help me someone, help me!"

Prior to hospitalization, Eleanor had been living in her home and though she was weaker because of the cancer treatments, she was still independent in all activities of daily living, including the management of her finances. Her granddaughter, Jane, had recently moved in to help with some of the heavier tasks and errands while she attended college nearby.

PHYSICAL EXAMINATION

Temperature: 37°C, blood pressure: 142/78, heart rate: 110, respiratory rate: 22

CNS: Oriented to self only, hyper alert, startles easily, agitated, visual hallucinations, seeing and speaking to people in her room that are not there, distracted and unable to complete coherent thoughts

Head, eyes, ears, nose, throat: Cream-colored coating on tongue, buccal mucosa red, inflamed; Sclera nonicteric, pupils equal, reactive to light

Cardiovascular: Regular rate and rhythm, tachycardic, no murmurs, no S3 or S4, strong pedal and radial pulses, no lower extremity edema

Pulmonary: Clear bilateral anterior and bases, no cough, no wheezing, mildly tachypneic on room air, mildly labored, SpO$_2$ 90% on 3 liters/minute per nasal cannula

Gastrointestinal: Soft, nontender, hypoactive bowel sounds

Genitourinary: Foley catheter in place, cloudy amber urine with some sediment noted.

Extremities: Decreased muscle mass but not cachectic, skin intact, no rashes or deformities, cool, clammy

DIAGNOSTICS

Pertinent labs:

Hematology: White blood cells: 2,700, hematocrit: 49%, hemoglobin: 8.9

Chemistries: Sodium: 135, potassium: 5.0, blood urea nitrogen: 40, creatinine: 1.35, glomerular filtration rate: 55

Microbiology: Urine analysis on admit: cloudy, "many" bacteria, "small" occult blood, and greater than 100 white blood cells

Urine culture: Positive on admission, now no growth

Blood cultures: positive on admission with gram-positive cocci-clusters; staphylococcus coagulase negative, now no growth

Head CT scan: Emerging encephalopathy/delirium, rule out possible brain metastases: negative

MEDICATIONS

Lorazepam 1 mg IV Q six hours PRN agitation, restlessness, anxiety; morphine 2 to 4 mg IV Q two hours PRN pain; rocephin 1 gram IV Q 12 hours; odansetron 4 mg IV Q six hours, pantoprozole 40 mg IV QD

? CLINICAL QUESTION

How should agitated delirium be treated?

✓ DISCUSSION

Natural History of Delirium

Although delirium is often referred to as a "waxing and waning" condition, more specifically it is the alertness and vigilance that fluctuate.[1] Delirium is defined as "a neurobehavioral syndrome caused by the transient disruption of normal neuronal activity secondary to systemic disturbances.[1] In a state of delirium, a person receives external stimuli but is not interpreting and integrating them correctly. Nurses identify this misinterpretation as inappropriate behavior and often describe the patient as being "confused," but this is a vague and nonspecific label for what is a serious medical complication. In fact, an expert panel of geriatric specialists described delirium as "a medical emergency in which the demands of acute management require frequent reassessment of treatment response and rapid dose adjustment."[2]

Although there is good understanding of the risk factors that contribute to the development of delirium, the actual pathophysiology is unclear. Basically, what is clear is that there is a common neural pathway that exists for the various causes of delirium. There are several proposed theories but according to Maldonado, they are complementary rather than competing.[1] A sampling of theories propose cerebral dysfunction from lack of oxygen; excess releases of dopamine, norepinephrine, and glutamate; too much or too little serotonin; and increased anti-inflammatory agents, such as cytokines, as the underlying cause of delirium.[1]

The incidence of delirium in the acute care setting is high. In hospitalized elderly patients, the overall incidence is 11% to 42%, with up to

53% for surgical patients on a regular floor and greater than 80% for those in an ICU.[1,3] In the palliative care setting, delirium is present in up to 85% of patients in the final weeks of life.[4] Unfortunately, despite a long held medical belief, it is not a condition that necessarily improves with time in the setting of acute illness, nor is it an inevitable state at the end of life. The adverse outcomes of delirium can be long-lasting and devastating and include:[1,5]

- Increased morbidity and mortality
- Increased cost of care and prolonged hospital stays,[6] with one study demonstrating health care costs for patients who developed delirium in the ICU as 31% higher than for patients with similar medical problems but without delirium[7]
- Increased hospital-acquired complications[1] such as infections, falls, and skin breakdown
- Poor functional and cognitive recovery. Once delirium begins, only 4% of patients are discharged with the condition fully resolved, and at six months, only 40% have recovered completely[8]
- For patients with evidence of dementia before hospitalization, delirium can accelerate the course of cognitive decline[9]
- Increased necessary placement at skilled nursing facilities[1]
- Decreased quality of life

Risk Factors

The etiology of delirium is usually multifactorial with many clearly identified risk factors:[6]

- Advanced age: For each additional year after 65, the probability of developing delirium increases by 2%.[6]
- Pre-existing/underlying dementia
- Medications: In particular, opioids, benzodiazepines, and anticholinergics greatly increase risk
- Sleep deprivation, which can cause, aggravate, and perpetuate delirium. One study showed that the average ICU patient gets less than two hours of sleep in a 24-hour period.[1]
- Hypoxia/anoxia
- Metabolic abnormalities
- History of substance abuse, especially with hepatic involvement
- Acute illness, surgery, trauma
- Prolonged sedation with intubation
- Brain lesions (primary tumors or metastases, stroke, carcinomatosis)

Assessment and Diagnosis

Delirium is not easily identified and is often misdiagnosed as dementia or depression. One study found that more than 40% of patients referred to psychiatry for suspected depression actually had hypoactive delirium.[10]

The American Psychiatric Association's Diagnostic and Statistical Manual of Mental Disorders (DSM-IV-TR) 4 provides the gold standard for diagnosis of delirium as evidenced by the following four hallmark criteria:

- Disturbance of consciousness with reduced ability to focus, sustain, or shift attention
- A change in cognition or perceptual disturbance not attributed to dementia
- Acute onset (hours to days) and fluctuating course (unlike dementia and depression, which generally develop slowly over an extended period of time)
- History, physical examination, and/or lab results demonstrate direct physiological consequences related to the general medical condition that results in the behavioral changes

Delirium is further subcategorized into three types:[4] In hyperactive delirium, the patient is visibly agitated, restless, disoriented, or delusional, and often presents with visual and/or auditory hallucinations. Hypoactive delirium is the most difficult type of delirium to identify and is often misdiagnosed as depression, given the withdrawn, inattentive, and disengaged patient presentation. The patient is lethargic, somnolent, undemanding, and unable to maintain arousal. Also difficult to diagnose is the mixed type (hyper/hypoalert) delirium, in which the patient presents with alternating levels of consciousness.

Diagnostic tools may help the provider to differentiate whether the patient is suffering from delirium, depression, or dementia, and some tools rate severity. The Confusion Assessment Method (CAM)[11] is widely used to diagnosis delirium. Developed in 1992, it is a quick, accurate, and reliable tool that assesses delirium according to the following four criteria:

- Acute onset and fluctuating course
- Inattention
- Disorganized thinking
- Altered level of consciousness

Additionally, information obtained from interviewing family and other care providers who are familiar with the patient's baseline behavior is invaluable in identifying delirium.

Prevention

As Ben Franklin said, "An ounce of prevention is worth a pound of cure," and this is certainly true with delirium. The first critical step to prevent delirium is to identify patients at high risk for developing it and then incorporate prevention strategies into the plan of care. There is overlap between measures taken to prevent delirium and measures to take when delirium develops. The following interventions can be applied to both prevention and treatment:[3,5–7,12,13]

- Follow orientation protocols to include environmental adjustments: opening shades during the day and closing them at night, having clocks and calendars visible, encouraging family presence and/or pictures and familiar items at the bedside.
- Encourage early mobilization with physical and occupational therapies, and encourage the patient to be as independent as possible in self-care activities.
- Use glasses, hearing aids, and other assistive devices.
- Support early and adequate nutrition.
- Correct electrolyte abnormalities, particularly sodium, potassium, and glucose.
- Detect and treat fluid imbalances (dehydration or overload).
- Minimize or discontinue use of benzodiazepines, opioids, and anticholinergics.
- Be alert to possible drug interactions and adverse effects and modify or discontinue potentially harmful medications.
- Use analgesics for pain control appropriately: nonopioids as the first line and if opioids are necessary, as low dose as possible. There is no role for meperidine, other than for management of rigors.
- Be alert to routine situations that may contribute to iatrogenic complications:
  - Avoid use of physical restraints.
  - Discontinue urinary catheters and other tubes and lines as soon as feasibly possible.
  - Implement bowel regimens.
  - Monitor oxygen saturation level and use supplemental oxygen as needed.
  - Use appropriate anticoagulation protocols.
  - Incorporate strategies to promote restful sleep: reduce noise levels and lights and schedule medications and treatments to avoid waking during the night.

Although studies are limited, it is noteworthy that there is currently insufficient evidence that supports the prophylactic use of neuroleptics, such as haloperidol.[5]

Treatment

The course of delirium depends largely on early diagnosis, identifying possible etiologies, and promptly treating the underlying cause (or causes) if possible. Correcting electrolyte abnormalities and fluid imbalance, initiating antibiotics for infection, eliminating high-risk medications, or providing supplemental oxygen are all examples of interventions that may quickly resolve delirium.

However, like pain, it is not necessary to determine the exact etiology before treating the distressing symptoms of delirium. The use of neuroleptics is the first-line pharmacological treatment for delirium.[14] The exception to this is if the delirium is clearly due to drug or alcohol withdrawal, in which case a benzodiazepine is indicated.[6] Of the neuroleptics, the first choice is the butyrophenone antipsychotic haloperidol (Haldol®).[14] It has been studied most extensively, has a favorable side effect profile, and can be administered via several routes. A typical starting dose is 0.5 to 1 mg oral or parenteral, titrating by 2 to 5 mg every hour until a daily dose requirement is established, which can then be administered as scheduled every six, eight, or 12 hours.

Oral administration of haloperidol has been noted in some studies to cause more extrapyramidal symptoms (EPS), making IV the preferred route.[6] It is also important to consider that haldoperidol can cause prolongation of the QTc interval so it may be appropriate to obtain a baseline electrocardiogram before or soon after starting. Haloperidol should be used with caution in patients with a QTc greater than 440 msec.[6]

Second-line neuroleptics include the newer atypical antipsychotics, including quetiapine, risperidone, and olanzapine.[4] These are recommended when the patient is at high risk for EPS or has an underlying neurological disorder such as Parkinson's disease. While effective, atypical antipsychotics have drawbacks including expense and limited administration routes.

Common errors include waiting too long before adjusting the regimen or discontinuing effective treatment too early. Given that delirium is considered a medical emergency, it is recommended that the dose or medication regimen be changed if there is no response to the treatment within 24 hours. Also, treatment should be continued for one week after the patient has a beneficial response.[2]

Other non-neuroleptic agents have been found to be effective in treating delirium. Melatonin may be useful in regulating the sleep/wake cycle.[1] Flumazenil has been shown to reverse coma from hepatic encephalopathy and cirrhosis.[1] Odansetron, the common antiemetic, has been shown to be effective by reducing high levels of serotonin, which are associated with hypoactive delirium and hepatic encephalopathy.[6]

Delirium in the Actively Dying Patient

Delirium is common in the end stages of life, occurring in 28% to 83% of terminally ill patients, and because it is so prevalent, it is often considered an unavoidable and inevitable condition.[15] Delirium is especially difficult to diagnose at the end of life, and because of physiological changes occurring due to the disease, it may not be possible to correct. However, delirium can be a very distressing symptom to both the patient and the family, negatively affecting the quality of time remaining for them, and it may respond to some fairly basic interventions.

The decision whether to aggressively treat delirium in the actively dying patient depends on several factors. First, as is the case with every clinical decision, the patient's goals of care should guide the treatment plan. Some patients prioritize being as alert and oriented as possible; others wish for comfort at the expense of being more awake and able to interact. Treatments that may help clear the delirium may also act to prolong life, and this may be at odds with the patient's goals.

Second, one should assess how distressing the delirium is for the patient and family. It is one thing to watch a loved one having hallucinations that involve calm conversations with deceased friends and relatives, and quite another to witness that person in an agitated and restless state, screaming in terror.

Like pain, the presentation of delirium does not require a clear identification of the cause before the symptom is treated, and in the case of someone who is dying, the benefit of any diagnostic work-up must be balanced with the burden of invasive and painful labs and tests. Although prevention is the best approach, when delirium develops in the dying patient, and it is determined that it is appropriate to treat with the goal of improving cognitive function, the interventions, both pharmacological and behavioral as discussed previously, should guide the treatment plan.

↻ BACK TO OUR CASE

Eleanor had several potential reasons for developing delirium including age, cancer diagnosis, and status post highly toxic chemotherapy, acute critical illness, infection, renal insufficiency, sleep deprivation in the ICU, hypoxia during the hypotensive period in the ICU, possible underlying early dementia, and medications including opioids and benzodiazepines.

Upon finding Eleanor, the nurse called the attending physician to report her behavior. Eleanor had pulled her intravenous access, and was too agitated and frightened to allow another to be placed. The physician considered the options, which included IM Haldol® or an oral neuroleptic that would be absorbed either orally or sublingually. Wanting to avoid the painful intervention of an injection, the physician ordered olanzapine oral dissolving tablet (Zydis™) 5 mg, which is absorbed on the tongue and has the advantage of being somewhat sedating. Though it took a bit of persuasion, the nurse was able to administer the medication, and within 30 minutes, Eleanor was calm and resting, cooperative, and following commands, though she remained disoriented to time and place. An IV was placed and Haldol® was scheduled 0.5 to 2 mg Q six hours and 0.5 to 1 mg Q two hours PRN delirium, agitation.

Eleanor's mentation improved over the next several days, returning to her baseline. She was ambulating in the halls and her room with stand-by assists only for safety. The IV Haldol® was switched to scheduled olanzapine 5 mg at 6 pm. With additional support of family, she was able to discharge to home with home care follow-up. She was discharged on a maintenance dose of olanzapine, at 2.5 mg each evening, with a plan to re-evaluate in the clinic a week after hospital discharge.

! TAKE AWAY POINTS

- Delirium is a medical emergency with potentially dire outcomes. When the patient presents with the four hallmark features of acute onset, inattention, disorganized thinking, and altered level of consciousness, treatment must not be delayed.
- Assess for risk factors and incorporate preventive strategies into the plan of care.
- When delirium develops at the end of life, the decision to treat is based on the patient's goals of care, balancing comfort with potential burdens of diagnostic work-up and intervention.

REFERENCES

[1] Maldonado JR. Pathoetiological model of delirium: a comprehensive understanding of the neurobiology of delirium and an evidence-based approach to prevention and treatment. *Crit Care Clin*; 2008; 24:789–856.
[2] Alexopoulos GS, Streim J, Carpenter D, Docherty JP. Using antipsychotic agents in older adults. Introduction: methods, commentary and summary. *J Clin Psychiatry*; 2004; 65[suppl 2]:1–105.
[3] Messinger-Rapport B. What's new in treating older adults? *Cleveland Clinic J of Med*; 2010; 77(11):770–783,790.
[4] Walsh TD, et al., eds. *Palliative Medicine*. Philadelphia: Saunders Elsevier; 2009.
[5] Holroyd-Leduc JM, Khandwala F, Sink KM. How can delirium best be prevented and managed in older patients in hospital? *CMAJ*. 2010; 182:465–470.
[6] Maldonado JR. Delirium in the acute care setting: characteristics, diagnosis and treatment. *Crit Care Clin*; 2008; 24:657–722.
[7] Milbrandt EB, Deppen S, Harrison PL, et al. Costs associated with delirium in mechanically ventilated patients. *Crit Care Med*; 2004; 32(4):955–962.
[8] Leukoff SE, Evans DA, Liptzin B, et al. Delirium. The occurrence and persistence of symptoms among elderly hospitalized patients. *Arch Intern Med*; 1992; 152(2):334–340.
[9] Fong TG, Jones RN, Shi P, et al. Delirium accelerates cognitive decline in Alzheimer disease. *Neurology*; 2009; 72:1570–1575.

[10] Farrell KR, Ganzini L. Misdiagnosing delirium as depression in medically ill elderly patients. *Arch Intern Med*; 1995; 155(22):2459–2464.

[11] Inouye SK, vanDyck CH, Alessi CA, et al. Clarifying confusion: the confusion assessment method. A new method for detection of delirium. *Ann Intern Med*; 1990; 113:941–948.

[12] Lundström M, Olofsson B, Stenvall M, et al. Postoperative delirium in old patients with femoral neck fracture: a randomized intervention study. *Aging Clin Exp Res*; 2007; 19:178–186.

[13] Gillis AJ, MacDonald B. Unmasking delirium. *Canadian Nurse*; 2006; 102(9):19–24.

[14] Quijada E, Billings JA. Pharmacologic management of delirium; Update on newer agents, 2nd edition. Fast Facts and Concepts. July 2006; 60. http://www.eperc.mcw.edu/fastfact/ff_060.htm. Accessed April 10, 2011.

[15] Casarett DJ, Inouye SK. Diagnosis and management of delirium near the end of life. *Ann Intern Med*; 2001; 135:32–40.

Section 3

Family Care Case Studies

Case 3.1	**Caring for the Family Expecting a Loss**	259
	Patricia A. Murphy and David M. Price	
Case 3.2	**Anticipatory Grief and the Dysfunctional Family**	266
	Rita J. DiBiase	
Case 3.3	**Acute and Uncomplicated Grief after an Expected Death**	277
	Rita J. DiBiase	
Case 3.4	**Bereavement after Unexpected Death**	289
	Garrett K. Chan	
Case 3.5	**Complicated Grief**	300
	Rita J. DiBiase	

Overview

Grief is the emotional and physical reaction to a loss, a normal process expressed in individual ways. The term anticipatory grief is used to describe the emotional and physical reactions to an impending loss that intensifies as the time of death approaches.

Acute grief occurs at the time of death, and is experienced by the patient's survivors; intensity is expected to decrease over time. Mourning is the outward display of the physical and emotional feelings associated with the loss. Religious beliefs, cultural norms, and customary rituals characterize mourning behaviors. There is no universal grief experience. Individuals vary even within the same family or community.

Caring for the family is challenging for clinicians for a number of reasons. Families often need a great deal of the clinician's time to have explanations and re-explanations of the patient's condition, assurances about patient comfort, and assurances that the right decisions were made about treatment goals. In addition, families have questions about caregiving, how to recognize imminent death, and tasks to accomplish at the time of death.

Caring for a grieving family can evoke anxiety as clinicians see parallels in their own experiences or anticipated experiences of personal loss. Clinicians also may fear saying the wrong thing during family interactions.

The cases in this last section provide clinicians with tools for caring for the family during a time of loss. Principles for caring for the family, including children, anticipating a loss are described in Case 3.1. Maladjusted families struggling with the strong emotions from grief and the unique care guidelines can be found in Case 3.2.

Grief characteristics vary when the patient's death is unexpected compared to when the death was expected. Cases 3.3 and 3.4 provide distinctions in family behaviors and care needs and interventions. Case 3.5 guides the clinician about recognizing complicated grief and making referrals for continuing care.

❗ TAKE AWAY POINTS

- Caring for the family can be as time-consuming, yet meaningful, as caring for the patient.
- Grief begins with anticipation of a loss and continues with varying emotional intensity during and after the patient's death.
- A range of expected grief behaviors requires patience and compassion from clinicians.

Case 3.1 Caring for the Family Expecting a Loss

Patricia A. Murphy and David M. Price

HISTORY

Joseph ("Joey"), an otherwise healthy 54-year-old, was admitted to the intensive care unit (ICU) with closed head trauma and multiple, newly stabilized orthopedic injuries. He had not regained consciousness since an out-of-control truck upended his lunch wagon parked in its usual spot on a downtown street. He was sedated and on a ventilator.

His daughter Emmaline, 31, also working in the lunch wagon, was brought by ambulance to the same hospital, but was found to have suffered only cuts and bruises. She and her mother, Joey's wife, followed Joey's stretcher to the ICU from the surgical waiting area. Mrs. Williams shuffled, supported by Emmaline and the neighbor who had brought her to the hospital several hours ago. Emmaline appeared concerned and somewhat frantic.

Janet, the nurse assigned to Joey, had just taken a summary of her patient's condition by telephone when the stretcher arrived, trailed by the wife, daughter, and family friend. The appearance of the wife and daughter prompted Janet to ask a colleague, Sue, whose patients were not in immediate distress, to attend to them. Sue steered Mrs. Williams to a chair near her husband's room. Sue noted that Mrs. Williams was breathing rapidly and that her eyes were wide but unseeing. She asked Emmaline, "What do you think is going on with your mother?" Emmaline replied, "I don't know, I haven't seen her like this before." Then she added "I have to go to my children, but I'm afraid to leave her." Sue asked about

---

Case Studies in Palliative and End-of-Life Care, First Edition. Edited by Margaret L. Campbell.
© 2012 John Wiley & Sons, Inc. Published 2012 by John Wiley & Sons, Inc.

Mrs. Williams' medical history and determined that Mrs. Williams did not have any medical problems that would account for her appearance.

Sue held Mrs. Williams by the shoulders and, speaking firmly, said, "Mrs. Williams, look at me! I need to make sure you are OK. Your daughter needs you. Your grandchildren need you." Mrs. Williams met Sue's gaze for the first time and her breathing slowed. A determined look came into her face. She squared her shoulders. "I'll be OK," she said, reaching for her daughter's hand. Sue said, "Your husband's nurse will soon finish settling him. Then, she will take you to be with him. Are you ready for that? Good." Then Sue turned to Emmaline. "Now, tell me about these children."

Over the next several hours, the staff gathered the following information: Mr. and Mrs. Williams had been married for 33 years. They had two children, Emmaline and her younger brother Leroy, who died in an automobile crash twelve years ago at the age of 17. Emmaline has two children, a girl, 9, and a boy, 7. All three have lived with Emmaline's parents since her husband left soon after his son was born. Mr. and Mrs. Williams established "Joey's Lunch Wagon" after their children started school and it soon became a fixture among downtown office workers. In recent years, Mrs. Williams has worked the breakfast and coffee break crowds before being replaced by Emmaline prior to the long lunch period. Mrs. Williams is always home when the children return from school and all three adults are home by 4:30 pm to share oversight of the children's play and homework. They have supper together every weeknight and spend every Wednesday evening at the First Baptist Church for supper and a family-oriented service of prayer and gospel singing.

On hospital day four, Joey remained unresponsive to all but painful stimuli and was still dependent on the ventilator. His Glasgow Coma Scale was 5/15. There had been some variability in his blood pressure and temperature, but no signs of infection. Mrs. Williams insisted on remaining at her husband's bedside, except for two hours each afternoon when she went home to bathe and watch the children after school. At various times during the day she was joined by friends and neighbors, many of whom were seen praying with her. Reverend Jackson, her pastor, visited each morning.

Meanwhile, Emmaline had managed to keep the lunch wagon open for lunch with a menu of cold sandwiches and salads that a friend helped her prepare each morning. She came to the hospital every evening and for a few minutes in the morning. She had yet to bring the children, despite encouragement from the nursing staff.

? CLINICAL QUESTION

What interventions are important when supporting a multigenerational family that is anticipating a loss?

TABLE 3.1.1. Tasks of mourning: children vs. adults.

Adult tasks of mourning	Child's tasks of mourning
Accept the reality of the loss	Understand that someone has died
Experience the pain or emotional aspects of the loss	Face the psychological pain of the loss, cope with periodic resurgence of pain
Adjust to an environment in which the deceased is missing	Invest in new relationships, develop a new sense of identity that includes experience of the loss
Emotionally relocate the deceased (this relocation process allows continuing bonds to the deceased)	Reevaluate the relationship to the dead person and return to age-appropriate developmental tasks

Murphy P, Mosenthal A. Death from trauma—management of grief and bereavement and the role of the surgeon. In: Asensio JA, Trunkey DD (eds). *Current Therapy of Trauma and Surgical Critical Care.* Philadelphia: Mosby; 2008; 748–751. Reprinted with permission from Elsevier.

✓ DISCUSSION

The rather straightforward medical facts should be familiar to experienced staff members in any ICU where patients are, even occasionally, brought after a motor vehicle crash or serious fall.

Because patients in these circumstances are often unconscious, exhibiting no signs of distress or awareness, the challenges of palliative care are focused exclusively on the family. Thus, at the outset, we are reminded of a basic principle of palliative care: The family is the unit of care.

Children and Anticipated Loss

Both adults and children experience grief after a loss, but the manifestations of grief are developmentally determined (Table 3.1.1). It is important to recognize the different ways that children express grief. The age of the child is an important determinant and should be taken into account when information is shared and support provided. In working with children, one must remember that a child's understanding of illness and death is determined by his cognitive capacity to understand that death is permanent. This occurs in children at about the age of 5, though developmental variability suggests the need for individual assessment.

Simple, clear information about the young child's reaction to the death should be given to the primary caregiver. Printed, easily understandable information should be readily available in the unit to be given to the responsible adults to take home. Iverson has published a simple, complete list of adult behaviors that are helpful to young children.[1]

It is essential that the child be told the truth in words that he can understand. "Real" words should be used to describe what has happened: "Your grandpa was in a terrible accident. The doctors have worked really hard to try and fix him, but his body just stopped working and he died." As in all matters, young children take their cues from their adult caregivers. They closely watch the reaction of adults, particularly in new situations. Thus, effective support for adult caregivers is also a help for their children.

Useful information and advice for caregivers of children includes:

- Children as young as 3 years can understand the concept of death.
- Do not tell children the dead person has "gone away" or is "sleeping." This will only confuse the child.
- Use simple, down-to-earth words to describe the death. Avoid euphemisms and indirect language.
- Answer the questions that the child asks. When a death occurs, young children often worry about three issues: Did I make it happen? Will it happen to me? Who will take care of me? Do not be surprised or judgmental about such questions. Simply answer them.
- Give the child the opportunity to attend family rituals surrounding death. If the child asks to attend, that usually means he is old enough to do so.

Anticipating Death

Anticipatory grief is the emotional and physical reaction to an impending loss and is experienced by family members as it becomes clearer that the patient will probably die soon. Some trauma patients spend days in the surgical ICU hovering near death. During this time the family is often desperate for any information that gives them hope. They ride a roller coaster of hope and despair with every conversation they have with the various health care professionals. They are exhausted and frequently ignore their own needs for rest and food. When their loved one finally dies it is perceived as a sudden event, even if weeks have gone by since the trauma. This is often due to their coping through an almost exclusive dependence on denial, frequently encouraged by staff members. The death shatters that defense.[2]

Complicating Effects of Sudden Death

Theorists have suggested that many issues are inherent in sudden, unanticipated death that complicate mourning.[3] Those relevant to trauma and sudden-onset, immediately life-threatening illnesses are:

- The capacity to cope is diminished as the shock effects of the death overwhelm the self.
- The assumptive world of the mourner is violently shattered (the world as orderly, predictable, and meaningful), causing intense reactions of fear, anxiety, and loss of control.
- The loss does not make sense and cannot be absorbed.

- Symptoms of acute grief and of physical and emotional shock persist for a long time.
- The mourner obsessively reconstructs events in an effort to comprehend the event.
- The mourner experiences a profound loss of personal security and confidence resulting in increasing anxiety.
- The death tends to leave mourners with relatively more intense emotions, along with a strong need to affix blame.

It is important for the health care team to understand these issues and be prepared to assess and intervene with reality-based information. There are no words that will "make it better" for families. Rather, families need the caring presence of others. Also, the nurse should ask the family about any religious or cultural rituals that are important to them.

Palliative care is about caring for the family as a unit. Events that occur around the death will stay with the family forever, becoming family memories. The acute care nurse's role includes giving permission to the family to sit vigil, bathe the patient, pray, cut a lock of hair, and do whatever else they need to do at this most difficult time. Doing so with empathy and basic knowledge minimizes the risks of and blunts the severity of long-term, complicated grief.

BACK TO OUR CASE

For our purposes, the important medical facts are:

- The patient has suffered a blow to the head, rendering him unconscious.
- The prognosis is uncomplicated by previous medical or surgical history. Long-term neurological recovery is unlikely.
- He remained stable on the ventilator, at least during the first four days of ICU care.

Early on in the case presentation there is clear evidence that Joey's nurse "gets" this fundamental feature of palliative care. As Janet saw her new patient being wheeled into the unit, her initial visual appraisal took in the family members who closely followed the stretcher. Seeing signs of distress, she immediately recruited a colleague to attend to them while she focused on her patient. That her initial, quick appraisal of her patient included his family members demonstrates her understanding that care for the family is an essential aspect of excellent intensive care nursing.

Sue, the colleague delegated by Janet to temporarily "cover" the family members, proved to be an apt choice for this assignment. She guided Mrs. Williams to a chair, presumably because the woman appeared unstable on her feet. Anyone would probably do the same. But note that Sue took her not to the nearest chair but to a chair near her husband's room. This shows that she was aware that separating the wife from her husband might have exacerbated the woman's distress. Then Sue went to eye level with Mrs. Williams to continue her assessment in the most face-to-face way possible. Sue's efficient examination suggested that Mrs. Williams' appearance was probably due to hyperventilation secondary to the emotional distress of the day's events.

Based on this assessment and on Emmaline's statement that she "has to get back to the children," Sue moved quickly to an excellent intervention. She challenged Mrs. Williams to demonstrate that Emmaline does not have to worry unduly about her. The form of the challenge was very smart, suggesting both that Sue knew that acute grief can produce a shock-like picture and that she hypothesized that Mrs. Williams was a caring mother and grandmother. Looking Mrs. Williams in the face, she held her by the shoulders and spoke firmly. "Mrs. Williams, look at me! I need to know that you are OK. Your daughter needs your help. Your grandchildren need you." Mrs. Williams met the challenge, simultaneously confirming Sue's hypothesis, reassuring Emmaline, and allowing the palliative care assessment to proceed to a focus on Emmaline and her children.

Experienced, confident palliative care professionals can often use this sort of direct appeal to a family member's sense of responsibility. Particularly in the case of parents, it is often possible to turn a "problem" person into a supportive ally by appealing to the needs of another, especially a child (of any age).

As the staff discovered, this family is very engaged with the grandchildren. The staff noted that the children have not visited their grandfather, despite encouragement to bring them in. The nurses are correct in thinking it was important to encourage Emmaline to include the children in the family crisis. One could reasonably hypothesize that Emmaline's reluctance was due either to her impulse to protect them from a painful experience or to her own feeling that she does not know how to help them deal with it. In either case, seasoned palliative care professionals and a growing number of ICU nurses are learning how to assure and support parents.

This family is very close and has included the grandchildren in all family activities. It is important to encourage Emmaline to include the children in these events as they unfold. Thus, Emmaline brought the children to the hospital to see their grandfather. Janet, the primary nurse, carefully explained all the tubes and machines surrounding him and the children hung up the pictures that they had drawn for him. They asked some questions and kissed him goodbye.

Mrs. Williams was very sad and maintained a vigil at her husband's bedside. The night nurse included her in selected aspects of patient care. As they worked together to bathe him, the nurse encouraged Mrs. Williams to tell her all about her husband: where they met, how long they have been together, how it was for them to have Emmaline and her children move in with them, how they coped with the death of their son. This informal life review was meant to help Mrs. Williams prepare for her husband's impending death. Incidentally, it brought the two women closer together and enriched the nurse's growing and richly rewarding experience of such late-night intimacies.

Mrs. Williams needed to be reminded to eat and to take occasional "breaks," even for short periods. The nurses did not encourage her to go home, correctly sensing that doing so might make her more anxious and fearful that she would not be there when he dies.[2] Because they know that people in Mrs. Williams' situation are often ambivalent, the nurses continue to assess her understanding of the fact that her husband will die and to educate her about the process. They include all the family members in their explanations of the signs of impending death. They correctly see it as part of their support for the family.

Joey was removed from the ventilator while his wife and daughter held his hands. He was given adequate medication to control even the appearance of distress. He died within an hour. The family was very sad, but profoundly grateful to the nursing staff for supporting them through this most difficult time. They were given phone numbers to call with any questions that might occur later. Janet, the nurse who most often cared for them, walked them to their car. She was also sad, but was comforted by the fact that she and her colleagues knew enough about palliative care to make a lasting difference in the lives of these family members.[2]

! TAKE AWAY POINTS

- The family is the unit of care.
- Human variability suggests that individual assessment guided by general knowledge be continual and ongoing in any case.
- Asking lots of personal questions leads to more than good clinical decisions. People also fascinate, amaze, amuse, inspire, and renew us.
- People usually remember in vivid detail and forever the people, events, and feelings associated with the sudden, unexpected death of a loved one. The importance of what we do and how we do it lives on.

REFERENCES

[1] Iverson K. *Grave Words: Notifying Survivors about Sudden, Unexpected Deaths.* Tucson: Galen Press; 1999.
[2] Campbell M. Nurse to nurse palliative care. New York: McGraw Hill; 2009; 119–125.
[3] Stroebe M, Hansson R, Stroebe W, Schut H. *Handbook of Bereavement Research.* Washington, DC: American Psychological Association; 2001.

Case 3.2 Anticipatory Grief and the Dysfunctional Family

Rita J. DiBiase

HISTORY

Helen, a 60-year-old woman with metastatic pancreatic cancer, was admitted with decreased level of consciousness, jaundice, and cachexia. Her husband Jack and children Sophie, Colin, and Trisha stayed close. Helen's condition was tenuous and the family was told she may only have days to live. The palliative team assessed Helen, discovering she had inadvertently taken her long-acting opioids for breakthrough pain. She received hydration, an opioid rotation, supportive medications, and care. Jack had spoken privately with the palliative team, stating that Helen made him promise her life wouldn't be extended. He asked if she could be given something to save her dignity and help her be free. The team reassured Jack that with intensive symptom management and support, Helen would be comfortable and her dignity maintained. It was explained that the treatment plan would focus on comfort with death not being hastened but instead a natural process.

Jack grudgingly agreed, then left the hospital intermittently, making funeral arrangements, organizing banking matters, and buying prepared meals to keep in the freezer. Sophie would not leave her mother's bedside, even though nurses had encouraged her to take breaks. Colin called Sophie a few times a day to check in and visited in the evenings. No one had seen Trisha for days and Jack finally found her painting in her art studio. She had refused to go to the hospital.

Case Studies in Palliative and End-of-Life Care, First Edition. Edited by Margaret L. Campbell.
© 2012 John Wiley & Sons, Inc. Published 2012 by John Wiley & Sons, Inc.

The family had anticipated Helen's death; however, over the next few days she slowly became oriented and alert. Jack was shocked when he walked in and saw Helen sitting up in bed, talking and drinking a beverage. He immediately went to the desk and asked why his wife was being given juice. He yelled, "She didn't want to be kept alive. You people are adding to her suffering!" Sophie overheard her father and accused him of wanting her mother dead. Colin came to visit his mother and began spending more time at the hospital. Trisha refused to visit, stating, "I've lost my mother already; I can't stand the pain of going through it all over again!"

Helen became quiet and withdrawn. Jack visited only for short periods. Sophie argued with her father, and the nurses had to intervene. Sophie and Colin supported each other and when Helen asked for Trisha, they said she was ill. They called Trisha and accused her of being heartless. Several of the staff were upset. They asked for another assignment, stating that Jack was being cold and the children were arguing instead of spending precious time with their mother.

?   CLINICAL QUESTION

What interventions are important when supporting a dysfunctional family who have experienced a loss and are grieving?

✓   DISCUSSION

Anticipatory grief is defined as a form of normal grief which is experienced in anticipation of or prior to a future loss.[1-3] The concept includes mourning, coping, interaction, planning, and psychosocial reorganization in response to the impending loss. There is a concurrent tenuous balance between holding on, drawing closer, and letting go of a loved one.[4] Anticipatory grief was initially described by Erich Lindemann in relation to family members of military personnel who attempted to adjust to the constantly looming threat of death, in essence confronting grief and letting go as reality.[5] They experienced depression and preoccupation with the absent family member, envisioning potential modes of death and anticipation of readjustment to life without their loved one. In some cases, detachment was so complete that marriages failed upon return of the soldiers. In 1984, Rando again described the phenomenon in relation to high divorce rates of POW soldiers who returned from Vietnam.[1]

Aldrich's[6] seminal paper, The Dying Patient's Grief, cited the presence of ambivalence associated with anticipatory grief, not usually present with post death grief. The longer the anticipation, the more risk of ambivalence and a wish for the inevitable to occur, placing patients in a vulnerable situation.[1] Early work by Fulton and Fulton delineated four aspects of anticipatory grief: depression, heightened concern for the terminally ill person, rehearsal of the death, and attempts to adjust to consequences.[7] Anticipatory grief, a multidimensional syndrome, is host to a myriad of emotions including anxiety, sadness, guilt, anger, loss, rage, fear, and difficulty functioning as usual.[8] Because anticipatory grief is reported to be unconscious and often unrecognized, clinicians must be aware of this facet to provide guidance to patients and their families.[1,9–11]

Forewarning and Preparedness

Fulton emphasizes that forewarning of loss refers to the perception that death is likely to occur.[11] It cannot be assumed that anticipatory grief will necessarily follow. It is important not to confuse forewarning of loss with anticipatory grief.[2] Whereas anticipatory grief is unconscious, forewarning is a conscious process.[10,12] Families of individuals who are forewarned of a grim prognosis will not necessarily react to it nor assimilate the information.[2,9,12]

Preparedness is the caregiver's perception or degree of readiness for the death.[13] The concept, in its infancy, has not been fully defined, conceptualized, or studied. Hebert, Prigerson, Schulz, and Arnold reviewed the literature, exploring uncertainty, determinants of preparedness, its multidimensional nature, and communication between caregivers and health care providers.[13] They propose that better communication about death and bereavement among significant parties will improve preparedness and ultimately clinical outcomes for the caregivers. Their framework incorporates discussions about end of life (EOL) as a primary focus, while discussions about medical, psychosocial, spiritual, and practical and other relevant issues can be embedded into conversations. Topics of conversation are identified in the model as: discussing prognosis; advance care planning; dealing with conflict; withdrawal of life support; addressing cultural or spiritual concerns; and discussing grief and loss. Clinical outcomes are identified as: caregiver satisfaction; caregiver mental health and adjustment; and surrogate decision making. This framework is relevant when considering the opportunity for communication and the uniqueness of each person and family during the period of anticipatory grief.[13] Health care providers who understand the differences and relationship between anticipatory grief, forewarning, and preparedness can address needs of individuals and families during an arduous time.

Negative Impact

Some family members may distance themselves in response to overwhelming sorrow and anxiety; however, if the detachment is too strong, the separation may be too complete.[1,5] This may be witnessed when family members appear impassive or stay away from the dying individual, causing distress for the patient, other family, and staff.[1] This unconscious coping strategy can be a disadvantage, with grief work done so effectively that individuals readjust and focus on new interactions.[5] The result may be lost opportunities for communication, physical presence, and emotional engagement.

When family members have grieved in anticipation and have emotionally detached but the patient experiences a remission or rallies and lives on, an intriguing and noteworthy phenomenon transpires. The Lazarus syndrome is based on the biblical character who returned from the dead.[1] Caregivers may feel like they are on a roller coaster and dread having to go through it all again, with the patient on the receiving end of those feelings.

Another challenge is family members' varying reactions, namely disbelief, emotional exhaustion, or dread, or on the other end of the spectrum, joy or even thoughts of a miracle.[3] The pain of grief can increase as the period of anticipation is prolonged and death draws closer. Caregivers may become so conscious of the impending loss they are unable to leave their loved one.[2] In extreme cases these behaviours may be due to feelings of guilt, loss, or ambivalence, especially in tumultuous relationships.[3]

With prolonged anticipation, overt manifestations of grief at the time of death may be absent. Resulting feelings may include shame, guilt, and being judged by others, including clinicians.[10] Families may not feel the need for a funeral, thus losing the opportunity for a healing ritual while also removing the ability for others to acknowledge the loss and support the family.

Positive Impact

The anticipatory period before death may be an opportunity for individuals to gradually deal with loss, handle unfinished business, resolve conflicts, and assimilate role changes that will occur.[4,10] Anticipatory grief shares some of the same characteristics as post-death grief; however, grief following the death is no less painful.[10] In preparing for expected losses, individuals and families develop coping strategies.[12] The designated time may draw people closer together, allowing for enhanced communication while planning special ways to say goodbye.[1,3,14] Psychosocial and existential distress can also be addressed. The use of dignity therapy,[15] a form of life review that engages patients in individualized psychotherapeutic intervention through a series of interviews, enables them to leave a legacy.

Limitations of Research

The concept of anticipatory grief has caused some stir among researchers and death studies scholars. Some suggest the concept does not exist, because grief cannot truly be experienced until the actual death.[17,18] Others have focused on the description and meaning of the concept itself.[1,2,7] Rando proposed the term anticipatory mourning because grief is only one component of a complex multidimensional phenomenon.[4] Studies that examined whether anticipatory grief helped with post-death bereavement reported conflicting findings.[3,11,19] Qualitative studies focused on experiences of families of adult or pediatric patients and spouses either pre or post death.[19]

Fulton published a critique, contrasting the terms forewarning of loss, anticipatory grief, and anticipatory mourning.[11] He discussed evolution of Lindemann's[5] original definition, asserting that the focus of early research had shifted. Lack of uniformity, variety in populations and scenarios, and incongruent operational definitions and concepts, along with methodological issues, were cited as factors leading to contradictory and inconsistent findings.[11,16] Fulton pointed out that the experts themselves can't agree, creating controversy, and thus prompting his colleagues to open a discussion and go beyond earlier works of pioneers.[11] In spite of opposing ideas, many see the time before an expected death as an opportunity to assist caregivers and patients.[11]

Interventions

National Principles and Norms of Practice

Health care providers can draw upon national evidence-based frameworks such A Model to Guide Hospice Palliative Care: Based on National Principles and Norms of Practice, developed in Canada.[20] The term hospice palliative care is used to validate convergence into one movement. One aspect of the model is the "square of care," which has two main components: guiding delivery of patient and family care. The first is essential and basic steps during a therapeutic encounter, which include categories of assessment, information sharing, decision-making, care planning, care delivery, and confirmation. The other component is the domains of issues associated with illness and bereavement, which guides professional caregivers toward addressing the multifaceted and complex issues faced by each patient and family (Figure 3.2.1).

Communication

Identifying and normalizing anticipatory grief with acknowledgement and validation can stimulate discussion, clarify future plans, and promote life review.[9] Clinicians optimize care by using an interdisciplinary approach and a theoretical framework promoting consistent messages for end-of-life conversations (Figure 3.2.1).[13] It is essential to address anxiety and uncertainty surrounding a situation that challenges individuals to separate yet remain connected.[13] Byock's book *The Four Things that Matter Most* delineate four simple but powerful statements: "Please forgive me," "I forgive you," "Thank you," and "I love you."[21] These decla-

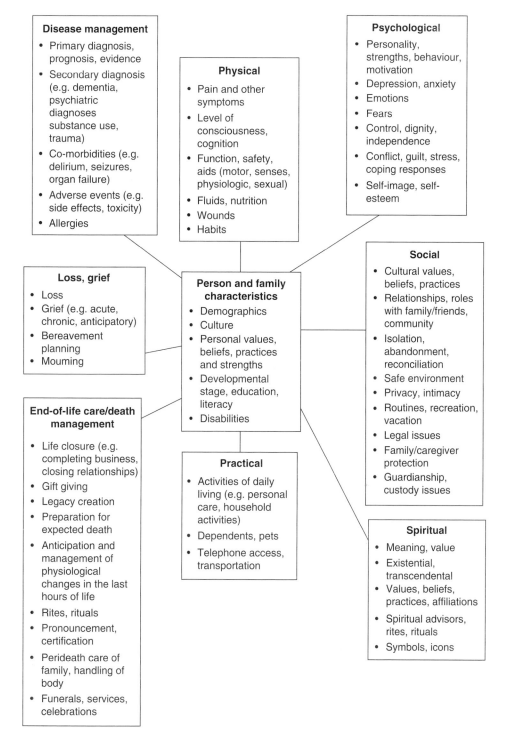

Figure 3.2.1. Domains of issues associated with illness and bereavement. Ferris FD, Balfour HM, Bowen K, Farley J, Hardwich M, Lamontagne C, Lundy M, Syme A, West P. *A Model to Guide Hospice Palliative Care*. Ottawa, ON: Canadian Hospice Palliative Care Association; 2002. Reprinted with permission from the Canadian Hospice Palliative Care Association.

rations may be catalysts to opening dialogues and easing suffering. Although psychosocial or spiritual professionals may be most comfortable discussing these scenarios, other team members who have trusting relationships with patients and caregivers can introduce the topic.

Dealing with Unfinished Business and Conflict

A recurring theme in the literature is that of unfinished business. Clinicians can play a powerful role in assisting patients and families dealing with this emotionally charged topic.[1,3,19,21,22] Heightened feelings may cause families to revisit past disputes and unresolved issues, creating conflict with family or staff. [22] A perception of neglect linked to the illness is more likely to lead to signs of aggression. Continual loss, role changes, and stifling of strong emotions may lead to frustration, helplessness, and outbursts. When family members wish for it to be over, then guilt may rear its ugly head.[1,10] Health care providers can reframe phrases such as "losing control" to "emotional liberation" or "intense emotions."[1] Coaching patients and caregivers to express themselves can help avoid stifling strong emotions that may eventually explode. Providing privacy, encouraging expression of emotions, and using a calm, supportive tone to validate distress displays empathy, reassurance, and acceptance.

Family Assessment, Support, and Family-Centered Interventions

Learning about roles and how families coped in the past avoids asking them to adapt in a manner to which they are not accustomed.[1,22] Nonjudgmental, supportive assessments of family relationships, roles, and dynamics are integral to identifying strengths, barriers, and customizing interventions.[1,22] Although professional counselors provide specialized care, all health care providers can contribute to assessments and support. Structured family meetings with the interdisciplinary team, patient, and family can provide updated information and education and build trust.[23] Support groups are also beneficial for some individuals.[3] Clinicians in all settings can use the family-centered interventions for EOL care and anticipatory grief by addressing cognitive, emotional, and social processes as described by Coombs (Table 3.2.1).[24]

Dignity Therapy

Dignity therapy provides those facing death with an opportunity for legacy making and generativity.[15] Patients are asked structured questions about what matters most, memories, and messages they wish to share. Audiotaped sessions are used to create a narrative, which is then edited and approved by the patient. The final written document is given to loved ones. Participants reported a heightened sense of dignity, meaning, and purpose and will to live while also showing significant improvement in suffering and reduction of depressive symptoms. Individuals found the document was appreciated by their loved ones.[15] Family members' perspectives endorsed the use of dignity therapy as

TABLE 3.2.1. Anticipatory grief and family-centered end-of-life care interventions.

Cognitive processes: Help the family to understand that death is imminent and be able to make decisions regarding end-of-life care. Role of the health care team:
- Provide consistent, timely, and honest information
- Demonstrate that the patient is being given strong collaborative care
- Make use of regular family conferences and communication tools such as written documentation
- Allow time during patient treatment discussions for family input
- Ask for and acknowledge patient and family preferences and concerns

Emotional processes: Help the family to be able to bring meaning and closure to the patient's life. Role of the health care team:
- Acknowledge the patient as a person and attempt to understand their life using Value Tool*
  - Valuing family statements
  - Acknowledging their emotions
  - Listening to the family
  - Understanding who the patient is as a person
  - Eliciting questions
- Empathize with the family about the impact of their loss
- Support the patient and the family and be present for them
- If possible, give reassurance that the family member will be kept free of pain and comfortable

Social processes: Help the family to maintain relationships and re-establish new ones after their bereavement. Role of the health care team:
- Assist the family in identifying sources of social support in the short and long term
- Provide the family with spiritual/cultural and physical resources (in the form of interventions for family centered care)

*Lautrette A, Darmon M, Megabane B, Joly L, Chevret S, Adrie C, et al. A communication strategy and brochure for relatives of patients dying in the ICU. *New England Journal of Medicine*; 2007; 356(5):469–480.
Coombs MA. The mourning before: can anticipatory grief theory inform family care in adult intensive care? *International Journal of Palliative Nursing*; 2011; 16(12):580–584.
Reprinted with permission from Mark Allen Group.

an intervention that lessened suffering and helped the patient retain dignity and other variables reported previously by patients.[25] In situations in which it is not feasible to provide a structured program of dignity therapy, if patients are open to the idea, elements of the intervention can be incorporated by health care teams in any setting.

BACK TO OUR CASE

Julia, the unit manager, called a staff meeting, inviting the palliative team and social worker. Nurses expressed their concerns about Helen and frustration with the family. Education about anticipatory grief, the Value Tool, EOL communication framework, and Domains of Issues were circulated and discussed. The group went over the documents, identifying domains in which there were issues. They all realized that Helen and the family would benefit from guidance and support. Helen's nurse met with her alone, providing an opportunity to express her sorrow and discuss her hopes and wishes. The social worker met with Jack and he wept, stating he was just trying to fulfill his wife's dying wishes. He expressed guilt at wishing the pain was over. The nurse, social worker, and palliative physician met with Jack and Helen to discuss feelings, unresolved issues, and a plan for the next weeks. Helen was asked to voice her hopes for her remaining time with her family. They were asked how they had managed as a couple and family during difficult times. Jack and Helen agreed that a family meeting would be helpful but were worried about Trisha attending. The social worker suggested Helen write Trisha a letter asking her to come.

The palliative nurse practitioner and primary nurse met with Sophie and Colin. They were initially reluctant but with coaching and validation of feelings, were able to express their frustration and sadness. They were also asked about family dynamics and to describe each of their roles in the family. They decided to talk with Trisha together and agreed to bring their mother's letter. Helen also asked to see her chaplain alone.

Trisha read her mother's letter alone. The social worker called her and she said she needed more time. After a few days, Trisha called her siblings and agreed to a come to the hospital for a family meeting. The palliative team, social worker, and primary nurse met with Helen and the family. Discussion addressed Helen's current health status, her hopes for her time with the family, family dynamics, and roles. The team went over some of the aspects of anticipatory grief, validating their experiences and helping the family normalize the process. Jack reminded everyone of how they had managed during difficult times. Although Sophie and Colin were able to give input, Trisha remained very quiet, withdrawn, and tearful. Helen told the family that she liked the idea of dignity therapy and the social worker agreed to set up the interviews. As discussed privately with the social worker and her chaplain, Helen asked Trisha if she could provide artwork for the finished booklet. Trisha quietly nodded.

Helen participated in dignity therapy and Trisha painted the finished booklet at her mother's bedside. Jack, Sophie, and Colin were also able to be with Helen and support each other. Helen lived two more weeks, remaining alert until her final days. An interdisciplinary team approach, education, resources, and support enabled the staff to provide comprehensive compassionate person- and family-centered care and support. Helen was able to treasure time with her husband and family, say goodbye, and leave a legacy.

! TAKE AWAY POINTS

- There are a number of evidence-based interventions health care providers can use to support patients and families experiencing anticipatory grief.
- An interdisciplinary team approach with inclusion of the patient and family is an effective means of providing compassionate person- and family-centered care.
- Communication and structured family meetings can help address intense emotions, unfinished business, and conflict experienced by those anticipating the death of their loved one.

REFERENCES

[1] Rando TA. *Grief, Dying, and Death: Clinical Interventions for Caregivers*. Champaign, IL: Research Press; 1984.
[2] Fulton R, Gottesman, DJ. Anticipatory grief: a psychosocial concept reconsidered. *British Journal of Psychiatry*; 1980; 137:45–54.
[3] Worden JW. *Grief counselling and Grief Therapy: A Handbook for the Mental Health Practitioner*, 3rd edition. New York: Springer Publishing Company Inc.; 1991.
[4] Rando TA, ed. *Clinical Dimensions of Anticipatory Mourning*. Champaign, IL: Research Press; 2000:1–13.
[5] Lindemann E. Symptomatology and management of acute grief. *Am J Psychiatry*; 1944; 101:141–148.
[6] Aldrich CK. The dying patient's grief. *Journal of the American Medical Association*; 1963; 184:329–331.
[7] Fulton R, Fulton JA. A psychosocial aspect of terminal care: anticipatory grief. *Omega*; 1971; 2:91–99.
[8] Theut SK, Jordan L, Ross LA, Deutsch SI. Caregiver's anticipatory grief in dementia: a pilot study. *International Journal Aging Human Development*; 1991; 33:113–118.
[9] Cassarett D, Kutner JS, Abrahm J. Life and death: a practical approach to grief and bereavement. *Ann Intern Med*; 2001; 134:208–215.
[10] Corless IB. Bereavement. In: Ferrell BA, Coyle N (eds). *Textbook of Palliative Nursing*, 3rd edition. New York: Oxford University Press; 2010; 597–612.
[11] Fulton R. Anticipatory mourning: a critique of the concept. *Mortality*; 2003; 8(4):342–351.
[12] Corr CA. Anticipatory grief and mourning: an overview. In: Doka KJ (ed). *Living with Grief: Before and After the Death*. Washington, DC: Hospice Foundation of America; 2007; 5–19.
[13] Hebert RS, Prigerson HG, Schulz R, Arnold RM. Preparing caregivers for the death of a loved one: a theoretical framework and suggestions for future research. *Journal of Palliative Medicine*; 2006; 9(5):1164–1171.

[14] Zilberfein F. Coping with death: anticipatory grief and bereavement. *Generations/care at the end-of-life: restoring a balance.* Spring 1999; 69–74.

[15] Chochinov HM, Hack T, Hassard T, Kristjanson LJ, McCleent S, Harlos M. Dignity therapy: a novel psychotherapeutic intervention for patients near end of life. *Journal of Clinical Oncology*; 2005; 23(24):5520–5525.

[16] Reynolds L, Botha D. Anticipatory grief: its nature, impact, and reasons for contradictory findings. *Counselling, Psychotherapy, and Health*; 2006; 2(2):15–26.

[17] Glick IO, Weiss RS, Parkes CM. *The First Year of Bereavement.* New York: Wiley; 1974.

[18] Silverman PR. Anticipatory grief from the perspective of widowhood. In: Schoenberg B, Carr AC, Kutscher AH, Petz D, Golderberg IK (eds). *Anticipatory Grief.* New York: Columbia University Press; 1974; 320–330.

[19] Kehl KA. Recognition and support of anticipatory mourning. *Journal of Hospice and Palliative Nursing*; 2005; 7(4):206–211.

[20] Ferris FD, Balfour HM, Bowen K, Farley J, Hardwich M, Lamontagne C, Lundy M, Syme A, West P. *A Model to Guide Hospice Palliative Care.* Ottawa, ON: Canadian Hospice Palliative Care Association; 2002.

[21] Byock I. *The Four Things that Matter Most.* New York: Free Press, Simon and Schuster Inc.; 2004.

[22] Kramer BJ, Boelk AZ, Auer C. Family conflict at the end of life: lessons learned in a model program for vulnerable older adults. *Journal of Palliative Medicine*; 2007; 9(3):791 801.

[23] Lautrette A, Darmon M, Megabane B, Joly L, Chevret S, Adrie, C, et al. A communication strategy and brochure for relatives of patients dying in the ICU. *New England Journal of Medicine*; 2007; 356(5):469–480.

[24] Coombs MA. The mourning before: can anticipatory grief theory inform family care in adult intensive care? *International Journal of Palliative Nursing*; 2011; 16(12):580–584.

[25] McClement S, Chochinov HM, Hack T, Hassard T, Kristjanson LJ, Harlos M. Dignity therapy: family member perspectives. *Journal of Palliative Medicine*; 2007; 10(5):1076–1082.

Case 3.3 Acute and Uncomplicated Grief after an Expected Death

Rita J. DiBiase

HISTORY

Mary, a 55-year-old retired teacher, had rarely left her husband Jim's bedside since being told of his imminent death from pancreatic cancer. Laura, 25 years old, sat holding her father's hand and crying. Danielle, 27 years old, ran errands and tended to funeral arrangements and other instructions provided by her father. She had been matter of fact and efficient, taking notes and assuring her mother she would take care of things.

Gail, Jim's favorite nurse, had returned to work, saddened to hear the news of his imminent death. Amy, a new nurse, had been caring for Jim the past two days. Amy reported that Jim was "palliative" with only days to live, not needing much intervention. She described Jim's wife and daughter, Mary and Laura, as being sad, often tearful and resigned, while Laura was acting odd, bustling around doing things with no visible signs of sadness. She mentioned that Jim reminded her of her own father and found it too sad to be in the room for long. She had provided care quickly and efficiently, mostly when she was called in.

When Gail entered the room, she was struck by how quiet and dark it was. Usually Jim had the curtains wide open, sunshine spilling in and music playing. She had quickly assessed Jim's unresponsiveness, Cheyne-Stokes respirations, and cool mottled lower extremities. Mary had been resting her head on Jim's bed. She looked bewildered, then

Case Studies in Palliative and End-of-Life Care, First Edition. Edited by Margaret L. Campbell.
© 2012 John Wiley & Sons, Inc. Published 2012 by John Wiley & Sons, Inc.

recognizing Gail, exclaimed how relieved they were to see Gail. She and her daughters had questions regarding what would happen next, whether Jim was in pain, how long it would be, and whether they should they call their chaplain and other family members. Mary began crying and Gail pulled a chair close, sitting silently and holding Mary's hand, with her other hand touching Jim. She nodded to the girls and after a few moments of silence, began to explain what was happening and what to expect in the next few hours. She asked if each of them had an opportunity to speak to Jim alone and they all nodded. After answering their questions she asked if they considered playing the music Jim had spent his career teaching to high school students. Gail also asked them if there was anything else Jim loved and they remembered his love of the outdoors and sunshine. She had offered to call their chaplain and did so from the room. Gail also told them that Sandy, the social worker, could come in and they all agreed.

Gail left the room to update the team. Within a short time, the oncologist, social worker, and chaplain had all been in to see Jim and the family. That afternoon, as Jim had taken his final breaths, Mary looked around with disbelief. She gasped and grabbed on to Jim, holding him tight and weeping. Laura sobbed loudly, holding her father's hand. Danielle stood near them, shaking her head and visibly trying to hold on to her composure. Gail stroked Jim's hand and remained silent. After a period of time, Mary looked up at Gail, bewildered. She began sobbing and saying "This can't be happening. He can't be dead. What will we do without him? We can't just leave him."

? CLINICAL QUESTION

What interventions are important when supporting a family during their bereavement?

✓ DISCUSSION

Unlike sudden or unexpected deaths, more than 90% of patients die after a prolonged illness, providing an opportunity for families and caregivers to spend time with their loved one.[1] When a death is expected, health care professionals play an integral role in those precious last days and hours, because circumstances and care provided at the end of life (EOL) are what loved ones recall.[2] Families and caregivers identify the need for information and sensitive and effective communication as priorities.[3,4] The perspectives of family members and close friends regarding EOL care have been examined.[3] The review of 186 responses revealed almost two-thirds of patients and families reported unmet EOL care needs, a finding supported in other studies.[4,5] Valued communication from clinicians included listening, explanation of what to expect, sensitivity, concern, and availability. Non-verbal communication such as body language and facial expressions was emphasized. Families were frustrated when communication included conflicting advice, mixed messages, insensitive delivery, or poor timing. Some reported that health care providers did not listen and withdrew when a patient's resuscitation status was changed to comfort care. During such a distressful time, families often don't communicate their needs; therefore, it is essential that clinicians initiate dialogue to individualize care and address personal and cultural components.[4,6] Family values and preferences[3] included:

- A supportive environment to secure peaceful death with dignity and respect.
- The wish to be present at time of death.[2,7]
- Attending to the needs and wishes of the dying individual and family. As death draws near, the focus of care shifts more substantially toward the family.[2,7]

Although families are aware that death is imminent, when it actually occurs there may be a sense of numbness, shock, disbelief, and denial.[6,7] Shear describes acute grief as occurring early after the death, marked by powerful prevalent emotions including sadness, crying, anguish, and seemingly relentless despair, which lessen into waves or bursts.[8] Immediately following the death of a loved one, acute grief reactions may vary among cultures, sub-cultures, and individuals within families. Grief manifestations may range from minimal to significant, affecting individuals emotionally, cognitively, socially, and behaviorally.[6]

The death of a loved one is among life's most stressful and painful events, typically causing profound sorrow and anguish for those experiencing the loss.[3,6] As professionals working in palliative care it is critical to have knowledge and resources related to grief, mourning, and bereavement.[2,5,9] With the premise of maintaining clinical practice based on evidence and expertise, the International Work Group on Death, Dying and Bereavement[10] published a statement proposing that members of a health care team and human services professionals receive substantial and relevant education about death, dying, and bereavement. Without this education clinicians cannot care for and support the imminently dying patient and their loved ones at perhaps the most vulnerable times in their lives.

Definitions

It has been noted that the terms "grief," "mourning," and "bereavement" are often used inconsistently and interchangeably in the literature in the field of thanatology.[7,11,12] To provide some clarity, the following brief descriptions acquired from selected literature are a foundation for this case. Loss, defined as absence of a possession or future possession, is often used in relation to the death of a person, but can also be applied to objects, relationships, situations, health, and changes in roles and attributes.[6] Losses may be physical or symbolic.[7] Grief is an individual's reaction or personal response to a significant loss. Grief has emotional, physical, behavioral, cognitive, social, cultural, and spiritual dimensions.[9,11] Mourning is the outward, social expression of grief. It includes cultural norms, customs, and rituals.[6] Bereavement is the experience or state of having lost a loved one to death. It is influenced primarily by culture. Bereavement also refers to the period after the loss and includes both grief and mourning.[11,12]

Models/Theories of Bereavement

In his 1944 landmark article The Symptomatology and Management of Acute Grief, Eric Lindemann presented the following common patterns reported in the bereaved:[13]

- Somatic or bodily distress occurring in waves, 20 minutes to one hour at a time, choking, shortness of breath, sighing, an empty feeling in the abdomen, lack of muscular power, an intense subjective distress described as tension or mental pain
- Preoccupation with the image of the deceased
- Guilt, either in relation to the deceased or around the circumstances of the death
- Hostile behaviors or reactions including responding with irritability and anger, loss of warmth in relationships, and a wish for others not to bother them
- The inability to function in the manner prior to the death

Intriguingly, more than 50 years later Worden reported that he and his colleagues saw very similar behaviors and patterns in grieving individuals.[9] Citing the diverse and expansive range of normal grief responses, he listed the most common in four categories: feelings, physical sensations, cognitions, and behaviors (Table 3.3.1).

Models and theories of grief and bereavement have evolved over the years. Although not exhaustive, a summary of models that have shaped perspectives is provided in Table 3.3.2. Worden discusses how theories range from Freud's early grief work to stages and phases.[9] Worden developed Tasks in Mourning, which he revised in 2009, with the major change being that the fourth task no longer addressed withdrawing from previous relationships but instead discusses a form of enduring connection while moving into a new life.[9] Rando illustrated six "R" processes that grievers manage, describing a more active approach to mourning.[7] Previous works are significant in that current theories have frequently drawn from them. Stroebe and Schut describe the Dual

TABLE 3.3.1. Manifestations of normal grief.

Feelings	• Sadness, with or without crying
	• Anger: frustration, regression, blaming, turned inward can lead to depression
	• Guilt a self-reproach: usually not warranted
	• Anxiety: insecurity, worrying about managing, personal death awareness
	• Loneliness: fatigue, usually self-limiting; if persists may be sign of depression
	• Helplessness
	• Shock
	• Yearning or pining
	• Emancipation
	• Relief: if person suffered, may feel guilt, may occur with difficult relationships
	• Numbness: worry about lack of feelings, usually early in process, protective
Physical sensations	• Hollowness in stomach
	• Tightness in chest
	• Tightness in throat
	• Oversensitivity to noise
	• Sense of depersonalization
	• Breathlessness or shortness of breath
	• Muscle weakness
	• Lack of energy
	• Dry mouth
Cognitions	• Disbelief
	• Confusion
	• Preoccupation
	• Sense of presence
	• Hallucinations
Behaviors	• Sleep disturbances: insomnia or early morning waking
	• Altered appetite: undereating and weight loss, less commonly overeating
	• Absentminded behavior: may lead to inconvenience or harm
	• Social withdrawal: usually short lived, may worry about it, may avoid news
	• Dreams: commonly about deceased, comforting or distressing, resolution
	• Avoid reminders: avoid memory triggers, places, objects, photos
	• Give away objects: may do so quickly then regret action later
	• Searching and calling out
	• Sighing
	• Restless overactivity
	• Crying
	• Visiting special places or carrying symbolic objects
	• Treasuring objects of the deceased

Created from information found in Worden JW. *Grief Counseling and Grief Therapy: A Handbook for the Mental Health Practitioner*, 3rd edition. New York: Springer Publishing Company Inc.; 1991.

TABLE 3.3.2. Models of bereavement.

Model/theory	Author	Components
Psycho-analytic Stages	Freud Lindemann Three stages	Grief work: Need to break attachment bond, face reality 1. Shock and disbelief 2. Preoccupation with image of the deceased 3. Reenters daily life
	Kubler-Ross 5 stages	1. Shock and denial 2. Anger 3. Bargaining 4. Depression 5. Acceptance
Phases	Bowlby Parkes	Grief is a psychological process to relinquishing deceased 1. Numbness and shock 2. Yearning and searching 3. Disorganization and despair 4. Reorganization
	Sanders	1. Shock 2. Awareness of loss 3. Conservation withdrawal 4. Healing 5. Renewal

	Rando
	Six ®
	Processes
		Early attachment patterns a adult attachment styles
		1. Avoidance phase
		  • Recognizes the loss
		2. Confrontation phase
		  • React to the separation
		  • Recollect, re-experience relationship and deceased
		  • Relinquish attachment and relationship to deceased
		3. Accommodation phase
		  • Re-adjust to new world without forgetting the old
		  • Re-invest in new relationships

Task	Worden	1. Accept reality of loss 2. Work through the pain of grief 3. Adjust to an environment without the deceased 4. Find connection with deceased, move on to new life
Two-Track Model of Bereavement	Rubin	Track I focuses on bereaved bipsychosocial functioning Track II bereaved ongoing relationship
Dual Process Model	Stroebe and Schut	Adaptive coping with bereavement Loss-orientation Restoration-orientation

Ferris FD, von Gunten CF, Emanuel LL. Competency in end-of-life care: last hours of life. *Journal of Palliative Medicine*; August 2003; 6(4):605–613.
Corless IB. Bereavement. In: Ferrell BA, Coyle N, eds. *Textbook of Palliative Nursing*, 3rd edition. New York: Oxford University Press; 2010; 597–612.
Rando TA. *Grief, Dying, and Death: Clinical Interventions for Caregivers*. Champaign: IL; Research Press; 1984.
Worden JW. *Grief counseling and Grief Therapy: A Handbook for the Mental Health Practitioner*, 3rd edition. New York: Springer Publishing Company Inc.; 1991.
Corr CA, Coolican MB. Understanding bereavement, grief, and mourning: implications for donation and transplant professionals. *Progress in Transplantation*; June 2010; 20:169–177.
Buglass E. Grief and bereavement theories. *Nursing Standard*; June 2010; 24(41):44–47.
Lindemann E. Symptomatology and management of acute grief. *Am J Psychiatry*; 1944; 101:141–148.

Process Model drawn from Cognitive Stress Theory.[14] Coping is seen as a process while consequences of bereavement, whether adaptive or nonadaptive, are considered. There are two categories, loss-orientation and restoration-orientation, with the griever oscillating between the two. Rubin et al. explain the Two-Track Model of Bereavement, which has a bifocal perspective.[15] The model unites general functioning or bio-psychosocial changes with the significance or state of the relationship with the deceased. Both perspectives are highly significant, building on the strength of the other.

Another perspective is the expression of grief, with Martin and Doka identifying two primary grieving styles.[16] Intuitive grievers experience strong waves of openly expressed emotions. The outpouring of these feelings assists in adaptation to their grief. Men who are intuitive grievers may be judged within some circles. Instrumental grievers express grief more cognitively, physically, or behaviorally. They may think through their loss or respond by "doing." This style acknowledges the loss, which is different than keeping busy to avoid reality. Women who are instrumental grievers may be labeled as cold or unfeeling. Instrumental grievers may be judged early in the grief process if they show little outward emotion. Most people use a combination of both styles, with one being more predominant. Culture, age, and other variables are also important to consider.

Interventions

Health care providers who care for dying patients frequently witness loss and acute grief of family caregivers. With an expected death, a vigil occurs, allowing health care providers to further encompass families in the plan of care. Even those with clinical expertise and excellent interpersonal skills may not possess the knowledge or skills required for EOL care of patients and families. The benefits of a comprehensive EOL/palliative curriculums such as the End-of-Life Nursing Education Consortium (ELNEC) are reported.[17] Education in Palliative and End-of-Life Care (EPEC) is another valuable educational curriculum described in the literature.[2] Such programs also help clinicians face their own grief and deal with unresolved losses, providing them with some resources that allow them to continue to provide care without being destroyed in the process.[18]

Another strategy is the use of evidence-based guidelines for provision of quality palliative and EOL care. In 2004, the National Consensus Project (NCP)[19] for Quality Palliative Care released The Clinical Practice Guidelines for Palliative Care, which delineated eight domains of quality palliative care:

- Structure and processes of care
- Physical aspects of care
- Psychological and psychiatric aspects of care

- Social aspects of care
- Spiritual, religious, and existential aspects of care
- Cultural aspects of care
- Care of the imminently dying patient
- Ethical and legal aspects of care

The National Quality Forum (NQF),[20] using the eight domains, created 38 preferred practices which are based on evidence or expert opinion. Selected preferred practices[5] can guide care of the imminently dying patient and address the period of acute grief at time of death (Table 3.3.3).

The following interventions are derived from evidence, expert opinion, NCP, NQF, ELNEC, and EPEC. Comprehending the needs and preferences of families is integral to the care plan. The desire for communication and information has been a consistent theme in the literature.[4] Providing timely updates and describing signs and symptoms of imminent death can assist with the wish to be present at the time of death. Those who are unable to be present also require support, with clinicians perhaps serving as mediators when family members have different preferences.[2]

Family members may be reluctant to leave the room for fear that their loved one will die while they are gone. Providing snacks and drinks in the room or nearby allows family to leave the room for a short time but remain close in case things change quickly. Provision of a comfort cart or bereavement tray is a strategy in caring for families. Employing an interdisciplinary team approach with members from nursing, medicine, social work, spiritual care, and volunteers provides the patient and family with support. Inquire about cultural practices or rituals that can be facilitated by the staff and include caregivers as a means of instrumental grieving.

Acute care institutions are often busy and focused on treatment and care of the living. Providing a private, peaceful and homelike environment, with unrestricted visiting hours, is essential. Placement of a sign or symbol on the door can notify staff from all departments that death is near, or has occurred, avoiding interruptions or unnecessary intrusion. Ideally, health care providers who know the patient and family are assigned to their care at EOL. Clinicians can suggest that family members may want to speak to the patient individually, allowing for private conversations. Health care providers can serve as role models by speaking to an unresponsive patient, and if culturally acceptable, expressing caring through touch of the patient or caregivers. Reassessing the desire for setting during the final hours is important, because family members may change their minds.

When death occurs, a silent presence can be most therapeutic. It is important to support the expression of feelings and individualize the grief process in relation to age, personality, and grieving styles.[16] Some

TABLE 3.3.3. National Quality Forum Preferred Practices for Domain 7: Care of the Imminently Dying.

Preferred practice 26: Recognize and document the transition to the active dying phase and communicate to the patient, family, and staff the expectation of imminent death.

Preferred practice 27: Educate family in a timely manner regarding the signs and symptoms of imminent death in an age-appropriate, developmentally appropriate, and culturally appropriate manner.

Preferred practice 28: As part of the ongoing care planning process, routinely ascertain and document patient and family wishes about the care setting for site of death and fulfill patient and family preferences when possible.

Preferred practice 29: Provide adequate dosage of analgesics and sedatives as appropriate to achieve patient comfort during the active dying phase and address concerns and fears about use of narcotics and analgesics hastening death.

Preferred practice 30: Treat the body after death with respect according to the cultural and religious practices of the family and in accordance with local law.

Preferred practice 31: Facilitate effective grieving by implementing in a timely manner a bereavement care plan after the patient's death when the family remains the focus of care.

Lynch M, Dahlin CM. The national consensus project and national quality forum preferred practices in care of the imminently dying. *Journal of Hospice & Palliative Nursing*; Nov.-Dec. 2007; 9(6):316–322.
National Consensus Project for Quality Palliative Care. *Clinical Practice Guidelines for Quality Palliative Care*, 2nd edition. 2009. http://www.nationalconsensusproject.org.

may be bewildered by their own reactions. Support and comfort are required to help families through such a distressful time. Rituals may be implemented to provide meaning and structure, with staff facilitating or even participating. It is essential to treat the body with respect and ask family if they wish to participate in physical care.[2] Providers can explain what will happen to the body and cultural practices must be assessed and honored. Cultural, religious, or personal practices and beliefs emphasizing individuality are the impetus for the care plan.

Individuals may feel numb and unsure of the next steps; therefore, assisting with funeral arrangements or calling family members and engaging the chaplain or social worker for support strengthens the interdisciplinary approach.[17,19,20] Practical aspects such as transportation home also must be addressed. Facilitation of grieving is addressed by provision of contact numbers for grief support. Continuing with the family as the focus of palliative care includes bereavement. Attending a funeral is a personal decision made by the health care professional. Sending a sympathy card or making a follow-up phone call provides an opportunity to show compassion and continuity of care, as well as assess grief.[2,19]

⤺ BACK TO OUR CASE

When Gail entered Jim's room, she was surprised to see Jim in his final hours. She was also concerned about the family's inquiries and distress. She heard their unanswered questions and fears about what to expect at the time of death. Amy, having had little experience with EOL care, had not recognized the signs and symptoms of imminent death. Amy was not aware of different grieving styles and thus was confused by Laura's behavior. Amy was also affected by her own fears, and thus was unable to be truly present for the patient and family.

After consulting with the family, Gail promptly called the social worker, oncologist, and patient's own chaplain, emphasizing the strengths of an interdisciplinary approach. She also realized that the family had been very reluctant to leave Jim; therefore, she had a comfort cart brought in. The family was provided with drinks and snacks for sustenance without the fear of being gone when Jim died. Gail placed a symbolic bereavement sign on the door, notifying all hospital staff that the patient was imminently dying. The card also had instructions to check at the desk prior to entering so the staff could speak with the family before visitors entered, ensuring the family's acceptance. Gail brought a booklet for them to read reinforcing the education she provided about the dying process.

At the actual time of Jim's death, Mary conveyed a sense of numbness and initial disbelief. Recognizing the need for support and direction, Gail asked the family if they would like to stay with Jim. They were very appreciative and looked relieved when Gail stated she would return within a short time to provide care. She explained the physical changes that would occur to his body so they wouldn't be alarmed. Gail had inquired about special practices or rituals. Mary and the girls had decided to play Jim's favorite songs and sing along as he loved them to do. Sandy, the social worker, had inquired about people to notify and assisted Mary with some calls. Their chaplain returned, prayed with the family, and assured them that the funeral arrangements were taken care of.

When Gail left the room she again ensured that the sign remained on the door so no one would disturb the family. Gail returned 15 minutes later and Jim's daughters left the room. Mary stayed and lovingly washed Jim's face and hands while Gail completed the rest of his care. The family stayed for a short time and then decided to leave. They hugged Gail, thanking her for making Jim's last hours peaceful and dignified.

❗ TAKE AWAY POINTS

- Grief is an individual process that has emotional, physical, behavioral, cognitive, social, cultural, and spiritual dimensions.

- Health care providers need current knowledge of grief models, theories, and resources to provide support and assistance to those experiencing acute grief.
- Family members remember the circumstances of the death of their loved ones; health care providers are in the unique position of creating a memory of a peaceful and dignified death.

REFERENCES

[1] Field MJ, Cassel CK, eds. *Approaching Death: Improving Care at the End of Life*. Washington, DC: National Academy Press; 1997; 28–30.

[2] Ferris FD, von Gunten CF, Emanuel LL. Competency in end-of-life care: last hours of life. *Journal of Palliative Medicine*; August 2003; 6(4):605–613.

[3] Boucher J, Bova C, Kaufman D, et al. Next-of-kin's perspectives of end-of-life care. *Journal of Hospice & Palliative Nursing*; Jan.-Feb. 2010; 12(1):41–50.

[4] Lowey S. Communication between the nurse and family caregiver in end-of-life care: a review of the literature. *Journal of Hospice & Palliative Nursing*; Jan.-Feb. 2008; 10(1):35–48.

[5] Lynch M, Dahlin CM. The national consensus project and national quality forum preferred practices in care of the imminently dying. *Journal of Hospice & Palliative Nursing*; Nov.-Dec. 2007; 9(6):316–322.

[6] Corless IB. Bereavement. In: Ferrell BA, Coyle N, eds. *Textbook of Palliative Nursing*, 3rd edition. New York: Oxford University Press; 2010; 597–612.

[7] Rando TA. *Grief, Dying, and Death: Clinical Interventions for Caregivers*. Champaign: IL; Research Press; 1984.

[8] Shear MK, Mulhare E. Complicated grief. *Psychiatr Ann*; 2008; 39:662–670.

[9] Worden JW. *Grief counseling and Grief Therapy: A Handbook for the Mental Health Practitioner*, 3rd edition. New York: Springer Publishing Company Inc.; 1991.

[10] International Work Group on Death, Dying, and Bereavement. A statement of assumptions and principles concerning education about death, dying, and bereavement for professionals in health care and human services. *Omega*; 1991; 23(3):235–239.

[11] Corr CA, Coolican MB. Understanding bereavement, grief, and mourning: implications for donation and transplant professionals. Progress in Transplantation; June 2010; 20:169–177.

[12] Buglass E. Grief and bereavement theories. Nursing Standard; June 2010; 24(41):44–47.

[13] Lindemann E. Symptomatology and management of acute grief. Am J Psychiatry; 1944; 101:141–148.

[14] Stroebe M, Schut H. The dual process model of coping with bereavement: a decade on. Omega; 2010; 61(4):273–289.

[15] Rubin SS, Nadav OB, Malkinson R, Koren D, Goffer-Shnarch M, Michaeli E. The two-track model of bereavement questionairre (TTBQ): development and validation of a relational measure. Death Studies; 2009; 33:305–333.

[16] Martin TL, Doka KJ. *Men Don't Cry. . . Women Do. Transcending Gender Stereotypes of Grief*. Philadelphia: Brunner/Mazel.

[17] Malloy P, Virani R, Kelly K, Harrington-Jacobs H, Ferrell B. Seven years and 50 courses later: end-of-life nursing education consortium continues to provide excellent palliative care education. Journal of Hospice and Palliative Nursing; July-Aug. 2008; 10(4):233–239.

[18] Vachon MLS. Caring for the professional caregivers: before and after the death. In: Doka, KJ (ed). *Living with Grief: Before and After the Death.* Washington, DC: Hospice Foundation of America; 2007; 311–330.

[19] National Consensus Project for Quality Palliative Care. Clinical Practice Guidelines for Quality Palliative Care, 2nd edition. 2009. http://www.nationalconsensusproject.org.

[20] National Quality Forum. *A National Framework and Preferred Practices for Pallative and Hospice Care Quality.* Washington, DC: National Quality Forum; 2006.

Case 3.4 Bereavement after Unexpected Death

Garrett K. Chan

HISTORY

George, a 78-year-old man, was brought in by ambulance to the emergency department (ED) for a self-inflicted gunshot wound to the head. George's wife, who had advanced lung disease and lived on the first floor of their home, said that the patient had a history of colon cancer. She heard the gun go off on the second story of their home, but she could not climb the stairs to see what happened and called 911 immediately. The paramedics found the patient unconscious and unresponsive with his pupils fixed and dilated. They intubated the patient and brought him to the ED. The police detained the wife at the home for questioning. The wife told the paramedics that there was an advance directive with instructions of do not resuscitate (DNR) but could not find the paperwork in time to send it with the paramedics.

When the patient arrived in the ED, the patient had two open wounds to his head with small amounts of brain parenchyma around one of the open wounds. The patient's vital signs were poor (heart rate 60 to 80 beats per minute (bpm) blood pressure 50 to 90/30s). The trauma surgeon, ED physician, and nurses were informed that there was an advance directive with DNR instructions. However, there was no immediate presentation of the document that accompanied the patient. The trauma surgeon and the social worker were immediately on the phone to a local health care maintenance organization (HMO) to get a copy of the advance directives faxed to the ED. The advance

Case Studies in Palliative and End-of-Life Care, First Edition. Edited by Margaret L. Campbell.
© 2012 John Wiley & Sons, Inc. Published 2012 by John Wiley & Sons, Inc.

directives indicated that the patient did not want to be intubated and no life-sustaining measures were to be performed. The patient was extubated yet had a copious amount of blood pooling in the nasopharynx and needed frequent suctioning by the primary nurse. The patient was breathing on his own but the oxygen saturation was decreasing steadily. The systolic blood pressure was fluctuating around the 60s to 70s and the heart rate was steady at 60 to 70 bpm. The nurses obtained orders for fentanyl to provide pain relief and to ease their concern that the patient was suffering.

The police discovered that the patient had left a suicide note at home. He stated in the letter that he took his life to end the excruciating pain that he was in. One nurse asked the detective who was at the bedside if he could contact the police who were interviewing the wife if he would allow her to come to the hospital because the patient was dying. The detective agreed readily to call the officer. The officer at the home offered to drive the woman to the hospital but she declined. She said that she was in very poor health herself and she didn't think she could make it.

The social worker called the patient's son. He said that he was coming from 30 miles away, and it would be a while before he could make it to the hospital. He also said that he wanted to stop by his parents' home to see if his mother was OK. Once the son got to his parents' house, he called the hospital to say that his mother was in a lot of distress and they wouldn't make it to the hospital.

The staff heard from the social worker that neither the wife nor the son was going to be able to make it to the hospital. The patient began to go into runs of ventricular tachycardia (VT) with oxygen saturations in the low 30s to 40s. As the patient began to go into these runs of VT, four nurses and an ED technician gathered at the bedside, just standing there with him as he went into sustained VT, then into ventricular fibrillation, and then into asystole. The patient died two hours after he arrived at the ED.

? CLINICAL QUESTION

What interventions are important when supporting a family that is suffering from a sudden loss and acute grief?

✓ DISCUSSION

A sudden loss from acute illness or trauma and that occurs without warning can precipitate acute grief. Sudden cardiac death, motor vehicle crashes, suicide, and homicide fall into this category.[1] Miscarriage, pediatric death, and sudden infant death syndrome are examples of sudden death but are beyond the scope of this case due to the unique needs of those populations.

In America, we are a death-defying and rescue-oriented society.[2] Our culture actively works to stave off death. The American Heart Association and the American Red Cross teach thousands of people cardiopulmonary resuscitation (CPR) annually. Additionally, laws support the assumption that people want resuscitation unless they explicitly opt out in the form of DNR orders or other advance directives. Emergency medical systems are designed to respond quickly to requests for help with an expectation of resuscitation measures.[3] In a seminal article by Diem and colleagues, resuscitations on the television shows ER, Chicago Hope, and Rescue 911 demonstrated that in one television season, 65% of patients survived immediate arrest and 67% survived to discharge.[4] These figures are inflated compared with studies that demonstrate that survival after medical cardiac arrest is about 7% to 8% for arrests that occur outside the hospital[5] and around 17% for arrests that occur within a hospital.[6] The public may perceive that this dramatization reflects reality. These factors, among others, may contribute to the American perception of death.

Sudden unexpected deaths can often precipitate a crisis in the bereaved.[7] A crisis syndrome[8] has been proposed as a constellation of characteristics that include:

- A stressful event that presents a problem or perceived threat that is seen as insoluble in the immediate future.
- The situation taxes the individual's emotional resources, because it is beyond his or her traditional problem-solving methods.
- A person's marked behavioral changes make him less efficient than usual, diminishing prior levels of functioning.
- A person feels helpless, ineffective, anxious, fearful, guilty, numb, overwhelmed, and defensive.
- The individual sees the event as a threat to her life goals.
- The person feels a generalized physical tension, symptomatic of anxiety.
- The situation awakens unresolved problems from the near or distant past.

These feelings can impair the person's ability to cope with the situation. Therefore, one of the main goals of caring for the suddenly bereaved is to help restore coping, recognizing that the characteristics above may influence the reaction of the bereaved.

Definitions

Corless synthesizes the literature and presents succinct definitions of loss, mourning, grief, and bereavement that are presented below.[9]

Having clear definitions assists clinicians in identifying the areas for intervention when faced with a complex situation.

Loss is a generic term that signifies absence of a person, animal, position, object, ability, or attribute. The strength of the relationship between the person and the item that is lost contributes to how significant that loss will be on mourning, grief, and bereavement. According to Robinson and McKenna, there are three critical attributes to loss:[10]

- Loss signifies that someone or something one has had, or ought to have had in the future, has been taken away.
- That which is taken away must have been valued by the person experiencing the loss.
- The meaning of loss is determined individually, subjectively, and contextually by the person experiencing it.

For the palliative care provider, it is helpful to explore what has been lost, how it was valued, and the meaning to the individual to aid in the healing process.

Mourning is the outward social expression of a loss.[11] Rituals, traditions, social customs, cultural practices, as well as personal preferences influence individual and community expressions of mourning. Previous experiences and individual personality also contribute to the outward expression of the loss.[9]

Grief has many definitions. Conceptually, grief is the emotional response to a real or perceived loss that can also include a physical reaction. The process of grief has been studied extensively, and types of grief (e.g., anticipatory, uncomplicated, complicated) have been proposed and are outside the scope of this case.[9]

Bereavement is defined as the "state of having experienced the death of a significant other."[12] Bereavement includes both grief (the inner feelings) and mourning (the outward expression) and takes time to adjust to a world without the physical, psychological, and social loss of the other.[11]

Theories of Grief and Bereavement

Grief is a broad construct that occurs in many situations along a continuum of acute and sudden to slow and progressive loss, and had has many theories.[13] One of the classic models of grief was proposed by Lindemann[14] following the Coconut Grove nightclub fire. Lindemann, whose study is considered to be the seminal work of acute grief,[15] analyzed 100 survivors' grief experiences and described five almost universally experienced symptoms and associated features (Table 3.4.1).

Stroebe and Schut[16] propose a model of coping with bereavement that incorporates both traditional stage models of grief and loss such as Kübler-Ross[17] with behaviors needed to restore coping with that loss. This is known as the dual process model of coping with

TABLE 3.4.1. Symptoms of acute grief.

Symptom	Features
Somatic distress	• A feeling of throat tightness and choking with shortness of breath • An intense feeling of distress, described as tension or mental pain • A marked tendency to have sighing respirations. Hyperventilation may occur • Exhaustion. A feeling that the individual lacks strength and is profoundly exhausted, to the point of difficulty climbing stairs, lifting objects, or walking normal distances • Insomnia • Headaches • An empty feeling in the abdomen and an inability to eat or enjoy food, and sometimes diarrhea
Preoccupation with the image of the deceased	• A slight sense of unreality • A feeling of increased emotional distance from other people • An intense preoccupation with the image of the decedent
Guilt	• Self-blame • Marked guilt feelings, with a search of the time just prior to death for evidence that the individual failed the deceased person in some way. The individual usually accuses himself of negligence and exaggerates minor omissions
Hostile reactions	• Lack of warm relationships with others • Responds with irritability and anger • Does not want to be bothered during a time when friends and relatives are making a special effort to relate
Loss of normal patterns of conduct	• Restlessness, an inability to sit still, aimless movement, and a continual search for something to do • Pressured speech, especially when speaking of the deceased person • Inability to concentrate • Depression

Iserson KV. *Grave Words: Notifying Survivors About Sudden, Unexpected Deaths.* Tuscon, AZ: Galen Press; 1999.
Lindemann E. Symptomatology and management of acute grief. *Am J Psychiatry;* 1944; 101:141–148.

bereavement (Figure 3.4.1). Loss-oriented processes relate to the death experience, including grief work. Restoration-oriented processes relate to coping with the adjustment to the loss. This model is flexible, with cultural and individual differences, while acknowledging that loss-oriented and restoration-oriented processes happen concurrently and interchangeably.

Kent and McDowell outline the various manifestations of grief that can be seen in the acute and long-term phases (Table 3.4.2).[18] Palliative care clinicians need to assess for the presences of these manifestations of grief and provide resources to mitigate against persistent problems. In cases of emotional or physical stress, survivors may experience symptoms of chest pain and shortness of breath that

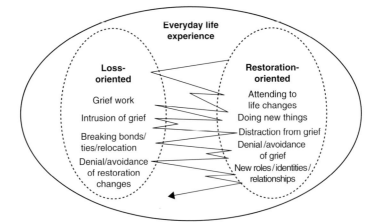

Figure 3.4.1. Dual process model of coping with bereavement. Stroebe M, Schut H. The dual process model of coping with bereavement: rationale and description. *Death Stud;* Apr.-May 1999; 23(3):197–224. Reprinted with permission from Taylor and Francis.

TABLE 3.4.2. Manifestations of grief.

Psychological reactions	• Anger • Anxiety • Apathy • Denial • Depression • Disbelief • Emotional lability • Guilt • Hallucinations of the deceased's presence (visual or auditory) • Helplessness • Impaired concentration • Irritability • Lowered self-esteem • Numbness • Sadness • Searching for the deceased
Physical reactions	• Anorexia • Change in weight • Chest pain • Fatigue • Gastrointestinal disorders • Hair loss • Headache • Immunodeficiency • Trouble initiating or maintaining sleep
Behavioral reactions	• Agitation • Crying • Fatigue • Social withdrawal

Reprinted from Bartrop R, et al. Depressed lymphocyte function after bereavement. Lancet. Apr 16 1977; 1(8016):834–836 with permission from Elsevier Ltd.

mimic an acute coronary syndrome (myocardial infarction or angina). There is a known pathology called takotsubo cardiomyopathy associated with emotional or physical stress.[19] Takotsubo cardiomyopathy is a severe, reversible, left ventricular dysfunction that can exhibit electrocardiogram changes, mild elevation of cardiac enzymes, and myocardial dysfunction in the absence of significant coronary artery occlusion or spasm. Takotsubo cardiomyopathy should be a diagnosis of exclusion.

Interventions

Brysiewicz and Uys propose a model (Figure 3.4.2) for dealing with sudden death in the ED; it can be applied in any setting where death is perceived to be sudden.[20] Interventions to help survivors cope with sudden death can be categorized in three stages: stage 1: before sudden death occurs, stage 2: during the death disclosure, and stage 3: after death notification.

In stage 1, the ED can establish a culture to support ethical and caring practices for survivors. The ED can prepare for these inevitable events by promoting good communication, reaching a consensus as to what is caring among the health care team, and being aware of colleagues' and one's own coping strategies during stressful events.[20] Being skillful at death disclosure (see Case 1.10: Notification of a Sudden Death),[21] developing a family presence during a resuscitation option program,[22] being clear about roles of all the health care team members during death disclosure, and preparing materials for aftercare instructions and resources readily available helps reduce clinician anxiety in Brysiewicz and Uys's stages 2 and 3.

Stage 2 starts when the patient arrives to the ED and ends when the patient has been declared dead. There are three ways to optimize caring in this stage: proximity (of the family to the patient), sensitive communication, and sensitive death notification.[20] If possible, the option for family presence during resuscitation should be given to the family. After declaration of death, the family should be offered the opportunity to view the body. Arrival of relatives or friends should be instructed where to go and who to ask for when they arrive to the hospital[18] (see Case 1.9 for additional information). When the first survivors arrive, health care providers should try to arrange for additional supportive friends or family to come to the hospital to support the bereaved.[23]

In stage 3, palliative care providers can help the bereaved family members and assist the health care providers. Information about the next steps, property, and follow-up care is vital to supporting the coping of the bereaved. Assistance to health care providers is vitally important when there is a particularly traumatic death, death of a child, or any other situation in which the provider identifies with the situation. Stress

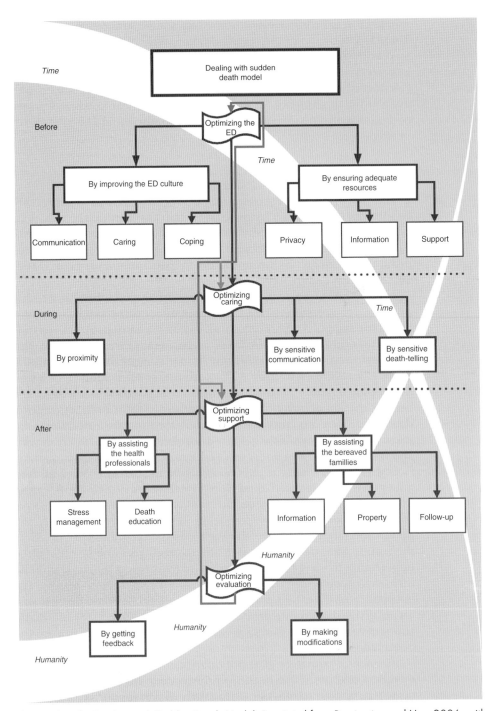

Figure 3.4.2. Dealing with Sudden Death Model. Reprinted from Brysiewicz and Uys, 2006, with permission from Lippincott Williams & Wilkins.

management and death education can support the coping of health care providers in this stage. Additionally in stage 3, leaders should obtain feedback and make necessary modifications to improve the experience of both survivors and health care providers when sudden death occurs.

BACK TO OUR CASE

The charge nurse wanted to keep the patient in the ED. She said that when the patient came in his blood pressure was in the 50s and that the team thought that once they removed the endotracheal tube he would not live very long. She expected that death would come soon and that perhaps the family would be able to come to the hospital. She said that she didn't want the patient to die alone or in transport to the medical/ surgical unit once they heard that the family was not going to be able to make it to the hospital. The primary nurse sat with the patient, gave him pain medications, and held his hand. She felt that it was important that people be around him as he died.

Once the patient was declared dead, the charge nurse called the wife and son said that she was sorry but that the patient had died. She was silent while the family absorbed the news. She asked if they wanted to hear what happened in the ED, and they said yes. She described the interventions with particular focus on pain medications and how three nurses were at his bedside the whole time until he died. The family was thankful for the call. The charge nurse gave the family the phone number to the coroner's office and described the next steps. She also gave the phone number to the ED and advised the family that they could call if they had any questions. As the charge nurse hung up the phone, she had tears in her eyes.

TAKE AWAY POINTS

- Bereavement includes both grief (the emotional response) and mourning (the outward expression).
- Reactions in acute grief commonly include somatic distress, preoccupation with the deceased person's image, guilt, hostile reactions, and loss of normal patterns of conduct.
- Preparation and skillful communication are essential to care for the suddenly bereaved. Brysiewicz and Uys'[20] Dealing with Sudden Death Model is helpful in creating a culture and process to care for the suddenly bereaved.

REFERENCES

[1] Kent H, McDowell J. Sudden bereavement in acute care settings. *Nurs Stand*; Oct. 20–26 2004; 19(6):38–42.

[2] Chan GK. End-of-life care models and emergency department care. *Academic Emergency Medicine*; 2004; 11(1):79–86.

[3] Iserson KV. Withholding and withdrawing medical treatment: an emergency medicine perspective. *Ann Emerg Med*; 1996; 28(1):51–54.

[4] Diem SJ, Lantos JD, Tulsky JA. Cardiopulmonary resuscitation on television: Miracles and misinformation. *New England Journal of Medicine*; 1996; 334(24):1578–1582.

[5] Sasson C, Rogers MA, Dahl J, Kellermann AL. Predictors of survival from out-of-hospital cardiac arrest: a systematic review and meta-analysis. *Circ Cardiovasc Qual Outcomes*; Jan. 2010; 3(1):63–81.

[6] Ebell MH, Afonso AM. Pre-arrest predictors of failure to survive after in-hospital cardiopulmonary resuscitation: a meta-analysis. *Fam Pract*; May, 18 2011; (28):505–515.

[7] Iserson KV. *Grave Words: Notifying Survivors About Sudden, Unexpected Deaths*. Tuscon, AZ: Galen Press; 1999.

[8] Eastham K, Coates D, Allodi F. The concept of crisis. *Can Psychiatr Assoc J*; Oct 1970; 15(5):463–472.

[9] Corless IB. Bereavement. In: Ferrell BA, Coyle N (eds). *Textbook of Palliative Nursing*, 3rd edition. New York: Oxford University Press; 2010; 597–612.

[10] Robinson DS, McKenna HP. Loss: an analysis of a concept of particular interest to nursing. *J Adv Nurs*; Apr. 1998; 27(4):779–784.

[11] Ferrell BR, Dahlin C, Campbell ML, Paice JA, Malloy P, Virani R. End-of-life nursing education consortium (ELNEC) training program: Improving palliative care in critical care. *Crit Care Nurs Q*; 2007; 30(3):206–212.

[12] Warren NA. Bereavement care in the critical care setting. *Crit Care Nurs Q*; Aug. 1997; 20(2):42–47.

[13] Buglass E. Grief and bereavement theories. *Nurs Stand* June 16–22 2010; 24(41):44–47.

[14] Lindemann E. Symptomatology and management of acute grief. *Am J Psychiatry*; 1944; 101:141–148.

[15] Edwards L, Shaw DG. Care of the suddenly bereaved in cardiac care units: a review of the literature. *Intensive and Critical Care Nursing*; June 1998; 14(3):144–152.

[16] Stroebe M, Schut H. The dual process model of coping with bereavement: rationale and description. *Death Stud*; Apr.-May 1999; 23(3):197–224.

[17] Kübler-Ross E. *On Death and Dying*. New York: Macmillan; 1969.

[18] Kent H, McDowell J. Sudden bereavement in acute care settings. *Nurs Stand*; Oct. 20–26 2004; 19(6):38–42.

[19] Akashi YJ, Goldstein DS, Barbaro G, Ueyama T. Takotsubo cardiomyopathy: a new form of acute, reversible heart failure. *Circulation*; Dec. 16 2008; 118(25):2754–2762.

[20] Brysiewicz P, Uys LR. A model for dealing with sudden death. *ANS Adv Nurs Sci*; July-Sep. 2006; 29(3):E1–11.

[21] Hobgood C, Harward D, Newton K, Davis W. The educational intervention "GRIEV_ING" improves the death notification skills of residents. *Academic Emergency Medicine*; Apr. 2005; 12(4):296–301.

[22] Walker WM. Sudden cardiac death in adults: causes, incidence and interventions. *Nurs Stand*; May 26-June 1 2010; 24(38):50–56; quiz 58.

[23] Benkel I, Wijk H, Molander U. Family and friends provide most social support for the bereaved. *Palliat Med*; Mar. 2009; 23(2):141–149.

Case 3.5 Complicated Grief

Rita J. DiBiase

HISTORY

George, a 75-year-old man, had been married to Brenda for almost 50 years when she died. George had been playing golf and when he returned home, he found Brenda sprawled at an odd angle on the kitchen floor. He had panicked when he realized she wasn't breathing and dropped the phone twice before being able to call 911. He had only a foggy memory of that day, only recalling that their daughter Jill had come to stay with him.

It was 13 months later when Jill called her childhood friend Robin, a nurse, to ask her advice. Her father rarely went out of the house, except to go to the cemetery daily. He spent hours at Brenda's grave, sometimes not returning until dark. Sometimes Jill saw him going from room to room as if looking for her mother. George had stopped golfing, an activity that had been a passion of his. He no longer attended church, stating that whatever faith he had was squashed when Brenda was taken so cruelly from him. He had lost 20 pounds and, previously well groomed, now always looked disheveled and bewildered. He cried often and became angry when Jill asked if he wanted to go on a trip with her. He told Jill that he didn't know what to do with himself and that he no longer had a purpose without Brenda. One night Jill had found him sitting on the floor at the spot where Brenda had collapsed. Sobbing, George told Jill that Brenda had asked him to take her to the market that fateful day but he had already made plans for golf. He no

Case Studies in Palliative and End-of-Life Care, First Edition. Edited by Margaret L. Campbell.
© 2012 John Wiley & Sons, Inc. Published 2012 by John Wiley & Sons, Inc.

longer spoke with Brenda's friends, saying that they had moved on without her. George had kept his lawn immaculate and Brenda had breathtaking flower beds; now George hired a young boy to do the yard work. When Jill cried and told George she needed her father back, he became angry and said she had a family and friends, while his life was empty.

| ? | **CLINICAL QUESTION** |

What interventions are important when supporting a family experiencing a complicated grieving process?

| ✓ | **DISCUSSION** |

Recognizing Uncomplicated Grief

Uncomplicated grief or normal grief is a natural human response that occurs in 80% to 90% of grievers in response to the loss of a loved one.[1-3] Uncomplicated grief is marked by an initial period of disbelief, with seemingly relentless emotions including sadness, crying, anguish, and despair, which lessen into waves or bursts.[1] At first there is no provocation; however, later feelings may be triggered by reminders. Preoccupation with memories and thoughts of the deceased are accompanied by difficulty concentrating. Grief manifestations may range from minimal to significant, affecting individuals emotionally, cognitively, socially, and behaviorally.[4] Visual or auditory hallucinations—seeing the loved one in a crowd, feeling her presence or touch or smelling a familiar scent—may occur and cause either comfort or distress.[5] Those who have never experienced such a roller coaster of emotions may be frightened by the intensity and unpredictability, wondering if they need professional help. There is a disinterest in others or daily life because the person's main role is to mourn his loved one.[4]

As the months pass, the deceased is more easily called to mind without the previous preoccupation that may have been disruptive. Significant dates, occasions, or stressful times may reawaken acute grief.[4] The griever integrates the new reality, forever changed but somehow adapting to a life without his loved one.[4] Eventually, the bereaved is able to participate in pleasurable activities, enjoying new interests and engaging in healthy relationships once again. The majority of individuals accept the reality of the death and foresee some promise in the future, even at six months post loss, which is viewed as a sign of resilience associated with positive outcomes.

Current theorists indicate that for most people grief diminishes but may never fully dissipate.[4] Notably, during the early months after a loss, many of the signs and symptoms of uncomplicated grief are very similar to those of complicated grief and depression. Individuals may meet the criteria for major depression within the first few months following a death; however, at one year the percentage drops dramatically.[4,5] Others note that with major depression there is a loss of self-esteem; anger is turned inward with the inability to imagine a life worth living without the deceased.[3,4]

Complicated Grief

There have been many variations of the term "complicated grief," namely pathologic grief, abnormal grief, atypical grief, pathologic mourning, and more recently prolonged grief disorder (PGD).[6] Complicated grief, which occurs in 10% to 20% of bereaved people, is marked by intense yearning, longing, bitterness, and difficulty accepting the loss.[5] There is a preoccupation with the deceased with an inability to imagine a future without her.[6,7] Rumination, intrusive thoughts about the loss and death, and regrets all create a cycle of mental anguish and engulfing sorrow. Grievers avoid painful reminders, are unable to trust others, and isolate themselves from family and friends.[3,4] Complicated grief symptoms significantly impair social, occupational, and other functioning.[6,7] Symptoms do not abate in frequency or intensity and last at least six months; however, if the grief is delayed the six-month period doesn't start immediately after the death.[7] Essentially grievers are stuck in a frightening labyrinth and they can't find their way out. There are typically four types of complicated grief described in the literature: chronic grief, delayed grief, exaggerated grief, and masked grief (Table 3.5.1).[5]

Complicated Grief, Posttraumatic Stress Disorder, and Major Depressive Disorder

Complicated grief is distinct from disorders of major depressive disorder (MDD), generalized anxiety disorder (GAD), and posttraumatic stress disorder (PTSD).[2-8] The following is a very brief and general description of the differences and overlaps between these disorders and complicated grief. Symptoms of depression include feelings of sadness, extreme weight loss, social withdrawal, delusions and fantasies involving the deceased, psychomotor retardation, feelings of worthlessness, and suicidal ideation.[9] Depressive manifestations may occur in some form early in grief but improve and resolve as time passes; therefore, a diagnosis of MDD is not made within the first two months post death.[9] If depression persists and a diagnosis of MDD is made, treatment involving medications and therapy are necessary for recovery.[4]

TABLE 3.5.1. Types of complicated grief.

Chronic or prolonged grief
- Does not subside over time
- Individual aware that he is not getting through the process
- Does not necessarily resolve on own
- May have confusing or ambivalent feelings
- May yearn for relationship he wishes was different
- May have had highly dependent relationship

Delayed grief
- Survivors' reactions are postponed or suppressed
- Individual consciously or unconsciously avoids the pain and reality of the death
- May have intense grief reaction later if pain of loss is carried forward
- Usually realizes her grief is out of proportion to timing
- May have lacked social support at time of loss
- Multiple losses can cause postponement of grief
- Intense feelings may be triggered by a social event, movie, etc.
- Intensity of feelings indicate unresolved grief of former loss

Exaggerated grief
- Intensification of normal grief reaction resulting in feeling overwhelmed
- May resort to maladaptive or self-destructive behaviors
- May become depressed
- Panic attacks
- Development of phobia
- Substance abuse
- After catastrophe may develop signs, symptoms of post-traumatic stress disorder (PTSD)
- May develop mania

Masked grief
- Behaviors cause person difficulty but they she does not recognize relation to loss
- Absent grief may play out as physical symptoms
- Absent grief may be exhibited via maladaptive behaviors
- Physical symptoms may mimic those of the loved one

Created from information found in Worden JW. Grief Counseling and Grief, 3rd edition. New York: NY: Springer Publishing Company Inc.; 1991.

Horowitz, who developed diagnostic criteria for posttraumatic stress disorder (PTSD), sees complicated grief as a stress response syndrome.[10] He developed the Impact of Events Scale which includes a subscale that measures severe grief. PTSD is characterized by symptoms of avoidance and horror not seen with complicated grief. Horowitz cites preoccupation with intrusive memories and avoidance of painful reminders as the common characteristics between PTSD and complicated grief.[10] The difference is that with PTSD, memories are painful, whereas with complicated grief, the

TABLE 3.5.2. Situations or factors associated with complicated grief.

- Traumatic death
- Sudden, unexpected death such as heart attacks, accidents
- Suicide
- Homicide
- Dependent relationship with deceased
- Patient with chronic illness after years of remission
- Death of a child
- Multiple losses
- Unresolved grief from prior losses
- Concurrent stressors (divorce, moving, children leaving home, other ill family members)
- History of mental illness or substance abuse
- Patient experienced poor pain management or psychosocial or spiritual suffering
- Limited or ineffective supports
- No faith system, cultural traditions, or religious beliefs to draw upon

Corless IB. Bereavement. In: Ferrell BA, Coyle N (eds). *Textbook of Palliative Nursing*, 3rd edition. New York: Oxford University Press; 2010; 597–612.
Prigerson H. Complicated grief when the path of adjustment leads to a dead end. *Healthcare Counselling & Psychotherapy Journal*; July 2005; 5(3):10–13.
Zisook S, Shear K. Grief and bereavement: what psychiatrists need to know. *World Psychiatry*; 2009; 8(2):67–74.
Worden JW. *Grief Counseling and Grief*, 3rd edition. New York: Springer Publishing Company Inc.; 1991.
Zhang B, El-Jawahri A, Prigerson HG. Update on bereavement research: evidence-based guidelines for the diagnosis and treatment of complicated bereavement. *Journal of Palliative Medicine*; 2006; 9(5):1188–1203.

memories are happy ones.[3] Of interest, one study reported that almost 75% of people experiencing complicated grief also met criteria for PTSD.[11]

Prigerson, who has contributed substantially to the body of evidence, proposes that complicated or prolonged grief is a disorder of attachment.[2,3,7,8] The symptoms unique to complicated grief are attachment-based and not seen in MDD or PTSD.[8] Complicated grief often occurs in conjunction with MDD and/or PTSD, making it essential that individuals are assessed for each disorder using relevant diagnostic criteria for treatment purposes. More recently referred to as prolonged grief disorder (PGD), this syndrome has been associated with increased risk of hypertension, cardiac events, immune dysfunction, increased smoking and alcohol consumption, suicidal ideations and attempts, hospitalizations, and deceased quality of life.[6,7]

Assessment of Complicated or Prolonged Grief

Some situations and variables associated with complicated grief are also related to circumstances surrounding illness, perception of care at end of life, mode of death, and other variables[12] (Table 3.5.2). Identifying those at risk for complicated or prolonged grief requires knowledge of relevant factors. Prigerson and her colleagues developed the Index of Complicated Grief (ICG) which can be used for assessment.[3] As related to attachments and relationships, Prigerson[7] identifies the following risk factors and clinical correlates:

- History of childhood separation anxiety
- Controlling parents
- Parental abuse or death
- A close relationship to the deceased
- Insecure attachment styles
- Marital supportiveness and dependency
- Lack of preparation for the death

Criteria for Prolonged Grief Disorder

A consensus panel of bereavement and mental health experts convened to develop a standardized criteria for prolonged grief disorder. The researchers used data analyzed from almost 300 people who lost a close family member. The findings of the study validated a diagnostic algorithm for PGD (Table 3.5.3).[7] The published criteria will be included in the American Psychiatric Association's *Diagnostic and Statistical Manual of Mental Disorders*, 5th edition (DSM-V) and in the World Health Organization's International Statistical Classification of Diseases and Related Health Problems, 11th edition (ICD-11). The significance of this breakthrough is the identification of PGD as a distinct mental disorder. This designation will help clinicians identify individuals who are at risk for PGD, as well as provide appropriate treatments for those experiencing PGD.[7] The inclusion of the validated criteria set into the DSM-V and ICD-11 is the result of years of research and advocacy by Prigerson[7] and other researchers.

Interventions

Bereavement researchers do not wish to deem uncomplicated grief pathological. It has been well established that grief therapy is not required for uncomplicated grief.[1-6] Individuals experiencing complicated grief require expert care. Antidepressant therapy, which has been effective for MDD, has been ineffective for PGD.[13] Health care professionals who are knowledgeable about evidence-based care related to grief and bereavement are in the position to assess those at risk for complicated or prolonged grief. By virtue of caring for their loved ones, clinicians have interactions with family members prior to the death, allowing them to identify risk factors predisposing them to PGD.[2-9] The invaluable role of the health care professional is to offer support and resources, and most importantly, to refer to a bereavement specialist. Involving social workers, chaplains, psychologists, psychiatrists, and

TABLE 3.5.3. Criteria for grief disorder proposed for DSM-V.

Category	Definition
A	Event: Bereavement (loss of a significant other)
B	**Separation distress**: The bereaved person experiences yearning (e.g., craving, pining, or longing for the deceased; physical or emotional suffering as a result of the desired but unfulfilled reunion with the deceased) daily or to a disabling degree
C	**Cognitive, emotional, and behavioral symptoms**: The bereaved person must have five (or more) of the following symptoms experienced daily or to a disabling degree: 1. Confusion about one's role in life or diminished sense of self (i.e., feeling that part of oneself has died) 2. Difficulty accepting the loss 3. Avoidance of reminders of the reality of the loss 4. Inability to trust others since the loss 5. Bitterness or anger related to the loss 6. Difficulty moving on with life (e.g., making new friends, pursuing interests) 7. Numbness (absence of emotion) since the loss 8. Feeling that life is unfulfilling, empty, or meaningless since the loss 9. Feeling stunned, dazed, or shocked by the loss
D	**Timing**: Diagnosis should not be made until at least six months have elapsed since the death
E	**Impairment**: The disturbance causes clinically significant impairment in social, occupational, or other important areas of functioning (e.g., domestic responsibilities)
F	**Relation to other mental disorders**: The disturbance is not better accounted for by major depressive disorder, generalized anxiety disorder, or posttraumatic stress disorder

Prigerson HG, Horowitz MJ, Jacobs SC, et al. Prolonged grief disorder: psychometric validation of criteria proposed for DSM-V and ICD-11. PLoS Med. 2009; 6(8): e1000121. Doi:10.1371/journal.pmed.1000121. Reprinted with permission from PLoS Medical.

other qualified team members solidifies the approach of advance preparation and ensuring comprehensive assessment, intervention, and referral. Identification of social support networks has been identified as an asset to the griever with lower risk of bereavement issues.

There has been progress in the treatment of complicated grief. Complicated grief therapy (CGT) uses the Dual Process Model of Grief[14] foundation to address both loss-restoration and restoration-orientation during a 16-session program. Other promising therapies, including Internet based approaches[15] and neuroimaging,[16] address specifically targeted interventions for complicated or prolonged grief. The future holds promise for further development of research and applicable interventions that will help those whose grief takes hold with such a fierce grip that they are unable to recover on their own.

BACK TO OUR CASE

Robin worked as a hospice nurse and was able to explain the signs of complicated grief to Jill. She gave Jill pamphlets for the bereavement resource center and some reading materials and websites. Jill made an appointment with a grief counselor and was able to talk about the loss of her mother and how she also felt she lost her father. She went to see George and told him what she had been doing, leaving the pamphlets on the counter. A week later George called Jill and told her he would be willing to see someone once. He said he dreamed of Brenda and she told him to take care of himself and Jill. Jill accompanied George the first time he went to the bereavement center. He worked with a therapist and received CGT. He attended all the sessions but it was weeks before he began to feel alive again. He wrote Jill a letter thanking her for her love, stating that even though he couldn't save Brenda, Jill had saved his life.

TAKE AWAY POINTS

- Some symptoms of early grief may resemble depression or complicated grief; therefore, diagnosis should not be made until six months has passed.
- Health care providers working in palliative and end-of-life care who can recognize the difference between uncomplicated grief and complicated or prolonged grief are able to assess, intervene, and refer when appropriate.
- Complicated or prolonged grief is distinct from major depressive disorder and posttraumatic stress disorder, and requires specialized therapy.

REFERENCES

[1] Buglass E. Grief and bereavement theories. *Nursing Standard*; June 2010; 24(41):44–47.
[2] Corless IB. Bereavement. In: Ferrell BA, Coyle N (eds). *Textbook of Palliative Nursing*, 3rd edition. New York: Oxford University Press; 2010; 597–612.
[3] Prigerson H. Complicated grief when the path of adjustment leads to a dead end. *Healthcare Counselling & Psychotherapy Journal*; July 2005; 5(3):10–13.
[4] Zisook S, Shear K. Grief and bereavement: what psychiatrists need to know. *World Psychiatry*; 2009; 8(2):67–74.

[5] Worden JW. *Grief Counseling and Grief*, 3rd edition. New York: Springer Publishing Company Inc.; 1991.

[6] Zhang B, El-Jawahri A, Prigerson HG. Update on bereavement research: evidence-based guidelines for the diagnosis and treatment of complicated bereavement. *Journal of Palliative Medicine*; 2006; 9(5):1188–1203.

[7] Prigerson HG, Horowitz MJ, Jacobs SC, et al. Prolonged grief disorder: psychometric validation of criteria proposed for DSM-V and ICD-11. *PLoS Med*. 2009; 6(8): e1000121. Doi:10.1371/journal.pmed.1000121.

[8] Prigerson HG, Maciejewski PK. A call for sound empirical testing and evaluation of criteria for complicated grief proposed for DSM-V. Omega; 2005; 2006;52(1):9–19.

[9] Love AW. Progress in understanding grief, complicated grief and caring for the bereaved. *Contemporary Nurse*; 2007; 27:73–83.

[10] Horowitz M, Siegel B, Holen A, et al. Diagnostic criteria for complicated grief disorders. *American Journal of Psychiatry*; 1997; 154(7): 904–911.

[11] Tolstikova K, Fleming S, Chartier B. Grief, complicated grief, and trauma: the role of the search for meaning, impaired self-reference, and death anxiety. *Illness, Crisis & Loss*; 2005; 18:293–313.

[12] Rando TA. *Grief, Dying, and Death: Clinical Interventions for Caregivers*. Champaign: IL: Research Press; 1984.

[13] Jacobs SC, Nelson JC, Zisook S. Treating depression of bereavement with antidepressants: a pilot study. *Psych Clin North America*; 1987; 10:501–510.

[14] Stroebe M, Schut H. The dual process model of coping with bereavement: a decade on. *Omega*; 2010; 61(4):273–289.

[15] Wagner B, Knaevelsrud C, Maercker A. Internet-based cognitive-behavioral therapy for complicated grief: a randomized controlled trial. *Death Studies*; 2006; 30:429–453.

[16] Gundel H, O'Connor MF, Littrel L, Fort C, Lane RD. Functional neuroanatomy of grief: An fMRI study. *American Journal Psychiatry*; 2003; 160:1946–1953.

Index

Anxiety 207–11
  Assessment 209
    Beck Depression Inventory 209
    Generalized Anxiety Disorder Tool 209
    Hospital Anxiety and Depression
      Scale 209
  Etiology 208
  Treatment 209–11
Ascites 241–5
  Assessment 243
  Etiology 241–2
  Treatment 243–5

Bowel obstruction 162–5
Brain death 43
  Religious beliefs 43

Communication
  Advance care planning 30
  Bad news 7
  Death notification 69–71, 74–5
    Affective Competency Score 76
    EASE 71
    Medicolegal investigation 78
    Telephone 79
  Diagnosis 6–10
  Do Not Resuscitate (DNR) 30
  Empathy 8

Family conference 36–7
Futility 55
Goals of care 36–7
Imminent death 13–16
Maladaptive family 63–5
Prognosis 6–10, 57
SPIKES 7
  Emotions 8
  Invitation 8
  Knowledge 8
  Perception 8
  Setting up interview 7
  Strategy/Summary 8
Constipation 192–6
  Assessment 191, 193–4
  Etiology 192–3
  Treatment 194–6
COPD 111–13
  Natural history 111–12
  Treatment 113
Cough 140–143
  Assessment 141
  Etiology 140
  Treatment 141–3
CPR 27–30
  AHA standards 28
  History 27–8
  Layperson estimates 30, 53

Case Studies in Palliative and End-of-Life Care, First Edition. Edited by Margaret L. Campbell.
© 2012 John Wiley & Sons, Inc. Published 2012 by John Wiley & Sons, Inc.

CPR (*cont'd*)
  National Registry of CPR 28
  Outcomes 28–9

Death
  Notifications 15–16, 69–71, 74–5
  Signs of 15
Delirium 249–54
  Assessment 250–251
    Confusion Assessment Method 251
  Etiology 249–50
  Prevention 251–2
  Risk Factors 250
  Treatment 252–4
Denial 22
Depression 199–202
  Assessment 200–201
    Beck Depression Inventory 201, 209
    Geriatric Depression Scale 201
    Hospital Anxiety and Depression
      Scale 200–201, 209
  Dignity Therapy 202
  Treatment 201–2
Dignity Therapy 202, 272–3
Donation after Cardiac Death 46–7
  Family care 47–8
  UNOS guidelines 46
Dyspnea 111–14, 121–5
  Assessment 112–13
  Benzodiazepines 114
  Opioids 114, 124–5
  Oxygen 114
  Positioning 114
  RDOS 114, 131
  Treatment 113–14

Family care
  Checklist of Family Relational
    Abilities 63–4
  Death vigil 264–5
  Family Resilience Framework 63
  Family Systems Illness Model 62–3
  Imminent death 15–16
  Maladaptive behaviors 61–2
  Organ donation 44–5
  Presence during CPR 76–8
  Relationship Centered Care 63–4
Futility
  AMA Code of Ethics 54
  Defined 54

Family requests 55–6
  State Laws 54

Grief
  Acute 278–85, 290–295
  Anticipatory 261–3, 267–73
  Complicated 301–7
  Death vigil 264–5
  Dignity therapy 272–3
  Index of Complicated Grief 305
  Prolonged Grief Disorder 305–6
  Treatment 270–273, 283–6, 295–7, 305

Heart failure 106–8, 119–25
  Assessment 121–2
    Echocardiogram 122
    EKG 122
    MUGA 122–3
  Classification 106, 120
  Dyspnea 121–5
  Natural history 119–21
  Pain treatment 107–8
  Seattle Heart Failure Score 105–6, 121
  Treatment 123
Hiccups 146–50
  Assessment 147–8
  Etiology 146–7
  Home remedies 148
  Treatment 148–50

Imminent death 13–14
  Signs of 13–14

Miracles 21–2
  Defined 22

Nausea 153–8, 162–5, 169–73
  Assessment 154, 163, 171–2
    Morrow Assessment of Nausea and
      Emesis 170
    Northern Alberta Renal Program 170
    Rhodes Index of Nausea and
      Vomiting 170
  Etiology 162–3, 170
  Palliative sedation 158
  Treatment 154–8, 164–5, 171–3

Opioids 92–3
  Breakthrough dosing 101
  Constipation 94–5, 192–6

Pruritus 177–81
  Rotation 100–101
  Titration 100
Organ donation 42–5
  Consent 43–4
  Designated requestor 43–4
  Family care 44–5
  History 42
Oxygen 114, 124

Pain
  Acute exacerbation 100–101
  Assessment 90–1
  Defined 89
  Malignant 89–95
    Etiologies 89–90
    Treatment 91–5
  Neuropathic 94
  Treatment 91–5
    Adjuvant medications 94–5
    Breakthrough dosing 101
    Constipation 93–4
    Intravenous titration 100
    Nonpharmacological 96
    Opioids 92–3
Palliative sedation
  Hiccups 150
  Nausea 158
Pressure Ulcers 231–6
  Assessment 233–5
    Staging 234
  Etiology 231–3
  Prevention 233
  Treatment 235–6
Pronouncing death 70

Pruritus 177–81, 183–7
  Etiology 177–8, 184–5
  Treatment 178–81, 186–7

Religiosity 19–22
  Defined 19
  Influence on decision-making 20
  Medical futility 20

Secretions 214–17
  Assessment 215
    Death Rattle Intensity Scale 215
  Etiology 214–15
  Treatment 216–17
Spirituality 19–22
  Assessment 21
  Defined 19
  Ethnic variations 20
  FICA 21
    Address in Care 21
    Community 21
    Faith 21
    Importance 21
  Professional boundaries 22
  Spiritual care professionals 22

Ventilator Withdrawal 129–33
  Algorithm 131–4
  Patient characteristics 130–131
  RDOS 131

Wounds 222–7
  Assessment 223–4
  Etiology 222–3
  Treatment 224–7